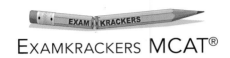

Examkrackers MCAT®

1001 QUESTIONS:
CHEMISTRY
GENERAL & ORGANIC CHEMISTRY

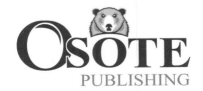

OSOTE
PUBLISHING

Major Contributors:
Kaitlyn Barkley, M.D.
Jennifer Birk Goldschmidt, M.S.
Daniel Campbell
Andrew Elson
Jay Li
Bryan Luu
Austin Mattox

Contributors:
Kirthi Bellamkonda
Matthew Buck
Daniel Huang
Michael Klug

Art Director:
Erin Daniel

Designer:
Dana Kelley

ISBN 13: 978-1-893858-96-1

To purchase additional copies of this book or other books of the 1001 Question series, call 1-888-572-2536.

Examkrackers.com
Osote.com

FAIR USE NOTICE. This book is an independent educational guide for students who are preparing to take the Medical College Admission Test® exam, also known as the MCAT® exam. This book has been prepared and published by Examkrackers, Inc. and is not endorsed or sponsored by, or otherwise affiliated with, the Association of American Medical Colleges (AAMC), which publishes the MCAT® exam and owns the foregoing trademarks. The trademarks owned by AAMC are used for information and identification only, and are not intended to claim or suggest any affiliation with AAMC.

Printed and bound in the United States of America.

Read this First

Practice with MCAT®-style materials is essential to success on the MCAT®. In fact, it is the single most important thing you can do to prepare for MCAT® day and ensure a high score.

The 1001 questions in this book were carefully designed to simulate the content, style, tone, and difficulty of the chemistry questions you will encounter on the MCAT®. Some questions are medically or biologically relevant, just like standalone MCAT® chemistry questions, and some are intended purely to reinforce the science. We have systematically created questions on every single tested topic and subtopic, paying special attention to challenging topics and high yield areas. We include a higher proportion of difficult research questions than you will find on the real MCAT® to ensure that you are well-prepared on MCAT® day.

How to Use This Book

The MCAT® is passage-based, so this book is not intended to provide simulation of full MCAT® sections. The MCAT®-style questions in this book are most useful for gaining familiarity with MCAT® standalone questions and for drilling and reinforcing science concepts.

Each chapter of *1001 Questions: Chemistry* tests the content covered by the corresponding chapter in Examkrackers *Chemistry* manual. To maximize your MCAT® preparation, use this book in tandem with Examkrackers *Chemistry* manual and Examkrackers *101 Passages: Chemistry book*.

As you study Examkrackers *Chemistry* manual and work through practice passages, use this book to reinforce your understanding of the science and shore up areas of weakness. Answering questions in topic areas you find challenging will increase your knowledge and confidence in a way that passive reading and review simply cannot.

Raising Your Score

Your goal as you work through the questions in this book should be to increase your raw score—the number of questions you answer correctly. Your raw score on the questions in this book cannot be translated into an MCAT® score, because the MCAT® is passage-based. In addition, we deliberately include a greater proportion of medium and hard questions than you will find on the real MCAT®. Do not worry about translating your raw scores from this book into an MCAT® score. Instead, focus on answering more and more questions correctly: more questions correct means a higher score on MCAT® day.

To ensure that you are gaining knowledge, confidence, and skill as you approach MCAT® day, you should build time into your study schedule not just for taking practice questions, but for reviewing the answers.

Effective review of practice questions means first marking questions you got wrong (or guessed at) without looking at the answer explanations. Review the science behind the question and retake the question. Check your answer again. If you still missed the question, read the answer explanation. Our answer explanations are thorough and process-oriented, meaning that we walk you through the answer choices one by one, showing you how to rule out each wrong answer choice and why the best answer choice is best.

Active, thoughtful review is key to what Examkrackers calls *Smart Practice*.

Smart Practice

There are two kinds of practice: practice that is repetitive and practice that is smart. Repetitive practice, in which you do the same thing over and over again, will reinforce skills that you already have, but it will not broaden your skills. It will also reinforce habits that are not working. Smart practice is active, thoughtful practice.

Smart Practice means:

1. Making plans and setting goals for your practice. What do you want to improve today? What science do you want to nail down; what skill or strategy do you want to master?

2. Being self-aware as you take practice questions. How are you approaching the questions? How do you feel as you work through them? Are you noticing any habits (negative thinking, daydreaming, nerves) you would like to break? Take notes on your habits and states of mind.

3. Immediately reviewing the questions and evaluating your progress after a practice session. Did you make the improvements you planned? Do you feel more confident in your grasp of the science?

4. Making specific commitments in light of your evaluation. What will your next goal be? What concrete action will you take the next time you fall into an unhelpful habit?

5. Document your goals, evaluations, and commitments. This will remind you of how far you have come in your practice, and help you identify areas where new commitments are needed.

When you engage in *Smart Practice* using this book together with other Examkrackers review and practice materials, you can feel confident that you are fully prepared for the MCAT®.

Full MCAT® Preparation

Examkrackers offers a full suite of manuals, practice materials, and study services to help you prepare fully for MCAT® day.

PREPARATION AND PRACTICE

Examkrackers Complete Study Package includes all six Examkrackers MCAT® preparatory manuals: *Reasoning Skills: Verbal, Research, and Math, Biology 1 Molecules: Biochemistry, Biology 2 Systems, Chemistry: General and Organic Chemistry, Physics*, and *Psychology and Sociology*. Each manual is packed with content review, MCAT® strategy, and guided practice.

Examkrackers 101 Passages series provides over 600 total simulated MCAT® passages to maximize your practice. The series includes *CARS, Biology 1 Molecules, Biology 2 Systems, Chemistry, Physics*, and *Psychology* and *Sociology*.

Our *1001 Questions* series reinforces science concepts and helps you gain familiarity with standalone, MCAT®-style questions. The series focuses on tackling challenging *Chemistry* and *Physics* questions.

Full-length, online *EK-Tests* provide an accurate simulation of the content, difficulty, style, and timing of the real MCAT®. Go to www.examkrackers.com to learn more.

Examkrackers offers in-person and online MCAT® prep courses. Go to www.examkrackers.com or call 1-888-KRACKEM to learn more about our Comprehensive MCAT® Courses.

SERVICES AND SUPPORT

Our free, online forum is available to you with the purchase of this or any other Examkrackers product. Access it at www.examkrackers.com. You can post questions and have them answered by experienced Examkrackers tutors and teachers.

Examkrackers Live MCAT® Hotline is a paid service that entitles you to call an expert, high-scoring MCAT® instructor and receive live, direct, one-on-one answers to your questions. The hotline is available ten hours a week.

Examkrackers live, online tutoring is available in 2, 10, 20, or 30 hour blocks. All of the MCAT® expertise of our seasoned course instructors can be available to you on your schedule.

Personal statement coaching is now available from Examkrackers. Coaching includes online, one-on-one meetings with an Examkrackers writer or instructor, and evaluation of multiple drafts of your personal statement.

Toward your success!

TABLE OF CONTENTS

LECTURE

1 **Introduction to General Chemistry** **1**

Atoms 2

Elements and the Periodic Table 2

Quantum Mechanics 10

Bonding 13

Reactions and Stoichiometry 14

Radioactive Decay 18

LECTURE

2 **Introduction to Organic Chemistry** **19**

Representations of Organic Molecules 20

Bonds and Hybridization 21

Resonance and Electron Delocalization ... 25

Functional Groups and Their Features 28

Stereochemistry 33

Substitution Reactions of Alkanes 42

LECTURE

3 **The Attackers: Nucleophiles** **43**

The Attackers: Nucleophiles 44

The Targets: Electrophiles 46

Substitution Reactions: Carboxylic Acids
and Their Derivatives 48

Addition Reactions: Aldehydes
and Ketones 59

Oxidation and Reduction of Oxygen
Containing Compounds 65

Carbonyls as Nucleophiles:
Aldol Condensation 66

Bonding and Reactions of
Biological Molecules 67

ANSWERS & EXPLANATIONS **159**

.... 160

.... 161

.... 167

.... 171

.... 172

.... 175

ANSWERS & EXPLANATIONS **177**

.... 178

.... 178

.... 181

.... 183

.... 187

.... 193

ANSWERS & EXPLANATIONS **195**

.... 196

.... 198

.... 199

.... 205

.... 210

.... 211

.... 211

LECTURE

4 **Thermodynamics and Kinetics** **71**

Physical Properties of Systems
and Surroundings 72

Chemical Kinetics 72

State and Path Functions: Internal
Energy, Heat, and Work........................78

Enthalpy and Entropy 82

Accounting for Energy: Gibbs Free
Energy and Hess's Law 86

Equilibrium................................ 90

Free Energy and Spontaneity................94

ANSWERS & EXPLANATIONS **215**

....216

....216

....219

....221

....223

....226

....229

LECTURE

5 **Phases** **97**

Behavior of Gases.................................. 98

Real Gases 110

The Liquid and Solid Phases................... 115

Calorimetry 116

Phase Changes 117

ANSWERS & EXPLANATIONS **231**

....232

....242

....245

....246

....247

LECTURE

6 **Solutions and Electrochemistry** **119**

Solution Chemistry 120

Vapor Pressure.................................... 123

Solubility 125

Chemical Potential and
Redox Reactions 129

Electrochemical Cells 132

ANSWERS & EXPLANATIONS **249**

....250

....252

....253

....256

....259

LECTURE

7 **Acids and Bases** **141**

Acids and Bases.................................... 142

Water and Acid-Base Chemistry 148

Titration 150

Salts and Buffers.................................... 155

ANSWERS & EXPLANATIONS **263**

....264

....268

....270

....272

Whoever holds this MCAT book, be he/she/they worthy, shall posses the power to slay the MCAT!

- I got into 2 great schools with a 3.2 undergrad GPA and a 504 MCAT. You're gonna be FINE!

PHYSICAL SCIENCES

DIRECTIONS. Most questions in the Physical Sciences test are organized into groups, each preceded by a descriptive passage. After studying the passage, select the one best answer to each question in the group. Some questions are not based on a descriptive passage and are also independent of each other. You must also select the one best answer to these questions. If you are not certain of an answer, eliminate the alternatives that you know to be incorrect and then select an answer from the remaining alternatives. A periodic table is provided for your use. You may consult it whenever you wish.

PERIODIC TABLE OF THE ELEMENTS

1 **H** 1.0																	2 **He** 4.0
3 **Li** 6.9	4 **Be** 9.0											5 **B** 10.8	6 **C** 12.0	7 **N** 14.0	8 **O** 16.0	9 **F** 19.0	10 **Ne** 20.2
11 **Na** 23.0	12 **Mg** 24.3											13 **Al** 27.0	14 **Si** 28.1	15 **P** 31.0	16 **S** 32.1	17 **Cl** 35.5	18 **Ar** 39.9
19 **K** 39.1	20 **Ca** 40.1	21 **Sc** 45.0	22 **Ti** 47.9	23 **V** 50.9	24 **Cr** 52.0	25 **Mn** 54.9	26 **Fe** 55.8	27 **Co** 58.9	28 **Ni** 58.7	29 **Cu** 63.5	30 **Zn** 65.4	31 **Ga** 69.7	32 **Ge** 72.6	33 **As** 74.9	34 **Se** 79.0	35 **Br** 79.9	36 **Kr** 83.8
37 **Rb** 85.5	38 **Sr** 87.6	39 **Y** 88.9	40 **Zr** 91.2	41 **Nb** 92.9	42 **Mo** 95.9	43 **Tc** (98)	44 **Ru** 101.1	45 **Rh** 102.9	46 **Pd** 106.4	47 **Ag** 107.9	48 **Cd** 112.4	49 **In** 114.8	50 **Sn** 118.7	51 **Sb** 121.8	52 **Te** 127.6	53 **I** 126.9	54 **Xe** 131.3
55 **Cs** 132.9	56 **Ba** 137.3	57 **La*** 138.9	72 **Hf** 178.5	73 **Ta** 180.9	74 **W** 183.9	75 **Re** 186.2	76 **Os** 190.2	77 **Ir** 192.2	78 **Pt** 195.1	79 **Au** 197.0	80 **Hg** 200.6	81 **Tl** 204.4	82 **Pb** 207.2	83 **Bi** 209.0	84 **Po** (209)	85 **At** (210)	86 **Rn** (222)
87 **Fr** (223)	88 **Ra** 226.0	89 **Ac⁼** 227.0	104 **Unq** (261)	105 **Unp** (262)	106 **Unh** (263)	107 **Uns** (262)	108 **Uno** (265)	109 **Une** (267)									

	58 **Ce** 140.1	59 **Pr** 140.9	60 **Nd** 144.2	61 **Pm** (145)	62 **Sm** 150.4	63 **Eu** 152.0	64 **Gd** 157.3	65 **Tb** 158.9	66 **Dy** 162.5	67 **Ho** 164.9	68 **Er** 167.3	69 **Tm** 168.9	70 **Yb** 173.0	71 **Lu** 175.0
*														
⁼	90 **Th** 232.0	91 **Pa** (231)	92 **U** 238.0	93 **Np** (237)	94 **Pu** (244)	95 **Am** (243)	96 **Cm** (247)	97 **Bk** (247)	98 **Cf** (251)	99 **Es** (252)	100 **Fm** (257)	101 **Md** (258)	102 **No** (259)	103 **Lr** (260)

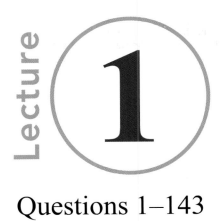

Lecture

(1)

Questions 1–143

Introduction to General Chemistry

Atoms
Elements and the Periodic Table
Quantum Mechanics
Bonding
Reactions and Stoichiometry
Radioactive Decay

LECTURE 1

Atoms

Refer to the hypothetical element E shown below to answer questions 1-6.

$$_{Z}^{A}E^{C}$$

Question 1

A on element E represents:

- ○ **A.** the number of neutrons.
- ○ **B.** the number of protons.
- ○ **C.** the number of neutrons plus protons.
- ○ **D.** the number of electrons.

Question 2

C on element E represents:

- ○ **A.** the number of electrons.
- ○ **B.** the number of protons.
- ○ **C.** the number of protons minus electrons.
- ○ **D.** the number of neutrons plus protons.

Question 3

The atomic number on the element E is represented by:

- ○ **A.** *A*.
- ○ **B.** *Z*.
- ○ **C.** *C*.
- ○ **D.** *A* + *Z*.

Question 4

Which of the following is always true of the relationship between *A* and *Z* on any stable element E?

- ○ **A.** *Z* is greater than *A*.
- ○ **B.** *A* is greater than *Z*.
- ○ **C.** *Z* is exactly half as great as *A*.
- ○ **D.** *A* minus *Z* gives the number of neutrons.

Question 5

Which of the following could NOT be true for any given element E?

- ○ **A.** There is more than one possible value for *A*.
- ○ **B.** There is more than one possible value for *C*.
- ○ **C.** There is more than one possible value for *Z*.
- ○ **D.** There is more than one possible value for *A* + *Z*.

Question 6

If two different atoms of element E have different values for *A*, they must be:

- ○ **A.** different elements.
- ○ **B.** ions of the same element.
- ○ **C.** isotopes of the same element.
- ○ **D.** isomers of the same element.

Question 7

When a bond is broken:

- ○ **A.** energy is always released.
- ○ **B.** energy is always absorbed.
- ○ **C.** energy is absorbed if the bond strength is positive.
- ○ **D.** energy is released if the bond strength is negative.

Elements and the Periodic Table

Question 8

Na and K belong to which family of elements?

- ○ **A.** The alkaline earth metals
- ○ **B.** The alkali metals
- ○ **C.** The transition metals
- ○ **D.** The halogens

Question 9

Which of the following elements has chemical properties most similar to K?

- ○ **A.** Ca
- ○ **B.** Cs
- ○ **C.** Ar
- ○ **D.** O

Question 10

Because of the ease with which it is oxidized, pure sodium sometimes catches fire when exposed to water. Which of the following pure elements is also most likely to catch fire when exposed to water?

- ○ **A.** Nitrogen
- ○ **B.** Beryllium
- ○ **C.** Titanium
- ○ **D.** Potassium

Question 11

Alkaline earth metals generally form ions with a charge of:

○ **A.** +1.

○ **B.** +2.

○ **C.** −1.

○ **D.** −2.

Question 12

Magnesium belongs to which of the following families?

○ **A.** The alkaline earth metals

○ **B.** The alkali metals

○ **C.** The transition metals

○ **D.** The noble gases

Question 13

Which of the following elements has the greatest electron affinity?

○ **A.** Chlorine

○ **B.** Barium

○ **C.** Tin

○ **D.** Silver

Question 14

When halogens make ions, they tend to:

○ **A.** lose one electron.

○ **B.** lose two electrons.

○ **C.** gain one electron.

○ **D.** gain two electrons.

Question 15

If X represents an alkali metal, and Y a halogen, what is the formula for the salt of X and Y?

○ **A.** XY

○ **B.** X_2Y

○ **C.** XY_2

○ **D.** The formula depends on X and Y.

Question 16

In organic chemistry halogens often function as:

○ **A.** leaving groups.

○ **B.** electrophiles.

○ **C.** reactive oxygen species.

○ **D.** gases.

Question 17

Iodine is often used as an antiseptic. Which of the following features of halogens may contribute to this property?

○ **A.** Halogens are highly electronegative.

○ **B.** Halogens have a strong electron affinity.

○ **C.** Halogens often exist as diatomic gases.

○ **D.** Halogens are strong enzyme inhibitors.

Question 18

Which of the following statements best characterizes Argon?

○ **A.** Ar is the most reactive of the elements in row 3.

○ **B.** Ar has two electrons in the $4p_x$ subshell.

○ **C.** Ar is isoelectronic with K^+.

○ **D.** Ar has a larger atomic radius than Kr.

Question 19

Liquid anesthetics are often packaged in vials with a narrow air layer to permit shaking by mixing. Manufacturers are most likely to utilize:

○ **A.** O_2.

○ **B.** N_2 and O_2.

○ **C.** Cl_2.

○ **D.** Ne.

Question 20

The electron configuration of Radon is:

○ **A.** $[Xe]4f^{14}5d^{10}6s^26p^6$.

○ **B.** $[Xe]4f^{10}5d^{12}6s^26p^6$.

○ **C.** $[Xe]6s^{10}6p^45d^{10}4f^{12}$.

○ **D.** $[Xe]6s^{10}6p^65d^24f^{14}$.

Question 21

Iron, silver, and mercury are:

○ **A.** representative elements.

○ **B.** halogens.

○ **C.** transition metals.

○ **D.** alkaline earth metals.

Question 22

Which of the following is more likely to have naturally occurring ions with two different charges?

- A. Na
- B. He
- C. V
- D. Sr

Question 23

Which solution is most likely to be colored?

- A. $Na_2CO_3(aq)$
- B. $NaCl(aq)$
- C. $KBr(aq)$
- D. $FeCl_3(aq)$

Question 24

Representative elements are defined based on:

I. group.
II. period.
III. family.

- A. I only
- B. II only
- C. I and III only
- D. II and III only

Question 25

Which of the following is FALSE with regards to the representative elements?

- A. They represent Groups 1, 2 and 13-18 of the periodic table.
- B. They become ions with electron configurations of noble gases to gain stability.
- C. They do not represent Groups 3-12 of the periodic table.
- D. They become ions with electron configurations of noble gases to gain instability.

Question 26

Chemically, what is the primary distinction between a metal and nonmetal?

- A. Metals are solid.
- B. Metals are lustrous.
- C. Metals tend to lose electrons.
- D. Metals are strong oxidizing agents.

Question 27

Which of the following only includes nonmetals?

- A. Table salt
- B. Glucose
- C. Hemoglobin
- D. Tap water

Question 28

Which feature is more common among nonmetals?

I. Loss of electrons when forming ions
II. Gain of electrons when forming ions
III. Formation of covalent bonds

- A. I only
- B. II only
- C. I and III only
- D. II and III only

Question 29

Which of the following two elements are in the same family?

- A. Cr and Fe
- B. O and Se
- C. B and C
- D. Ir and Pt

Question 30

Which of the following elements is found in the chalcogen group?

- A. Carbon
- B. Calcium
- C. Sulfur
- D. Argon

Question 31

The attraction of the nucleus on the outermost electron in an atom tends to:

- A. decrease moving from left to right and top to bottom on the periodic table.
- B. decrease moving from right to left and top to bottom on the periodic table.
- C. decrease moving from left to right and bottom to top on the periodic table.
- D. decrease moving from right to left and bottom to top on the periodic table.

Question 32

The nucleus of which of the following would exert the greatest electrostatic force on its outermost electron?

- **A.** Na
- **B.** Cs
- **C.** F
- **D.** Mg

Question 33

Removing an electron from which of the following would require the most energy?

- **A.** Na
- **B.** Na^+
- **C.** Na^{2+}
- **D.** Na^{3+}

Question 34

Removing an electron from which of the following would most likely require the most energy?

- **A.** Na
- **B.** Na^+
- **C.** Mg
- **D.** Mg^+

Question 35

Lithium's first and second ionization energies are 519 kJ/mol and 7300 kJ/mol, respectively. Element X has a first ionization energy of 590 kJ/mol and a second ionization energy of 1150 kJ/mol. Element X is most likely to be:

- **A.** oxygen.
- **B.** sodium.
- **C.** calcium.
- **D.** xenon.

Question 36

Fe^{2+} has a higher ionization energy than Fe. Which of the following is a reasonable explanation for this fact?

- **A.** Fe^{2+} is larger than Fe.
- **B.** Fe^{2+} is isoelectronic with chromium, which has a higher ionization energy than Fe.
- **C.** The outer electrons of Fe^{2+} experience a greater effective nuclear charge than those of Fe.
- **D.** Energy had to be put into Fe to ionize it to Fe^{2+}.

Question 37

Atom A and Atom B are in the same row of the periodic table. Atom A has a greater radius than Atom B. Atom A probably also has a greater:

   I. electronegativity.

   II. first ionization energy.

   III. atomic weight.

- **A.** III only
- **B.** I and III only
- **C.** I, II, and III only
- **D.** None of the above

Question 38

Researchers studying ionization energies of new elements wished to validate their technique by testing the ionization energy of known elements. Which of the following results would indicate a valid measure?

- **A.**

Element	Ionization energy
Carbon	1075 kJ/mol
Sodium	1000 kJ/mol
Phosphorus	500 kJ/mol

- **B.**

Element	Ionization energy
Carbon	500 kJ/mol
Sodium	1075 kJ/mol
Phosphorus	1000 kJ/mol

- **C.**

Element	Ionization energy
Sodium	590 kJ/mol
Nitrogen	500 kJ/mol
Calcium	1400 kJ/mol

- **D.**

Element	Ionization energy
Sodium	500 kJ/mol
Nitrogen	1400 kJ/mol
Calcium	590 kJ/mol

Question 39

Based on electron configuration, which of the following atoms would have the lowest ionization energy?

- ○ **A.** $1s^2$
- ○ **B.** $[He]2s^22p^1$
- ○ **C.** $[Kr]5s^1$
- ○ **D.** $[Kr]4d^{10}5s^25p^5$

Question 40

Which of the following correctly depicts the ionization energy for the first group of elements?

○ **A.**

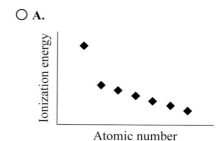

○ **B.**

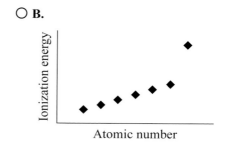

○ **C.**

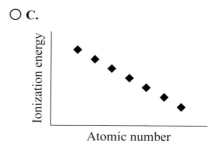

○ **D.**

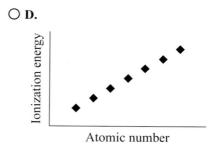

Question 41

Which of the following elements has the greatest electron affinity?

- ○ **A.** Chlorine
- ○ **B.** Barium
- ○ **C.** Tin
- ○ **D.** Silver

Question 42

Which of the following elements has the most negative electron affinity?

- ○ **A.** Calcium
- ○ **B.** Fluorine
- ○ **C.** Nitrogen
- ○ **D.** Argon

Question 43

Which of the following atoms is most likely to ionize to become an anion?

- ○ **A.** Oxygen
- ○ **B.** Iodine
- ○ **C.** Calcium
- ○ **D.** Hydrogen

Question 44

The trend for electron affinity has a few outliers, especially for atoms with nearly full *d* orbitals. Which of the following tables best depicts electron affinity?

○ **A.**

Element	Electron affinity
Calcium	−2.4 kJ/mol
Chlorine	−248.6 kJ/mol
Gold	−222.7 kJ/mol

○ **B.**

Element	Electron affinity
Calcium	−248.6 kJ/mol
Chlorine	−2.4 kJ/mol
Gold	−222.7 kJ/mol

○ **C.**

Element	Electron affinity
Calcium	−222.7 kJ/mol
Chlorine	−2.4 kJ/mol
Gold	−248.6 kJ/mol

○ **D.**

Element	Electron affinity
Calcium	222.7 kJ/mol
Chlorine	248.6 kJ/mol
Gold	2.4 kJ/mol

Question 45

Which of the following is the best definition for electron affinity?

○ **A.** The amount of energy needed to add an electron to an atom.

○ **B.** The amount of energy needed to add an electron to an element.

○ **C.** The amount of energy released when adding an electron to an atom.

○ **D.** The amount of energy released when adding an electron to an element.

Question 46

Which of the following elements would lose an electron with the least amount of energy input?

○ **A.** Li

○ **B.** F

○ **C.** Mg

○ **D.** N

Question 47

Electron affinity follows a general trend across the periodic table but some atoms deviate from expected values. Which of the following electron configurations represents an atom most likely to deviate from expected electron affinity such that the affinity is lesser than expected?

○ **A.** $[Kr]4d^9$

○ **B.** $[Kr]4d^{10}$

○ **C.** $[Kr]4d^{10}5s^1$

○ **D.** $[Kr]4d^{10}5s^2$

Question 48

Which of the following elements most easily accepts an extra electron?

○ **A.** Cl

○ **B.** Fr

○ **C.** He

○ **D.** Na

Question 49

An element within Group 1, when compared to an element from Group 7 in the same row, would possess:

○ **A.** a smaller atomic radius and energy of ionization, but greater electron affinity.

○ **B.** a smaller atomic radius, but greater energy of ionization and electron affinity.

○ **C.** a larger atomic radius and energy of ionization, but greater electron affinity.

○ **D.** a larger atomic radius, but less energy of ionization and electron affinity.

Question 50

Which of the following elements has the greatest electronegativity?

○ **A.** Lithium

○ **B.** Chlorine

○ **C.** Carbon

○ **D.** Fluorine

Question 51

Which of the following statements does NOT describe electronegativity?

○ **A.** Electronegativity is the probability of an atom accepting an additional electron.

○ **B.** Elements with significant electronegativity tend to have a stronger pull on electrons during a bond than elements with a lesser degree of electronegativity.

○ **C.** Electronegativity provides a system of predicting the type of bond expected to form between two atoms.

○ **D.** Elements with vast differences in electronegativity tend to form ionic bonds.

For questions 52-53, refer to the data collected below:

	EN (Pauling scale)
Element A	3.0
Element B	2.1
Element C	1.0
Element D	2.5
Element E	2.0

Question 52

Which two elements are most likely to form an ionic bond?

○ **A.** Elements A and C

○ **B.** Elements B and C

○ **C.** Elements A and D

○ **D.** Elements A and B

Question 53

Which two elements would form a nonpolar covalent bond?

○ **A.** Elements A and C

○ **B.** Elements B and D

○ **C.** Elements A and E

○ **D.** Elements A and B

Question 54

Many chemists consider the electronegativity of helium to be undefined. Why?

○ **A.** The small size of helium makes its electronegativity difficult to measure.

○ **B.** Helium does not have inner-shell electrons.

○ **C.** Helium atoms are electrically neutral.

○ **D.** Helium does not form bonds with other elements.

Question 55

The element with the greatest electronegativity is:

○ **A.** Cl.

○ **B.** Fr.

○ **C.** He.

○ **D.** F.

Question 56

Which of the following elements is the most electronegative?

○ **A.** Be

○ **B.** Br

○ **C.** Cs

○ **D.** Kr

Question 57

In a bond between H and any two of the following atoms, the bonding electrons would be most strongly attracted to:

○ A. Cl.

○ B. Rb.

○ C. He.

○ D. I.

Question 58

Fluorine is the most electronegative element. What is the second most electronegative element?

○ A. Nitrogen

○ B. Chlorine

○ C. Oxygen

○ D. Neon

Question 59

Which of the following elements has the largest atomic radius?

○ A. Cl

○ B. Ar

○ C. K

○ D. Ca

Question 60

An atom of phosphorous will be most similar in size to which of the following atoms?

○ A. O

○ B. Ge

○ C. As

○ D. Se

Question 61

Which of the following pairs has the greatest difference in atomic radius?

○ A. Sodium and cesium

○ B. Lithium and fluorine

○ C. Hydrogen and helium

○ D. Aluminum and antimony

Question 62

Which of the following figures correctly depicts the shape of the outermost electron shells when moving across period 3?

○ A.

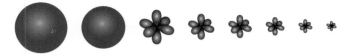

○ B.

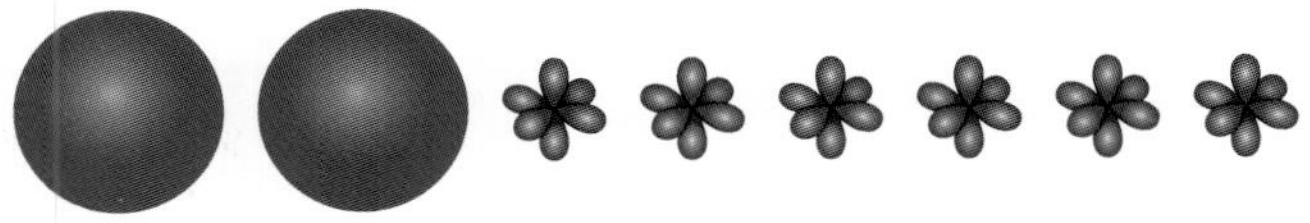

○ C.

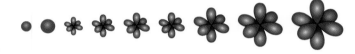

○ D.

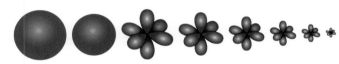

Question 63

Which of the following has the largest radius?

○ A. Cl⁻

○ B. Ar

○ C. K⁺

○ D. Ca²⁺

Question 64

Of the following atoms with the same electron configuration, which has the largest atomic radius?

○ A. O^{2-}

○ B. F^-

○ C. Na^+

○ D. Mg^{2+}

Question 65

Which of the following is ordered correctly in terms of atomic radius, from smallest to largest?

○ **A.** Al^{3+}, Al, S, S^{2-}

○ **B.** Al^{3+}, S, Al, S^{2-}

○ **C.** S, Al^{3+}, S^{2-}, Al

○ **D.** S, S^{2-}, Al^{3+}, Al

Question 66

Why is Mg^{2+} smaller than Na^+?

○ **A.** Mg^{2+} has fewer electrons than Na^+, and the size of an ion is determined by the size of its electron cloud.

○ **B.** Mg^{2+} has a greater mass than Na^+, and thus holds its electrons more tightly.

○ **C.** Mg^{2+} has a greater atomic number than Na^+, and thus holds its electrons more tightly.

○ **D.** Mg^{2+} has a smaller ionization energy than Na^+, and thus a smaller size.

Quantum Mechanics

Question 67

Which of the following is true of the energy levels for an electron in a hydrogen atom?

○ **A.** Since there is only one electron, that electron must be in the lowest energy level.

○ **B.** The spacing between the $n = 1$ and $n = 2$ energy levels is the same as the spacing between the $n = 4$ and $n = 5$ energy levels.

○ **C.** The energy of each level can be computed from a known formula.

○ **D.** The energy levels are identical to the levels in the He^+ ion.

Question 68

Which of the following statements is true of the Bohr atomic model?

○ **A.** Electrons rotate around the nucleus in a path characterized by a certain energy level.

○ **B.** Electrons can only occupy a specific energy level.

○ **C.** Nuclear radius shrinks as electrons are added.

○ **D.** Nuclear radius increases as electrons are added.

Question 69

Which of the following quantum systems defies the Pauli exclusion principle?

○ **A.** $n = 2$; $\ell = 1$; $m_l = 0$; $m_s = +\frac{1}{2}$ and $n = 2$; $\ell = 1$; $m_l = 0$; $m_s = +\frac{1}{2}$

○ **B.** $n = 1$; $\ell = 2$; $m_l = 0$; $m_s = +\frac{1}{2}$ and $n = 1$; $\ell = 2$; $m_l = 0$; $m_s = -\frac{1}{2}$

○ **C.** $n = 3$; $\ell = 2$; $m_l = 3$; $m_s = +\frac{1}{2}$ and $n = 1$; $\ell = 2$; $m_l = 3$; $m_s = -\frac{1}{2}$

○ **D.** $n = 6$; $\ell = 2$; $m_l = 0$; $m_s = +\frac{1}{2}$ and $n = 6$; $\ell = 2$; $m_l = 0$; $m_s = -\frac{1}{2}$

Question 70

Which of the following statements correctly describes the Pauli exclusion principle?

○ **A.** Two electrons must have opposite spins if they are orbiting the same atom.

○ **B.** Two photons cannot exist in the same quantum state.

○ **C.** Two fermions cannot exist in the same quantum state.

○ **D.** Electrons occupy the lowest energy orbitals.

Question 71

How many quantum numbers are necessary to describe a single electron in an atom?

○ **A.** 1

○ **B.** 2

○ **C.** 3

○ **D.** 4

Question 72

Which quantum number designates the shell level of an electron?

○ **A.** The principal quantum number

○ **B.** The azimuthal quantum number

○ **C.** The magnetic quantum number

○ **D.** The electron spin quantum number

Question 73

What is the maximum number of electrons that can fit in a shell with principal quantum number 3?

○ **A.** 2

○ **B.** 3

○ **C.** 10

○ **D.** 18

Question 74

Which of the following sets of quantum numbers describes the highest energy electron?

- **A.** $n = 3$; $\ell = 2$; $m_\ell = 2$; $m_s = -\frac{1}{2}$
- **B.** $n = 2$; $\ell = 1$; $m_\ell = 0$; $m_s = -\frac{1}{2}$
- **C.** $n = 1$; $\ell = 0$; $m_\ell = 0$; $m_s = -\frac{1}{2}$
- **D.** $n = 2$; $\ell = 1$; $m_\ell = 0$; $m_s = +\frac{1}{2}$

Question 75

Only one set of the following quantum numbers could exist. Which set is it?

- **A.** $n = 3$; $\ell = 3$; $m_l = 2$; $m_s = -\frac{1}{2}$
- **B.** $n = 2$; $\ell = 1$; $m_l = 2$; $m_s = -\frac{1}{2}$
- **C.** $n = 4$; $\ell = 2$; $m_l = 2$; $m_s = -\frac{1}{2}$
- **D.** $n = 1$; $\ell = 2$; $m_l = 3$; $m_s = +\frac{1}{2}$

Question 76

In what way is it inaccurate to picture an electron as a tiny particle orbiting a nucleus?

- **A.** An electron is actually much larger than a typical nucleus.
- **B.** The electron jumps from orbit to orbit more frequently than would be predicted by classical mechanics.
- **C.** Since it is impossible to know both the position and momentum of an electron simultaneously, it is inappropriate to consider the electron to be a localized particle with a definite orbit.
- **D.** It is difficult to determine the precise orbit experimentally.

Question 77

Does the Heisenberg uncertainty principle apply to macroscopic objects such as basketballs?

- **A.** Yes, but the large size of a basketball makes it difficult to determine its position with precision.
- **B.** Yes, but the large mass of a basketball makes the uncertainty in velocity very small even if the uncertainty in position is also very small.
- **C.** No, because the basketball is made up of very many atoms, and the uncertainties cancel out.
- **D.** No, because a basketball is constantly interacting with its environment.

Question 78

Which of the following is true with regards to elements within the same group of the periodic table that exhibit similar chemical properties?

- **A.** They have the same number of electrons in their outermost shell.
- **B.** They have the same number of electrons in their innermost shell.
- **C.** They have a similar number of electrons in their outermost shell.
- **D.** They have a similar number of electrons in their innermost shell.

Question 79

Which represents the generic electronic configuration for an alkali metal?

- **A.** $[X]ns^1$
- **B.** $[X]ns^2$
- **C.** $[X]ns^2np^3$
- **D.** $[X]ns^2(n-1)d^1$

Question 80

The graph below shows the melting points of the elements across Period 4.

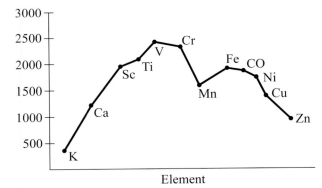

Melting points for period 4

Based on this figure, what should the melting point of cesium be compared to barium?

- **A.** Significantly higher than that of barium
- **B.** Significantly lower than that of barium
- **C.** Approximately equal to that of barium
- **D.** Not enough information provided

Question 81

Suppose an element X with n shells, atomic mass m, and atomic number k forms a $z+$ cationic charge. An ion with which characteristic would best be able to substitute element X in a buffering solution?

- ○ **A.** An element with atomic number $k + 1$ or $\ell - 1$
- ○ **B.** An element that forms a $z+$ cationic charge
- ○ **C.** An element with n shells
- ○ **D.** An element that forms an isotope with mass m

Question 82

What is the electron configuration of iron in the ground state?

- ○ **A.** $[Ar]4s^24d^6$
- ○ **B.** $[Ar]3s^23d^6$
- ○ **C.** $[Ar]3s^24d^6$
- ○ **D.** $[Ar]3d^64s^2$

Question 83

What is the electron configuration of the iodide ion in the ground state?

- ○ **A.** $[Kr]4d^{10}4d^{14}5s^25p^5$
- ○ **B.** $[Kr]3d^{14}4d^{10}5s^25p^6$
- ○ **C.** $[Kr]4d^{10}5s^25p^6$
- ○ **D.** $[Kr]5s^25p^5$

Question 84

What is the electron configuration of the Cr^{3+} ion?

- ○ **A.** $[Ar]4s^23d^4$
- ○ **B.** $[Ar]4s^23d^1$
- ○ **C.** $[Ar]4s^23d^7$
- ○ **D.** $[Ar]3d^3$

Question 85

Suppose electrons could have three possible spin states (up, down, and sideways), rather than just two. Assuming nothing else was different, which of the following would be the correct ground state electron configuration for an element with atomic number 16?

- ○ **A.** $1s^21p^62s^22p^6$
- ○ **B.** $1s^22s^23s^23p^64s^24p^2$
- ○ **C.** $1s^32s^32p^93s^1$
- ○ **D.** $3s^23p^63d^8$

Question 86

Which of the following represents an excited state of an atom?

- ○ **A.** $1s^22s^23s^1$
- ○ **B.** $1s^22s^22p^1$
- ○ **C.** $1s^22s^22p^6$
- ○ **D.** $1s^22s^22p^63s^1$

Question 87

Which of the following electron configurations could represent an atom that has absorbed light?

- ○ **A.** $1s^22s^22p^63s^23d^{10}$
- ○ **B.** $1s^22s^22p^63s^23p^64s^1$
- ○ **C.** $1s^22s^22p^63s^23d^33p^6$
- ○ **D.** $1s^22s^22p^63s^23p^63d^{10}4s^24p^6$

Question 88

If a sulfur atom is in its ground state, how many unpaired electrons does it have?

- ○ **A.** 0
- ○ **B.** 1
- ○ **C.** 2
- ○ **D.** 4

Question 89

Suppose an element in its ground state is capable of absorbing photons with energies of 2.3 eV and 4.1 eV, but no other intermediate energies. If the atom in its ground state absorbs a photon with an energy of 4.1 eV, it is found to sometimes later emit a single photon of 4.1 eV, but sometimes it emits a photon with an energy of:

- ○ **A.** 1.8 eV.
- ○ **B.** 2.0 eV.
- ○ **C.** 2.3 eV.
- ○ **D.** 4.1 eV.

Question 90

In order to be responsive to external magnetic fields, an element must have:

- ○ **A.** a complete subshell with each unpaired electron parallel to one another.
- ○ **B.** an incomplete subshell with each unpaired electron parallel to one another.
- ○ **C.** a complete subshell with no unpaired electrons.
- ○ **D.** an incomplete subshell with no unpaired electrons.

Question 91

The element diagrammed below would show the following qualities EXCEPT:

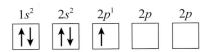

$1s^2 \quad 2s^2 \quad 2p^1 \quad 2p \quad 2p$

- ○ **A.** reactivity to an external magnetic field.
- ○ **B.** attraction or repulsion to similar compounds.
- ○ **C.** diamagnetism.
- ○ **D.** unpaired electrons.

Question 92

An electron in a certain element can have energies of -2.3, -5.1, -5.3, -8.2, and -14.9 eV. -14.9 eV is the ground state of the electron, and no other levels exist between -14.9 and -2.3 eV. Which of the following represents a partial list of photon energies that could be absorbed by an electron in the ground state of this atom? All energies are in electron volts.

- ○ **A.** $-2.3, -5.1, -5.3, -8.2, -14.9$
- ○ **B.** $0.2, 2.8, 2.9, 6.7$
- ○ **C.** $2.3, 5.1, 5.3, 8.2, 14.9$
- ○ **D.** $6.7, 9.6, 9.8, 12.6, 15.0, 16.1$

Question 93

Monatomic hydrogen gas is placed in a container of fixed volume, initially at STP. As the temperature is slowly raised, spectral lines corresponding to electrons in energy levels above the ground level appear. No matter how far the temperature is raised, however, no spectral lines for electrons above the $n = 7$ level are ever found. Which of the following is a possible explanation for this phenomenon?

- ○ **A.** No elements have electrons in levels above $n = 7$.
- ○ **B.** Energy levels above $n = 7$ correspond to orbitals so large that the hydrogen atoms would overlap, disrupting the spectral lines.
- ○ **C.** At the temperatures required to raise electrons to orbitals above $n = 7$, hydrogen nuclei would decompose.
- ○ **D.** Beyond $n = 7$, STP cannot be maintained.

Question 94

Which of the following is NOT an implication of the photoelectric effect?

- ○ **A.** Electrons can be excited to higher energy states.
- ○ **B.** Light frequency is proportional to the kinetic energy of emitted electrons.
- ○ **C.** Only metals are capable of experiencing the photoelectric effect.
- ○ **D.** Light is composed of particles.

Question 95

The following data were collected in an experiment by a chemist studying the photoelectric effect. Which of the following metals has the lowest energy work function?

Metal	Light color	Kinetic energy (eV)
Ca	Blue	0.3
K	Blue	0.8
Cr	Blue	0 (No ejection)
La	Red	0 (No ejection)

- ○ **A.** Ca
- ○ **B.** K
- ○ **C.** Cr
- ○ **D.** La

Bonding

Question 96

When sodium chloride melts, what kind(s) of bonds are breaking?

   I. Covalent

   II. Ionic

   III. Dipole-dipole

- ○ **A.** I only
- ○ **B.** II only
- ○ **C.** III only
- ○ **D.** II and III only

Question 97

Which of the following compounds lacks ionic bonds?

- ○ **A.** NaCl
- ○ **B.** NaH
- ○ **C.** HCl
- ○ **D.** $Ca_3(PO_4)_2$

Question 98

Hydrogen sulfide (H_2S) is a colorless gas with an odor of rotten eggs. Why is hydrogen sulfide gaseous but water is liquid at room temperature?

- A. Sulfur is less electronegative than oxygen, so intermolecular forces are weaker.
- B. Sulfur is less electronegative than oxygen, so intramolecular forces are weaker.
- C. Sulfur is more electronegative than oxygen, so intermolecular forces are weaker.
- D. Sulfur is more electronegative than oxygen, so intramolecular forces are weaker.

Question 99

Researchers measured the boiling points of four compounds. Data are presented in the table below.

Compound	Boiling point (°C)
H_2O	100.0
H_2S	−61.2
H_2Se	−42.3
H_2Te	28.1

Which of the following conclusions can be ascertained from the researchers' data?

- A. Hydrogen bonding increases the boiling points of all compounds.
- B. Molecular weight is directly correlated with boiling point.
- C. Maximized dipole-dipole interactions increase the boiling point.
- D. Greater quantities of *p* and *d* orbitals allow for greater induced dipole interactions.

Question 100

The structure of dimethylformamide is shown below.

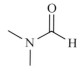

What are the primary interactions between molecules of dimethylformamide in the liquid phase?

- A. Dipole-dipole
- B. Covalent bonding
- C. Hydrogen bonding
- D. Induced dipole-induced dipole

Question 101

Iodine is required for the formation of thyroid hormone, but it is not an endogenously produced element. For this reason, salt is often iodized, and it is essential that food chemists understand how iodized salt functions in an aqueous environment. What is the predominating source of intermolecular interaction between molecules of I_2 in water?

- A. Dipole-dipole
- B. Induced dipole-induced dipole
- C. Hydrogen bonding
- D. Covalent

Question 102

Of the molecules listed below, which are likely to exhibit Van der Waals' forces?

    I. C_9H_{20}
    II. Br_2
    III. H_2O

- A. I only
- B. II only
- C. I and II only
- D. I, II, and III

Reactions and Stoichiometry

Question 103

What is the mass in kilograms of a single water molecule?

- A. $(18)(6.02 \times 10^{23})(1000)$
- B. $\dfrac{18}{(6.02 \times 10^{23})(1000)}$
- C. $\dfrac{(18)(1000)}{6.02 \times 10^{23}}$
- D. $\dfrac{18}{6.02 \times 10^{23}}$

Question 104

If the mass percent of nitrogen in a compound is 10% and there are two nitrogen atoms in each molecule of the compound, what is the molecular weight of the compound?

- A. 28 g/mol
- B. 70 g/mol
- C. 140 g/mol
- D. 280 g/mol

Question 105

The mass percent of a compound is as follows: 71.65% Cl; 24.27% C; and 4.07% H. If the molecular weight of the compound is 98.96 amu, what is the molecular formula of the compound?

- **A.** ClC_2H_2
- **B.** $ClCH_2$
- **C.** $Cl_2C_2H_4$
- **D.** $Cl_3C_3H_8$

Question 106

The mass percent of a compound is as follows: 43.64% P, and 56.36% O. If the molecular weight of the compound is 283.88 amu, what is the molecular formula of the compound?

- **A.** P_2O_3
- **B.** P_2O_5
- **C.** P_3O_7
- **D.** P_4O_{10}

Question 107

What is the mass of one molecule of water?

- **A.** 18 g
- **B.** 18 amu
- **C.** 18 moles
- **D.** 18 g/mol

Question 108

What is the percent by mass of chlorine in carbon tetrachloride?

- **A.** 50%
- **B.** 75%
- **C.** 80%
- **D.** 92%

Question 109

What is the mass percent of nitrogen in NO_2?

- **A.** 14.0%
- **B.** 20.5%
- **C.** 30.4%
- **D.** 33.3%

Question 110

What is the balanced reaction for the combustion of methane?

- **A.** $NH_3 + OH^- \rightarrow NH_4OH$
- **B.** $CH_3OH + 2O_2 \rightarrow CO_2 + 2H_2O$
- **C.** $CH_4 + OH^- \rightarrow CH_3OH$
- **D.** $CH_4 + 2O_2 \rightarrow CO_2 + 2H_2O$

Question 111

Which reaction gives the balanced reaction for the combustion of ethanol (C_2H_5OH)?

- **A.** $C_2H_5OH + O_2 \rightarrow CO_2 + H_2O$
- **B.** $C_2H_5OH + 2O_2 \rightarrow 2CO_2 + 2H_2O$
- **C.** $C_2H_5OH + 3O_2 \rightarrow 2CO_2 + 3H_2O$
- **D.** $4C_2H_5OH + 13O_2 \rightarrow 8CO_2 + 10H_2O$

Question 112

Which of the following represents the balanced double displacement reaction between copper(II) chloride and iron(II) carbonate?

- **A.** $Cu_2Cl + Fe_2CO_3 \rightarrow Cu_2CO_3 + Fe_2Cl$
- **B.** $CuCl_2 + Fe(CO_3)_2 \rightarrow Cu(CO_3)_2 + FeCl_2$
- **C.** $Cu_2Cl + FeCO_3 \rightarrow Cu_2CO_3 + FeCl$
- **D.** $CuCl_2 + FeCO_3 \rightarrow CuCO_3 + FeCl_2$

Question 113

The following is an unbalanced reaction:

$$C_{12}H_{22}O_{11}(l) + O_2(g) \rightarrow CO_2(g) + H_2O(g)$$

How many moles of oxygen gas are required to burn one mole of $C_{12}H_{22}O_{11}$?

- **A.** 1
- **B.** 6
- **C.** 12
- **D.** 24

Question 114

The following is an unbalanced reaction:

$$C_6H_{12}O_6(s) + O_2(g) \rightarrow CO_2(g) + H_2O(g)$$

How many moles of oxygen gas are required to burn one mole of $C_6H_{12}O_6$?

- **A.** 1
- **B.** 3
- **C.** 6
- **D.** 12

Question 115

The following is an unbalanced reaction for the combustion of hexane (C_6H_{14}):

$$C_6H_{14}(g) + O_2(g) \rightarrow CO_2(g) + H_2O(g)$$

How many moles of oxygen gas are required to burn 2 moles of hexane?

○ **A.** 6
○ **B.** 12
○ **C.** 14
○ **D.** 19

Question 116

Which of the following is true about the following equation?

$$2\ H_2O_2 + \text{Peroxidase} \leftrightarrow 2\ \text{Water} + \text{Oxygen}$$

○ **A.** It is appropriate to use words rather than formulas for a reaction.

○ **B.** A reverse arrow is acceptable in this case since H_2O and O_2 can be combined to make hydrogen peroxide.

○ **C.** Peroxidase should not be on the left side of this equation.

○ **D.** This reaction is missing a coefficient.

Question 117

Which of the following is true of notation convention for organic reaction?

○ **A.** A retrosynthesis should use a double headed arrow.

○ **B.** All solvents should be noted above the arrow in the case of a single reaction.

○ **C.** All solvents should be noted below the arrow in the case of a multi-step reaction.

○ **D.** Not all reactants need to be listed to the left of the arrow.

Question 118

Which of the following is a physical reaction?

○ **A.** Boiling of a liquid
○ **B.** Combustion of a gas
○ **C.** Dehydration of a solid
○ **D.** Elimination of a liquid

Question 119

Which of the following bonds could be broken in a physical reaction?

○ **A.** Hydrogen bonds
○ **B.** Peptide bonds
○ **C.** Covalent bonds
○ **D.** Intramolecular bonds

Question 120

$$CH_4(g) + 2O_2(g) \leftrightarrow CO_2(g) + 2H_2O(g)$$

The reaction shown above is NOT an example of a(n):

○ **A.** combustion reaction.
○ **B.** chemical reaction.
○ **C.** oxidation-reduction reaction.
○ **D.** physical reaction.

Question 121

A compound containing iron and chlorine is reacted to produce a salt of tetraethylammonium chloride. Which of the following is a plausible reaction to describe this?

○ **A.** $FeCl_2 + ((C_2H_5)_4N)Cl \rightarrow ((C_2H_5)_4N)_2[FeCl_2]$

○ **B.** $FeCl_3 + ((C_2H_5)_4N)Cl \rightarrow ((C_2H_5)_4N)[FeCl_4]$

○ **C.** $FeCl_2 + 2((C_2H_5)_4N)Cl \rightarrow ((C_2H_5)_4N)_2[FeCl_4]$

○ **D.** $FeCl_4 + 2((C_2H_5)_4N)Cl \rightarrow ((C_2H_5)_4N)_2[FeCl_4] + 2Cl^-$

Question 122

What is the best classification of the following reaction?

$$H_2O_2 \rightarrow 2H_2O + O_2(g)$$

○ **A.** Decomposition
○ **B.** Catalytic
○ **C.** Single replacement
○ **D.** Disproportionation

Question 123

Which of the following is true of the following reaction?

$$Cl_2 + H_2O \rightarrow HCl(aq) + HClO(aq)$$

○ **A.** Water is both oxidized and reduced.
○ **B.** Chlorine is both oxidized and reduced.
○ **C.** Water is oxidized.
○ **D.** Chlorine is oxidized.

Question 124

The following is an unbalanced reaction:

$$Fe(s) + O_2(g) \rightarrow Fe_2O_3(s)$$

If 2 moles of iron react to completion with 2 moles of oxygen gas, what remains after the reaction?

○ **A.** 1 mole of Fe_2O_3 only

○ **B.** 1 mole of Fe_2O_3 and 0.5 mole of oxygen gas

○ **C.** 1 mole of Fe_2O_3 and 0.5 mole of iron

○ **D.** 1 mole of Fe_2O_3, 1 mole of iron, and 1 mole of oxygen gas

Question 125

The following is an unbalanced reaction:

$$Au_2S_3(s) + H_2(g) \rightarrow Au(s) + H_2S(g)$$

If 1 mole of $Au_2S_3(s)$ is reacted with 5 moles of hydrogen gas, what is the limiting reagent?

○ **A.** $Au_2S_3(s)$

○ **B.** $H_2(g)$

○ **C.** $Au(s)$

○ **D.** $H_2S(g)$

Question 126

Fifteen moles of $N_2O_4(l)$ are reacted with $N_2H_3CH_3(l)$ to produce 36 moles of water via the equation shown below:

$$5N_2O_4(l) + 4N_2H_3CH_3(l) \rightarrow 12H_2O(g) + 9N_2(g) + 4CO_2(g)$$

How many moles of $N_2H_3CH_3(l)$ are used up in the reaction?

○ **A.** 4

○ **B.** 8

○ **C.** 10

○ **D.** 12

Question 127

Ten moles of $N_2O_4(l)$ are added to an unspecified amount of $N_2H_3(CH_3)(l)$ according to the equation shown below:

$$5N_2O_4(l) + 4N_2H_3(CH_3)(l) \rightarrow 12H_2O(g) + 9N_2(g) + 4CO_2(g)$$

If 23 moles of water are produced and the reaction runs to completion, what is the limiting reagent?

○ **A.** $N_2O_4(l)$

○ **B.** $N_2H_3(CH_3)(l)$

○ **C.** $H_2O(g)$

○ **D.** There is no limiting reagent.

Question 128

In the following reaction, which is run at 600 K, 4.5 moles of nitrogen gas are mixed with 11 moles of hydrogen gas:

$$N_2(g) + 3H_2(g) \rightarrow 2NH_3(g)$$

The reaction produces 6 moles of ammonia. What is the percent yield of ammonia?

○ **A.** 42%

○ **B.** 57%

○ **C.** 82%

○ **D.** 100%

Question 129

When the following reaction is run, a 75% yield is achieved:

$$PCl_3(g) + 3NH_3(g) \rightarrow P(NH_2)_3(g) + 3HCl(g)$$

How many moles of phosphorous trichloride are required to produce 328 grams of HCl?

○ **A.** 1 mol

○ **B.** 2 mol

○ **C.** 3 mol

○ **D.** 4 mol

Question 130

How much does a 3 mole sample of Na weigh?

○ **A.** 23 amu

○ **B.** 69 amu

○ **C.** 23 grams

○ **D.** 69 grams

Question 131

How many atoms of Mg are in a 48 g sample of solid Mg?

○ **A.** 2 atoms

○ **B.** 4 atoms

○ **C.** $2 \times 6.02 \times 10^{23}$ atoms

○ **D.** $4 \times 6.02 \times 10^{23}$ atoms

Question 132

Which of the following represents the charge on one mole of electrons?

○ **A.** 1 e

○ **B.** 6.02×10^{23} e

○ **C.** 1 C

○ **D.** 6.02×10^{23} C

Question 133

The charge on one mole of electrons is given by Faraday's constant ($F = 96,500$ C/mol). What is the total charge of all the electrons in 2 grams of He?

- ○ **A.** 48,250 C
- ○ **B.** 96,500 C
- ○ **C.** 193,000 C
- ○ **D.** 386,000 C

Radioactive Decay

Question 134

A half-life is:

- ○ **A.** the time required for half the amount of a substance to decay.
- ○ **B.** half the time required for half the amount of a substance to decay.
- ○ **C.** the time required for all of a substance to decay.
- ○ **D.** half the time required for all of a substance to decay.

Question 135

If 12 g of substance X remain from an original sample of 384 g, and substance X has a half-life of 10 hours, how much time has passed?

- ○ **A.** 20 hours
- ○ **B.** 50 hours
- ○ **C.** 100 hours
- ○ **D.** 320 hours

Question 136

Which of the following is an electron?

- ○ **A.** Neutrino
- ○ **B.** Gamma particle
- ○ **C.** Photon
- ○ **D.** Beta particle

Question 137

Which of the following most accurately describes radioactive decay?

- ○ **A.** Molecules spontaneously break apart to produce energy.
- ○ **B.** Atoms spontaneously break apart to produce energy.
- ○ **C.** Protons and neutrons spontaneously break apart to produce energy.
- ○ **D.** Electrons spontaneously break apart to produce energy.

Question 138

^{222}Rn decays once to form ^{218}Po. What type of particle is emitted?

- ○ **A.** A gamma particle
- ○ **B.** An alpha particle
- ○ **C.** A beta particle
- ○ **D.** A positron

Question 139

Neutron bombardment of ^{238}U results in ^{239}U, which spontaneously undergoes beta decay to produce the new element:

- ○ **A.** ^{239}Np.
- ○ **B.** ^{238}Np.
- ○ **C.** ^{239}Pa.
- ○ **D.** ^{238}Pa.

Question 140

^{11}C produces a positron to form:

- ○ **A.** ^{10}B.
- ○ **B.** ^{11}B.
- ○ **C.** ^{12}C.
- ○ **D.** ^{11}N.

Question 141

^{218}Po undergoes one alpha decay and two beta decays to make:

- ○ **A.** ^{214}Po.
- ○ **B.** ^{214}Pb.
- ○ **C.** ^{214}Bi.
- ○ **D.** ^{210}Pb.

Question 142

^{201}Hg undergoes electron capture to form:

- ○ **A.** ^{200}Au.
- ○ **B.** ^{201}Au.
- ○ **C.** ^{201}Tl.
- ○ **D.** ^{202}Tl.

Question 143

^{238}U undergoes seven alpha decays and six beta decays to make:

- ○ **A.** ^{210}Po.
- ○ **B.** ^{210}Pb.
- ○ **C.** ^{210}Bi.
- ○ **D.** ^{206}Pb.

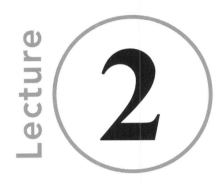

Lecture

2

Questions 144–286

Introduction to Organic Chemistry

Representations of Organic Molecules
Bonds and Hybridization
Resonance and Electron Delocalization
Functional Groups and their Features
Stereochemistry
Substitution Reactions of Alkanes

Representations of Organic Molecules

Question 144

The Lewis dot structure of CO_2 is shown. How many electrons exist in the pi bonds of CO_2?

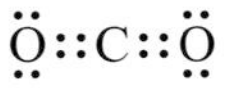

$$\ddot{O}::C::\ddot{O}$$

- A. 2
- B. 4
- C. 8
- D. Cannot be determined

Question 145

How many electrons are involved in the sigma bond between the carbon atom and the nitrogen atom?

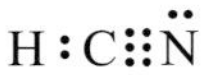

$$H:C\overset{\cdot\cdot}{\cdot\cdot}\ddot{N}$$

- A. 0
- B. 1
- C. 2
- D. 6

Question 146

What is the correct Lewis dot structure for CH_3CH_2CHO?

- A.

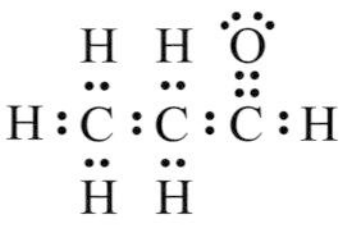

    H H O̤
    H:C:C:C:H
    H H

- B.

    H H O̤
    H:C:C::C:H
    H H

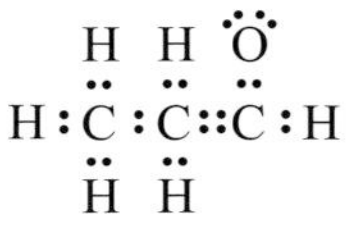

- C.

    H H O̤:H
    H:C:C:C:
    H H

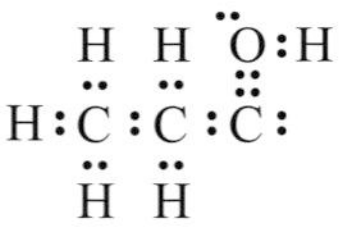

- D.

    H H
    H:C:C::C::O̤:H
    H H

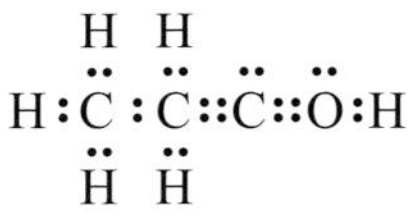

Question 147

What is the correct Lewis dot structure for HCN?

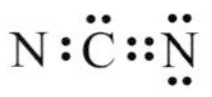

- A.

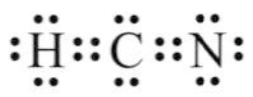

    :H::C::N:

- B.

    N:C::N̈

- C.

    H:C::H

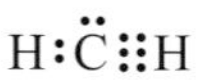

- D.

    H:C::N̈

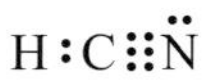

Question 148

A student discovers that a Lewis electron dot representation of an atom contains more than 8 electrons. These results best validate which of the following conclusions?

- A. The atom contains unoccupied d orbitals.
- B. The atom is in period 3 of the periodic table.
- C. The atom is more electronegative than its adjacent atoms.
- D. The student made a mistake, as atoms cannot break the octet rule.

Refer to the resonance structure of the nitrite ion (NO_2^-) for questions 149-151.

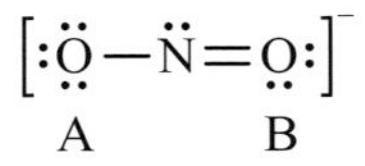

$$\left[:\ddot{O}-\ddot{N}=\underset{\cdot\cdot}{O}:\right]^-$$
$$\quad\ \ A \qquad\quad B$$

Question 149

What are the formal charges of Oxygen A, Nitrogen, and Oxygen B, respectively?

- A. $-1, 0, 0$
- B. $0, 0, -1$
- C. $-2, -3, -2$
- D. $-6, -2, -4$

Question 150

The structure of HCN is shown below.

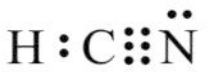

$$H:C\overset{\cdot\cdot}{\cdot\cdot}\ddot{N}$$

What is the formal charge on the nitrogen atom in HCN?

- A. 0
- B. 1
- C. 2
- D. 3

Question 151

In an attempt to determine the charge distribution of the nitrite ion, researchers chose to analyze the formal charges of atoms. Will their conclusions be adequately supported by these research results?

○ **A.** Yes, atoms with the most negative formal charges will have the greatest electron density.

○ **B.** Yes, summing the formal charges will then indicate the overall charge of the ion.

○ **C.** No, the researchers would need to further consider the electronegativities of the individual atoms.

○ **D.** No, x-ray crystallography is necessary to determine charge distribution.

▲

Question 152

What is the total charge on the Lewis dot structure displayed below?

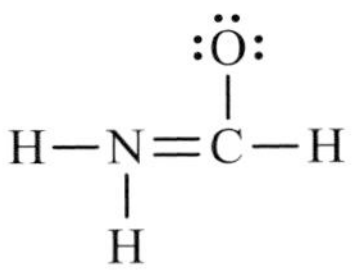

$$\overset{\displaystyle :\ddot{O}:}{\underset{\displaystyle H}{\overset{\displaystyle |}{H-N=C-H}}}$$

○ **A.** −2
○ **B.** −1
○ **C.** 0
○ **D.** Cannot be determined

Bonds and Hybridization

Question 153

The structure of Chlorophyll-a, a plant pigment, is displayed below. How many double bonds are contained in the conjugated system found in Chlorophyll-a?

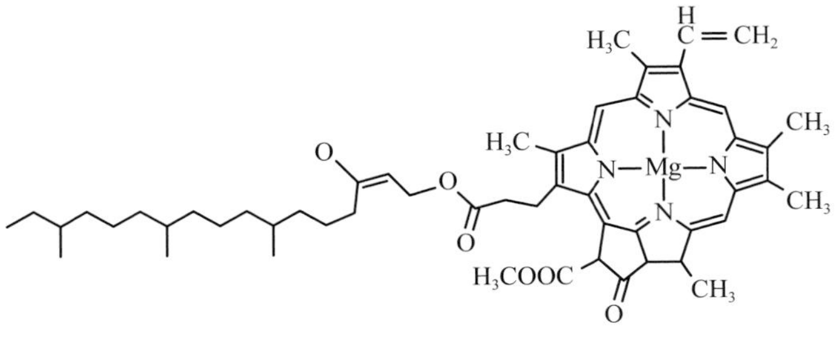

○ **A.** 10
○ **B.** 11
○ **C.** 12
○ **D.** 16

Question 154

Atoms in period 15 of the periodic table are expected to form which type(s) of bond(s) and still remain neutrally charged?

  I. Single bonds

  II. Double bonds

  III. Triple bonds

○ **A** I only
○ **B.** I and II only
○ **C.** I and III only
○ **D.** I, II, and III

Question 155

The overlap of which two orbitals form the pi bond between carbon atoms in an alkene?

○ **A.** Two p orbitals
○ **B.** Two sp^2 orbitals
○ **C.** Two sp^3 orbitals
○ **D.** Two s orbitals

Question 156

Which bond requires the most energy to break?

○ **A.** Sigma bond
○ **B.** Pi bond
○ **C.** Hydrogen bond
○ **D.** Dipole-dipole bond

▼

For questions 157-158, refer to the diagrams provided below:

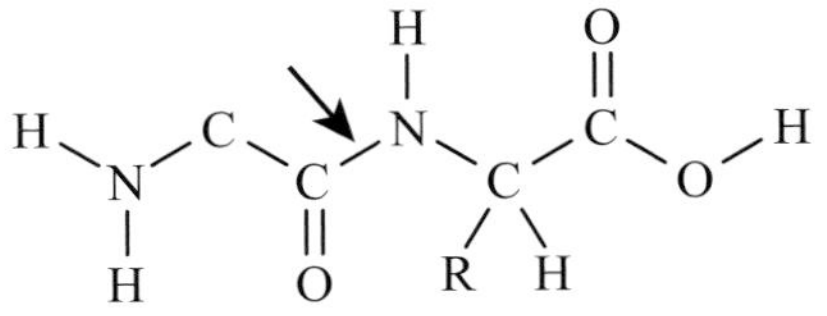

Compound A

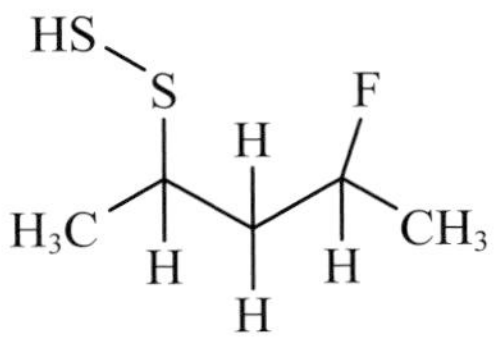

Compound B

Question 157

Which compound would display the most rigidity in its molecular structure?

○ **A.** Compound A due to the π bonds in its molecular structure.

○ **B.** Compound A due to a lack of π bonds in its molecular structure.

○ **C.** Compound B due to the π bonds in its molecular structure.

○ **D.** Compound B due to a lack of π bonds in its molecular structure.

Question 158

Which compound would display the LEAST amount of rigidity in its molecular structure?

○ **A.** Compound A due to the π bonds in its molecular structure.

○ **B.** Compound A due to a lack of π bonds in its molecular structure.

○ **C.** Compound B due to the π bonds in its molecular structure.

○ **D.** Compound B due to a lack of π bonds in its molecular structure.

▲

Question 159

Which of the following properties of estrogen allows it to bind its cytoplasmic receptor?

   I. Planar shape

   II. Nonpolar character

   III. Charged functional groups

○ **A.** I only

○ **B.** I and II only

○ **C.** II and III only

○ **D.** I, II and III

Question 160

Which of the following statements best explains why T_3, a thyroid hormone, is able to pass through both the plasma and nuclear membranes?

○ **A.** T_3 contains many hydroxyl and carbonyl groups.

○ **B.** T_3 contains an aromatic ring that maintains planar structure.

○ **C.** T_3 is highly flexible around its carbon-carbon single bonds.

○ **D.** T_3 contains F atoms that allow it to diffuse through the plasma membrane.

Question 161

A researcher designs an experiment to determine the volume of distribution (V_d) in adipose tissue of an intravenous anesthetic. The scientist would most likely measure the greatest V_d in a drug with:

   I. aromatic rings.

   II. hydroxyl side chains.

   III. prenyl functional groups.

○ **A.** I only

○ **B.** I and III only

○ **C.** II and III only

○ **D.** I, II, and III

Question 162

How much *s* character does an sp^3 hybridized orbital have?

○ **A.** No *s* character

○ **B.** 25%

○ **C.** 33.3%

○ **D.** 50%

▼

Cocaine is a stimulant that is isolated from coca leaves. Refer to the structure of cocaine shown below to answer questions 163-167.

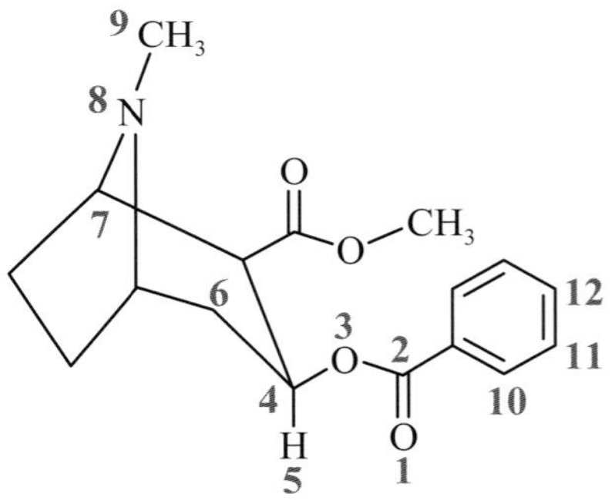

Question 163

The hybridization of the C9 carbon in cocaine is:

○ **A.** *sp*.

○ **B.** sp^2.

○ **C.** sp^3.

○ **D.** sp^3d.

Question 164

The hybridization of the N8 nitrogen in cocaine is:

○ **A.** *sp.*

○ **B.** sp^2.

○ **C.** sp^3.

○ **D.** sp^3d.

Question 165

The bond angle formed by C2, O3, and C4 in cocaine is:

○ **A.** 180°.

○ **B.** 120°.

○ **C.** 109°.

○ **D.** 90°.

Question 166

How much *s* character is in the hybridized orbital on the C2 carbon in the cocaine structure?

○ **A.** No *s* character

○ **B.** 25%

○ **C.** 33.3%

○ **D.** 50%

Question 167

How much *p* character is in the hybridized orbital on the N8 nitrogen in the cocaine structure?

○ **A.** 33.3%

○ **B.** 50%

○ **C.** 66.6%

○ **D.** 75%

Question 168

How much *p* character is in the hybridized orbital on the center carbon in acetone (CH_3COCH_3)?

○ **A.** 33.3%

○ **B.** 50%

○ **C.** 66.6%

○ **D.** 75%

Question 169

According to VSEPR theory, what is the molecular geometry of sulfur tetrafluoride?

○ **A.** Tetrahedral

○ **B.** Square planar

○ **C.** Seesaw

○ **D.** It depends on the relative electronegativity of sulfur and fluoride.

Refer to the structure of aspartame, an artificial sweetener, to answer questions 170-172.

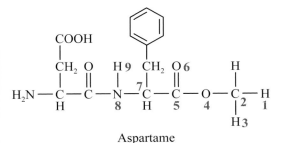

Aspartame

Question 170

The bond angle formed by H1, C2, and H3 in aspartame is:

○ **A.** 180°.

○ **B.** 120°.

○ **C.** 109°.

○ **D.** 90°.

Question 171

The bond angle formed by O4, C5, and O6 in aspartame is:

○ **A.** 180°.

○ **B.** 120°.

○ **C.** 109°.

○ **D.** 90°.

Question 172

The bond angle formed by C7, N8, and H9 in aspartame is:

○ **A.** 180°.

○ **B.** 120°.

○ **C.** 109°.

○ **D.** 90°.

Question 173

In formamide the nitrogen has a bond angle of 120°, indicating sp^2 hybridization rather than the expected sp^3 hybridization. The best explanation for this observation is:

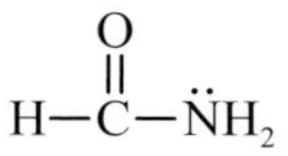

$$H-\overset{\overset{\displaystyle O}{\|}}{C}-\ddot{N}H_2$$
formamide

○ **A.** in one of the resonance structures the nitrogen has a double bond.

○ **B.** nitrogen always has sp^2 hybridization.

○ **C.** the lone pair of electrons on the nitrogen indicates sp^2 hybridization.

○ **D.** the nitrogen has three atoms attached therefore it must have sp^2 hybridization.

Question 174

Which bond requires the most energy to break?

○ **A.** Single bond

○ **B.** Double bond

○ **C.** Triple bond

○ **D.** Hydrogen bond

Question 175

What is the length of the bond between C1 and C2 in the structure shown below?

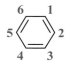

○ **A.** The length of a carbon-carbon bond in an alkane

○ **B.** The length of a carbon-carbon double bond in an alkene

○ **C.** Shorter than the length of a carbon-carbon double bond in an alkene

○ **D.** Between the length of a carbon-carbon bond in an alkane and the length of a carbon-carbon double bond in an alkene

Question 176

What is the length of the bond between C2 and C3 in the structure shown below?

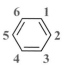

○ **A.** The length of a carbon-carbon bond in an alkane

○ **B.** The length of a carbon-carbon double bond in an alkene

○ **C.** Shorter than the length of a carbon-carbon double bond in an alkene

○ **D.** Between the length of a carbon-carbon bond in an alkane and the length of a carbon-carbon double bond in an alkene

Average bond energies are shown in the table below. Use the table to answer questions 177-178.

Bond	Average bond energy kcal mol^{-1}
C—C	83
C=C	146
C≡C	200

Question 177

Based on the values in the table, what is the approximate average bond energy for each sigma bond?

○ **A.** 60 kcal mol^{-1}

○ **B.** 80 kcal mol^{-1}

○ **C.** 150 kcal mol^{-1}

○ **D.** 200 kcal mol^{-1}

Question 178

Based on the values in the table, what is the approximate average bond energy for each pi bond?

○ **A.** 60 kcal mol^{-1}

○ **B.** 80 kcal mol^{-1}

○ **C.** 150 kcal mol^{-1}

○ **D.** 200 kcal mol^{-1}

Resonance and Electron Delocalization

Question 179

Which of the structures is NOT a resonance structure of benzene?

○ **A.**

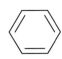

○ **B.**

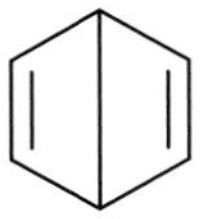

○ **C.**

○ **D.**

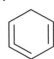

Question 180

Which of the following structures has delocalized electrons?

I. $H_3C-C=C-CH_3$ (with H, H below the double-bonded carbons)

II. (benzene ring with one double bond shown)

III. $H_2C=C-\overset{\overset{\displaystyle O}{\|}}{C}-CH_3$ (with H below)

○ **A.** I only
○ **B.** II only
○ **C.** I and III only
○ **D.** II and III only

Question 181

Which of the following structures has delocalized electrons?

I. $H_3C-C=C-CH_3$ (with H, H below the double-bonded carbons)

II. 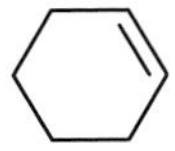 (cyclohexene ring with one double bond)

III. $H_2C=C-C-C=CH_2$ (with H, H_2, H below)

○ **A.** I only
○ **B.** II only
○ **C.** I and III only
○ **D.** None of the structures

Question 182

Which of the following is NOT a resonance structure of the phenol anion?

○ **A.**

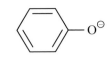

○ **B.**

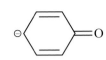

○ **C.**

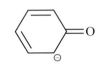

○ **D.**

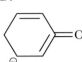

Question 183

Conjugation in a molecule will shift the IR absorption band to a lower energy. Which of the following structures will have IR bands at lower energies than that of a non-conjugated double bond?

I. $H_2C=C-C-C-CH_3$ (with H, H_2, H_2 below)

II. $H_2C=C-C-C=CH_2$ (with H, H_2, H below)

III. $H_2C=C-C=C-CH_3$ (with H, H, H below)

○ **A.** II only
○ **B.** III only
○ **C.** I and III only
○ **D.** II and III only

Question 184

Which of the following structures is a major resonance contributor for the structure shown below?

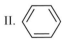

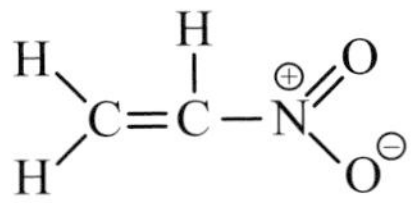

○ **A.**

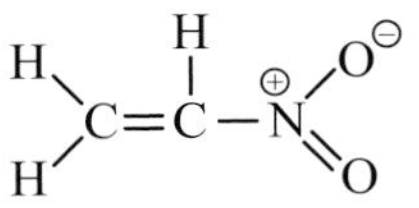

(structure A)

○ **B.**

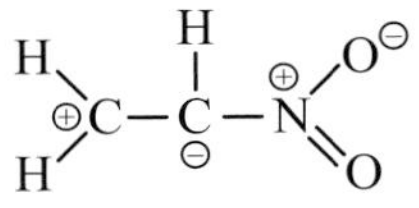

(structure B)

○ **C.**

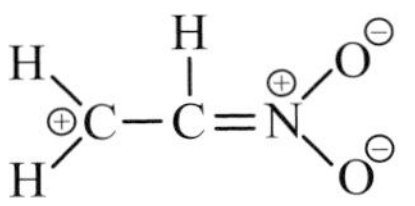

(structure C)

○ **D.**

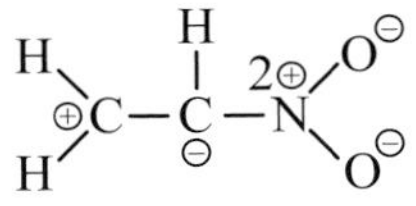

(structure D)

Question 185

Which one of the following structures is NOT a resonance structure of the cation shown below?

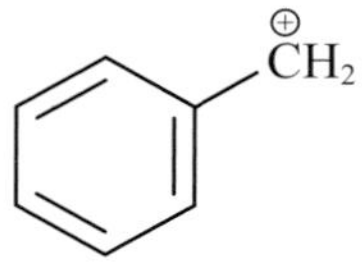

○ **A.**

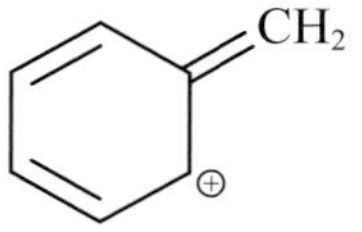

○ **B.**

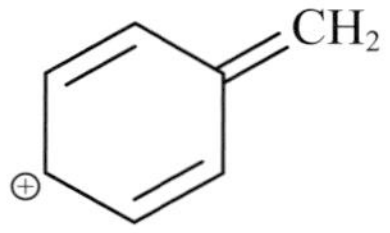

○ **C.**

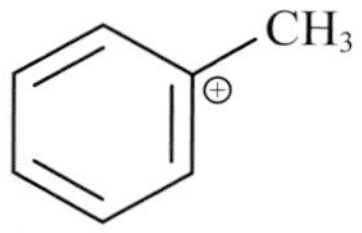

○ **D.**

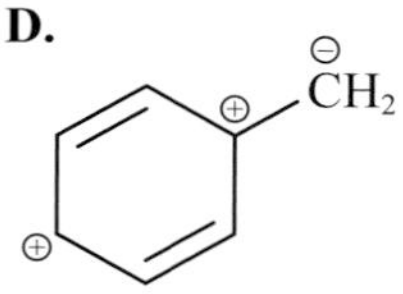

Question 186

Which of the following is a resonance structure of 2-pentanone?

○ **A.**

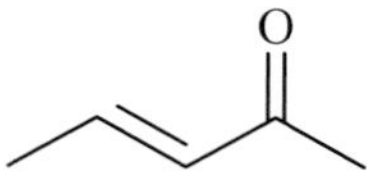

○ **B.**

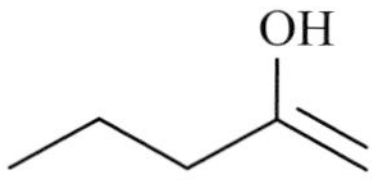

○ **C.**

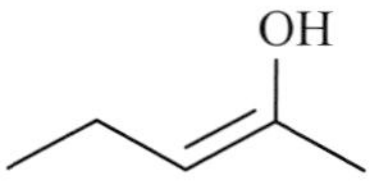

○ **D.**

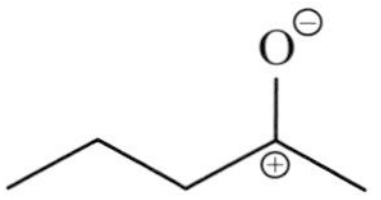

Question 187

Which of the following structures is the most minor resonance contributor of urea (H_2NCONH_2)?

○ **A.**

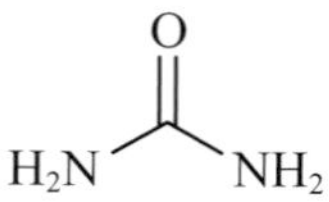

○ **B.**

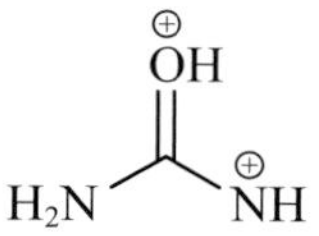

○ **C.**

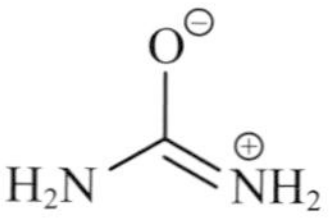

○ **D.**

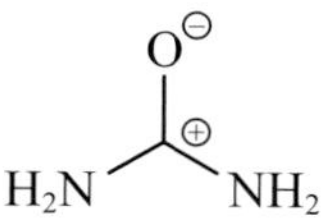

Question 188

Which statement is most likely true of the resonance contributor that makes up the greatest proportion of the actual molecular structure? This contributor:

○ **A.** has the lowest number of atoms with nonzero formal charges.

○ **B.** is the only structure found in nature.

○ **C.** contains the greatest separation of charge.

○ **D.** has a plane of symmetry.

Question 189

Which of the following resonance structures of NCO^- has the smallest resonance energy?

○ **A.**

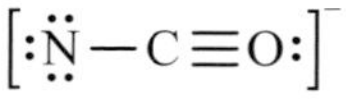

$$\left[:\ddot{N} - C \equiv O: \right]^-$$

○ **B.**

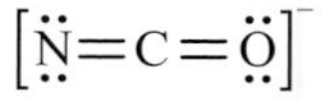

$$\left[\ddot{N} = C = \ddot{O} \right]^-$$

○ **C.**

$$\left[:N \equiv C - \ddot{O}: \right]^-$$

○ **D.**

$$\left[\ddot{N} = C = \ddot{O}: \right]^{2-}$$

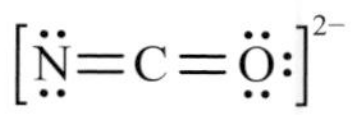

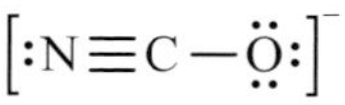

Question 190

Analysis of x-ray crystallographic data allowed researchers to determine structural properties of a molecule as presented in the table.

Resonance structure	Percentage of actual molecular structure
A	19%
B	72%
C	2%
D	8%

Resonance structure D most likely has:

○ **A.** unpaired electrons.

○ **B.** a greater separation of charge than resonance structure A.

○ **C.** a greater number of delocalized electrons than structure C.

○ **D.** a smaller number of nonzero formal charges than resonance structure B.

Question 191

After analyzing the resonance contributors of L-arginine, researchers determine that each of the individual contributors exists at a higher energy level than that of the actual molecule. What additional finding would best explain these results?

○ **A.** The actual molecule has the lowest absolute value heat of combustion.

○ **B.** The actual molecule has a small degree of intramolecular charge separation.

○ **C.** The actual molecule exists as the weighted average of every resonance contributor.

○ **D.** The majority of the actual molecule's electron delocalization occurs on its side chain.

Question 192

What force is responsible for the bonds between atoms?

○ **A.** Dipole-dipole

○ **B.** Hydrogen bonding

○ **C.** Gravitational

○ **D.** Electrostatic

Question 193

Researchers have determined that an enzymatic active site can be competitively inhibited by a benzene ring with an attached group. The greatest inhibition occurs when the bond of the side group has partial ionic character. Which of the following correctly depicts the K_M for the following four inhibitors?

I.   II.   III.   IV.

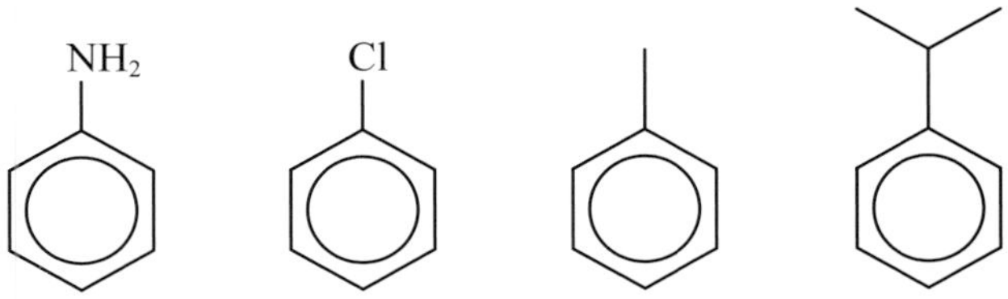

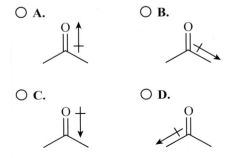

○ **A.**

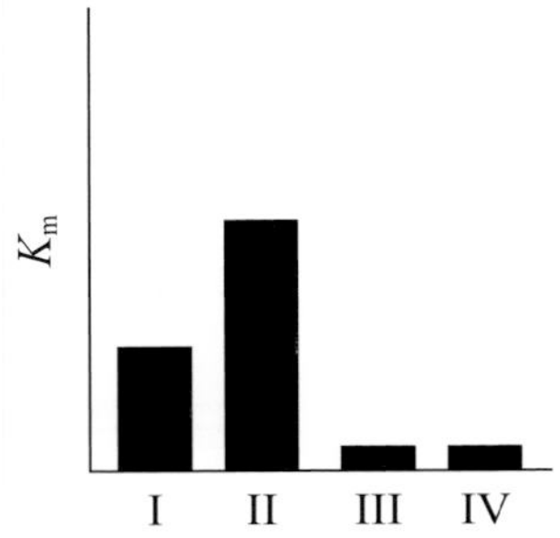

○ **B.**

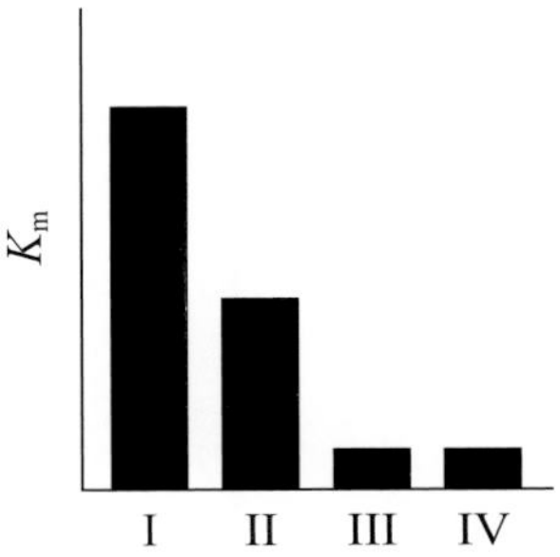

○ **C.**

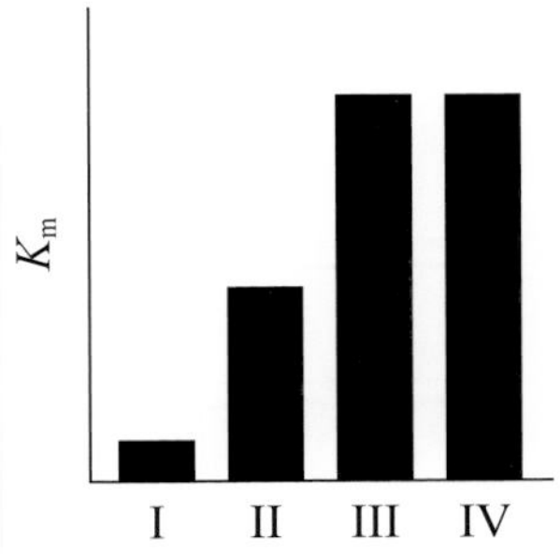

○ **D.**

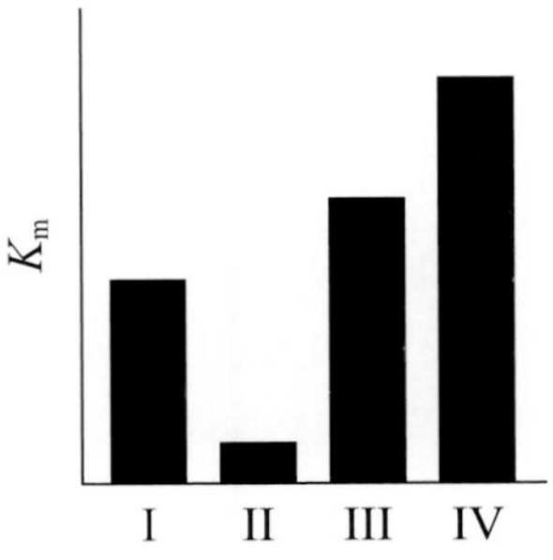

Question 194

Which of the following structures shows the correct net dipole moment for acetone?

○ **A.**   ○ **B.**

○ **C.**   ○ **D.**

Question 195

What is the correct net dipole moment for the structure shown below?

○ A.

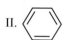

○ B.

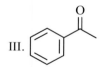

○ C.

○ D.

Question 196

In order to be IR active (have an absorption band in an IR spectrum), a molecule must have a dipole moment. Which of the following molecules are IR active?

I. CH_3CH_2OH

II.

III.

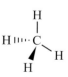

○ A. II only
○ B. III only
○ C. I and III only
○ D. II and III only

Question 197

Which of the three molecules pictured below contains a net dipole moment?

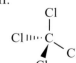

○ A. II only
○ B. III only
○ C. I and III only
○ D. II and III only

Question 198

Which structure has the correct bond dipole found in ethanol?

○ A.

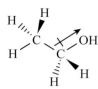

○ B.

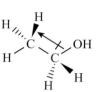

○ C.

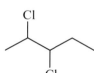

○ D.

Functional Groups and Their Features

Question 199

Which of the following is a haloalkane?

○ A.

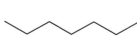

○ B.

○ C.

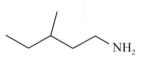

○ D.

○ A.

○ B.

Question 200

Which of the following is NOT an alkane?

○ A.

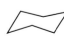

○ B.

○ C.

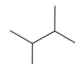

○ D.

Question 201

Which of the following is a geminal halide?

○ **A.**

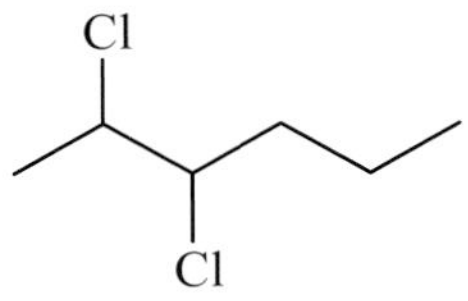

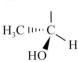

○ **B.**

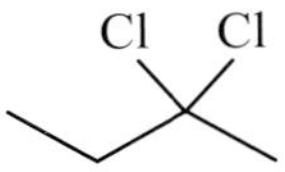

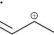

○ **C.**

○ **D.**

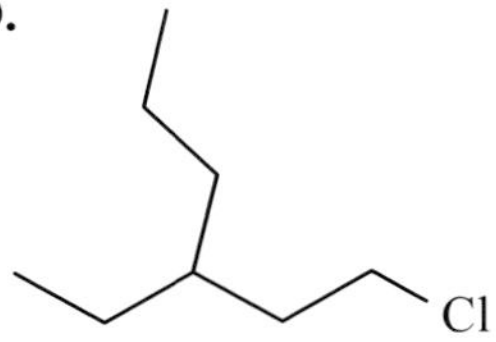

Question 202

Pharmaceutical researchers attempting to maximize the blood solubility of a novel chemotherapeutic agent choose to conjugate the drug with a haloalkane. Which of the following haloalkanes should the researchers choose?

○ **A.** 1-chlorohexane

○ **B.** 1-fluorohexane

○ **C.** 1,1,1-tribromopropane

○ **D.** 1,1,1-tribromopentane

Question 203

Which of the following alkenes is the most stable?

○ **A.**

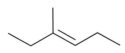

○ **B.**

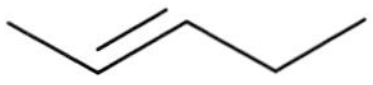

○ **C.**

○ **D.**

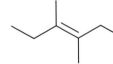

Question 204

Myrcene, a terpene found in bayberry, is shown below.

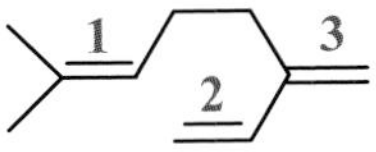

myrcene

How many geometric isomers of myrcene exist?

○ **A.** 0

○ **B.** 3

○ **C.** 6

○ **D.** 9

Question 205

Which of the following is the least stable cation?

○ **A.**

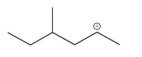

○ **B.**

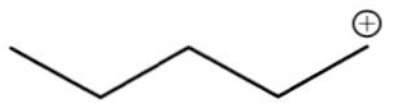

○ **C.**

○ **D.**

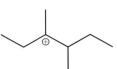

Question 206

Why is the following reaction impractical to use on an industrial scale to produce the given product?

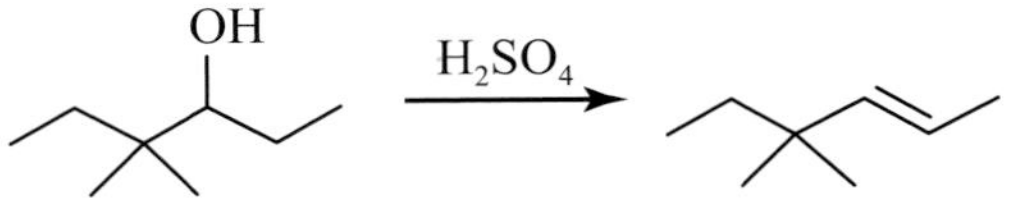

OH $\xrightarrow{H_2SO_4}$

○ **A.** The carbocation intermediate leads to multiple products.

○ **B.** Dehydration of alcohols is not acid catalyzed.

○ **C.** Alkenes cannot be formed from an alcohol.

○ **D.** The alcohol is not available in large quantities.

Question 207

Which of the following will promote hydration of an alkene to an alcohol?

○ **A.** Concentrated H^+ and heat

○ **B.** H_2 with Ni

○ **C.** O_3 and $(CH_3)_2S$

○ **D.** Dilute acid and cold conditions

Question 208

If 2-methyl-2-butanol is heated with sulfuric acid, what are the resulting products?

 I. 2-methyl-1-butene

 II. 2-methyl-2-butene

 III. 3-methyl-1-butene

○ **A.** I only

○ **B.** III only

○ **C.** I and II only

○ **D.** I, II, and III

Question 209

Which of the following is an electrophile?

- ○ **A.** OH⁻
- ○ **B.** NH₃
- ○ **C.** H⁺
- ○ **D.** CH₄

Question 210

What is the product when 2-methyl-2-pentene is reacted with HBr?

- ○ **A.** 2-bromo-2-methylpentane
- ○ **B.** 3-bromo-2-methylpentane
- ○ **C.** 2-bromo-pentane
- ○ **D.** 2-bromo-2-methylpentene

Question 211

Which of the following alkenes would react the fastest with HBr?

- ○ **A.** Ethene
- ○ **B.** 1-butene
- ○ **C.** 2-butene
- ○ **D.** 2-methyl-2-butene

Question 212

Why does benzene undergo substitution reactions rather than addition reactions?

- ○ **A.** Benzene does not have a double bond.
- ○ **B.** If benzene underwent an addition reaction, the aromaticity of the ring would be disrupted.
- ○ **C.** When benzene undergoes a substitution reaction, the aromaticity is disrupted.
- ○ **D.** Benzene is an alkene.

Question 213

Which of the following structures is an aldehyde?

○ **A.**   ○ **B.**

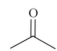

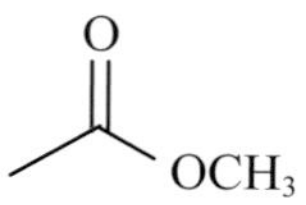

○ **C.**   ○ **D.**

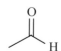

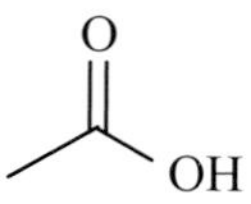

Question 214

Which of the following structures is a ketal?

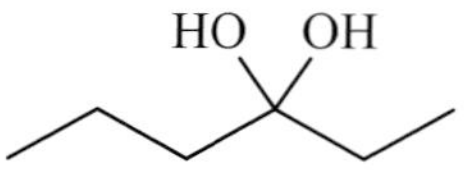

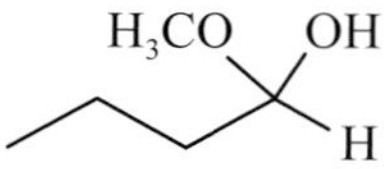

○ **A.**   ○ **B.**

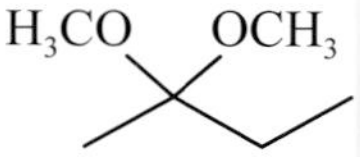

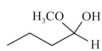

○ **C.**   ○ **D.**

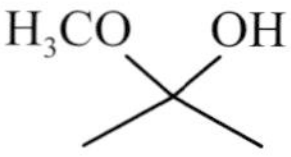

Question 215

Which of the following structures is a hemiacetal?

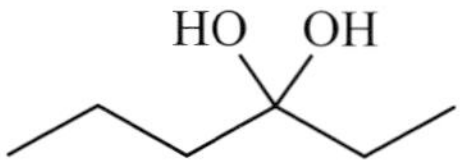

○ **A.**   ○ **B.**

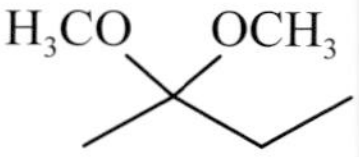

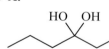

○ **C.**   ○ **D.**

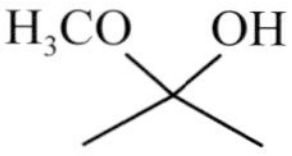

Question 216

Which of the following structures is a hemiketal?

○ **A.**   ○ **B.**

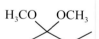

○ **C.**   ○ **D.**

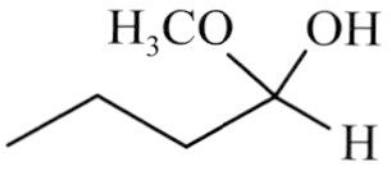

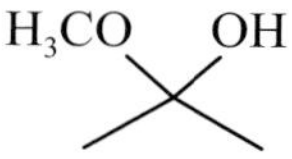

Question 217

A brightener that is used for white shirts is Calcofluor White MR. The structure of this whitener is shown below. How many amine functionalities are present in this molecule?

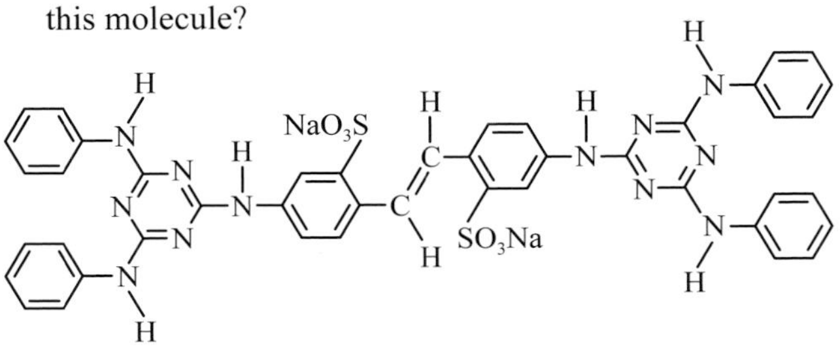

- ○ **A.** 0
- ○ **B.** 6
- ○ **C.** 12
- ○ **D.** 14

Question 218

The structure of piperazine, used to kill intestinal worms, is shown below. Piperazine is a:

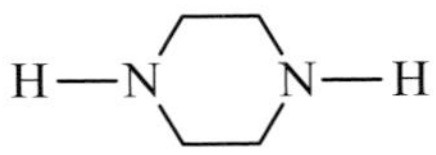

- ○ **A.** primary amine.
- ○ **B.** secondary amine.
- ○ **C.** tertiary amine.
- ○ **D.** quaternary amine.

Question 219

The reaction shown below favors the reactants. What is the best explanation for the energy relationship between the reactants and the products?

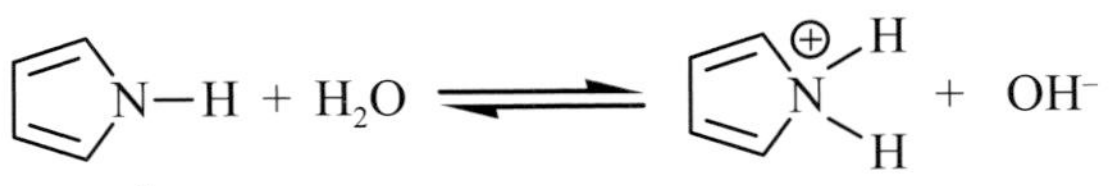

pyrrole

- ○ **A.** Secondary amines are more basic than primary amines.
- ○ **B.** Primary amines are more basic than secondary amines.
- ○ **C.** The product is stabilized by aromaticity.
- ○ **D.** The reactant is stabilized by aromaticity.

Question 220

Given the structures for p-nitroaniline (pK_b 13.0) and p-toluidine (pK_b 8.92) below, what is the best explanation for the relative pK_b values for the amines?

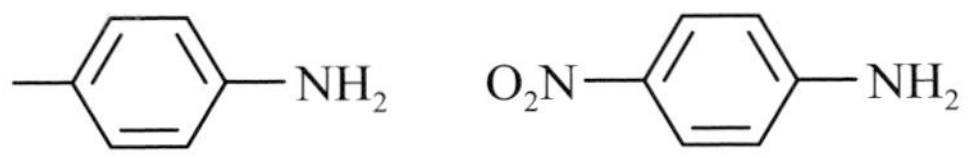

p-toluidine p-nitroaniline

- ○ **A.** *Para*-toluidine is more basic than p-nitroaniline because a methyl group is electron donating and a nitro group is electron withdrawing.
- ○ **B.** *Para*-toluidine is less basic than p-nitroaniline because a methyl group is electron donating and a nitro group is electron withdrawing.
- ○ **C.** *Para*-toluidine is more basic than p-nitroaniline because a methyl group is electron withdrawing and a nitro group is electron donating.
- ○ **D.** *Para*-toluidine is less basic than p-nitroaniline because a methyl group is electron withdrawing and a nitro group is electron donating.

Question 221

Given the information about the dipoles of given bonds shown below, which atom has the largest difference in electronegativity compared to carbon?

Bond	Dipole moment in debye
C—H	0.30 D
C—N	0.22 D
C—O	0.86 D
C—Cl	1.56 D

- ○ **A.** H
- ○ **B.** N
- ○ **C.** O
- ○ **D.** Cl

Question 222

What determines the polarity of a covalent bond?

- ○ **A.** Difference in atomic size
- ○ **B.** Difference in electronegativity
- ○ **C.** Difference in total number of protons
- ○ **D.** Difference in total number of valence electrons

Question 223

Which of the following molecules has the most even distribution of electrons in the 1s orbital?

- ○ **A.** HF
- ○ **B.** HBr
- ○ **C.** N_2
- ○ **D.** BH_3

Question 224

The greatest dipole moment is likely to be found in a bond where:

- ○ **A.** both bonding elements have high electronegativity.
- ○ **B.** both bonding elements have moderate electronegativity.
- ○ **C.** both bonding elements have low electronegativity.
- ○ **D.** one bonding element has high electronegativity and the other has low electronegativity.

Question 225

In a water molecule, oxygen has a partial negative charge because:

- ○ **A.** oxygen is more electronegative than hydrogen.
- ○ **B.** oxygen has more valence electrons than hydrogen.
- ○ **C.** oxygen is sp^3 hybridized.
- ○ **D.** water is bent.

Question 226

Which of the three molecules pictured below contains a polar bond?

I.  II.  III.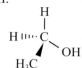

- ○ **A.** I only
- ○ **B.** III only
- ○ **C.** II and III only
- ○ **D.** I, II, and III

Question 227

A carbon-chlorine bond is characterized by:

- ○ **A.** equal sharing of electrons.
- ○ **B.** a dipole moment.
- ○ **C.** a zero energy bond.
- ○ **D.** a pi bond.

Question 228

A very electronegative leaving group:

- ○ **A.** decreases polarization of a bond.
- ○ **B.** is a poor leaving group.
- ○ **C.** makes the associated carbon a strong electrophile.
- ○ **D.** will favor E1 and E2 reactions.

Question 229

What is the chemical formula for ATP, shown below?

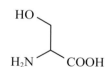

- ○ **A.** $C_5H_8N_5O_3P_3$
- ○ **B.** $C_{10}H_8N_5O_3P_3$
- ○ **C.** $C_{10}H_{16}N_5O_3P_3$
- ○ **D.** $C_{12}H_{16}N_5O_3P_3$

Question 230

A modified cysteine is used in some proteins and is encoded as a UGA codon. Which of the following structures depicts this unusual amino acid?

- ○ **A.**
- ○ **B.**
- ○ **C.**
- ○ **D.**

Stereochemistry

Isopulegols result as a side product from the oxidation of citronellol. Refer to the structure below to answer questions 231 and 232.

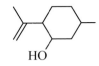

Isopulegols

Question 231

How many chiral centers are present in isopulegols?

○ **A.** 0
○ **B.** 1
○ **C.** 2
○ **D.** 3

Question 232

Pulegol can be synthesized from isopulegol. The structure of pulegol is shown below. How many chiral centers does pulegol have?

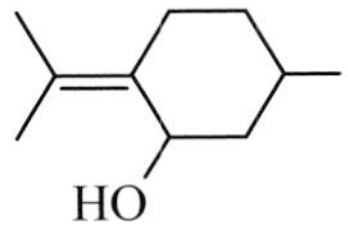

HO

○ **A.** 0
○ **B.** 1
○ **C.** 2
○ **D.** 3

Refer to the Fischer projection below to answer questions 233-234.

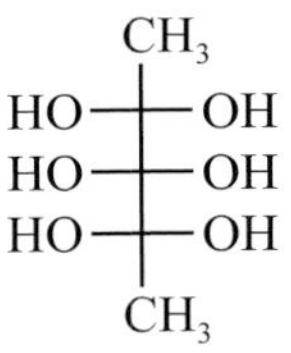

$$CH_3$$
HO——OH
HO——OH
HO——OH
$$CH_3$$

Question 233

In the Fischer projection, what do the intersections of the vertical and horizontal lines represent?

○ **A.** Rotation of the bond
○ **B.** Carbon atoms
○ **C.** Double bonds
○ **D.** Nothing

Question 234

In the Fischer projection shown, the hydroxyl groups are:

○ **A.** coming out of the page on the right side and into the page on the left.
○ **B.** coming out of the page on the left side and into the page on the right.
○ **C.** coming out of the page.
○ **D.** going into the page.

Question 235

In the Newman projection below, what does the circle represent?

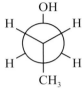

○ **A.** The largest carbon in the structure
○ **B.** The second carbon along the axis of the bond
○ **C.** The first carbon along the axis of the bond
○ **D.** The radius of the bond

Question 236

Which of the following molecules is chiral?

○ **A.** CH_2ClBr
○ **B.** CH_3CH_2OHCl
○ **C.** $CH_3CH(CH_2CH_3)Cl$
○ **D.** $CH_3CH(CH_3)Cl$

Question 237

The reduction of 1,2-dibromopentene is shown below.

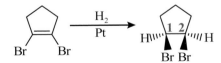

The 1,2-dibromocyclopentane is called a(n):

○ **A.** chiral compound.
○ **B.** anomeric compound.
○ **C.** meso compound.
○ **D.** enantiomer.

Question 238

Which structure is the Fischer projection for the structure shown below?

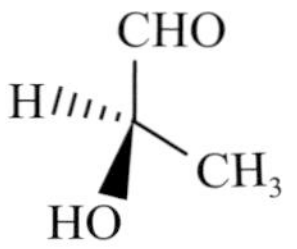

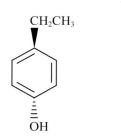

○ **A.**

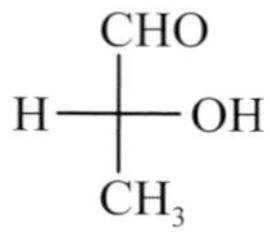

CHO

H ─┼─ OH

CH₃

○ **B.**

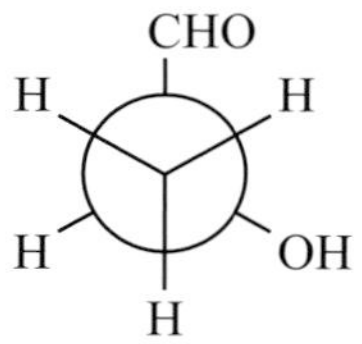

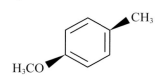

○ **C.**

CHO

HO ─┼─ H

CH₃

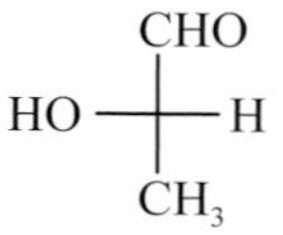

○ **D.**

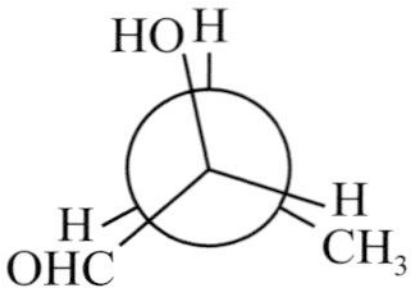

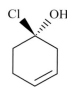

Question 239

Which of the following is an isomer of the compound below?

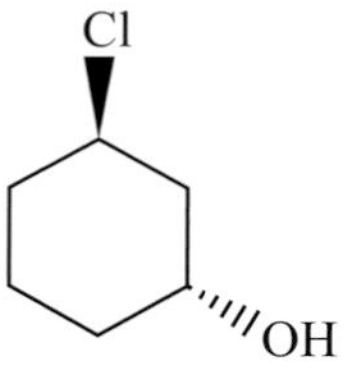

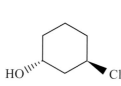

○ **A.**

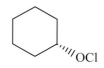

○ **B.**

Cl   OH

○ **C.**

⟨cyclohexane⟩''OCl

○ **D.**

CH₃CH₂─CH(Cl)─CH₂─CH(OH)─CH₃

Cl   OH

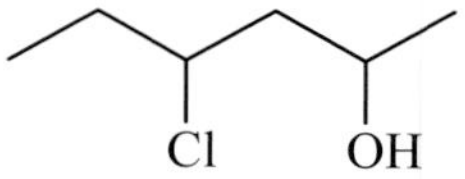

Question 240

Which of the following is NOT an isomer of the compound below?

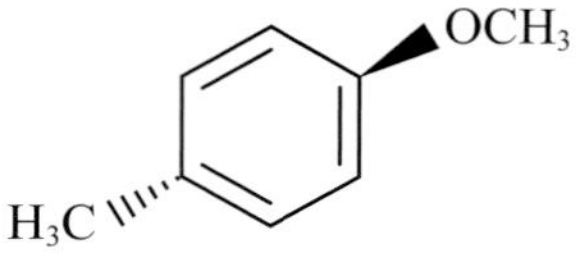

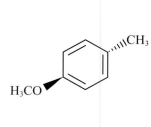

○ **A.**

CH₂CH₃

⟨benzene⟩

OH

○ **B.**

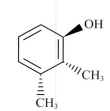

○ **C.**

H₃CO⟨benzene⟩CH₃

○ **D.**

OH

''CH₃

CH₃

Question 241

What is the relationship between structures A and B?

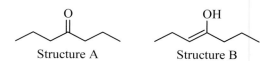

Structure A   Structure B

○ **A.** Geometric isomers
○ **B.** Stereoisomers
○ **C.** Tautomers
○ **D.** No relationship

Question 242

Which of the following statements, if true, would allow for a molecule to be classified as an isomer of the structure below? The molecule:

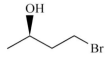

- ○ **A.** has an "*S*" absolute configuration.
- ○ **B.** has the same bond-to-bond connectivity but different number of atoms.
- ○ **C.** has the same bond-to-bond connectivity with an "*R*" absolute configuration.
- ○ **D.** has a molecular formula of C_4H_9OBr with a hydroxyl group on the same carbon attached to bromine.

Question 243

Combustion analysis allowed researchers to determine that the empirical formula of an unknown compound with a molar mass of 56 grams is CH_2. Which of the following compounds could be an isomer of the unknown compound?

○ **A.**   ○ **B.**

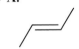

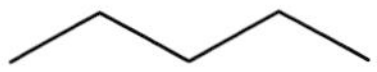

○ **C.** 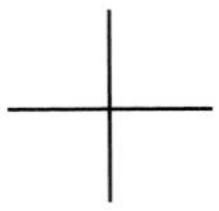   ○ **D.**

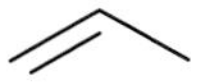

Question 244

Which of the following is a structural isomer of the molecule below?

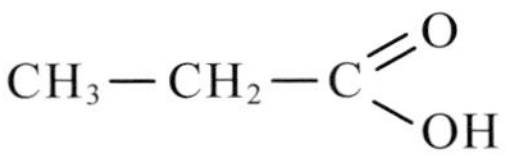

$$CH_3-CH_2-C\overset{\displaystyle O}{\underset{\displaystyle OH}{\big<}}$$

○ **A.**

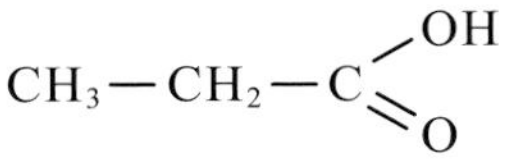

$$CH_3-CH_2-C\overset{\displaystyle OH}{\underset{\displaystyle O}{\big<}}$$

○ **B.**

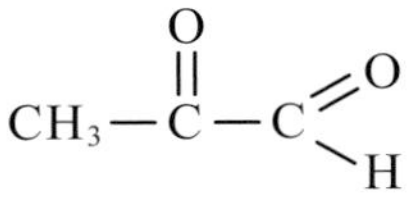

$$CH_3-\overset{\overset{\displaystyle O}{\|}}{C}-C\overset{\displaystyle O}{\underset{\displaystyle H}{\big<}}$$

○ **C.**

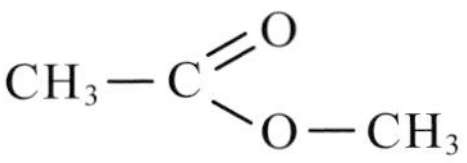

$$CH_3-C\overset{\displaystyle O}{\underset{\displaystyle O-CH_3}{\big<}}$$

○ **D.**

$$CH_3-CH_2-CH_2-C\overset{\displaystyle O}{\underset{\displaystyle OH}{\big<}}$$

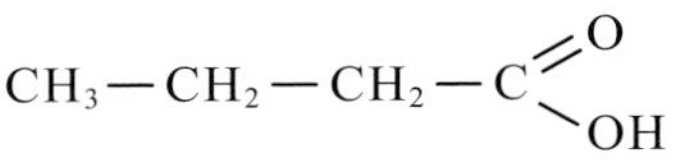

Question 245

How many structural isomers with the molecular formula $C_4H_{10}O$ are alcohols?

- ○ **A.** 2
- ○ **B.** 4
- ○ **C.** 5
- ○ **D.** 10

Question 246

How are the molecules shown below related?

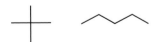

- ○ **A.** Conformers
- ○ **B.** Enantiomers
- ○ **C.** Structural isomers
- ○ **D.** Geometric isomers

Question 247

How are the pair of molecules shown below related?

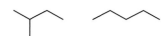

- **A.** Conformers
- **B.** Enantiomers
- **C.** Structural isomers
- **D.** Geometric isomers

Question 248

How are the pair of molecules shown below related?

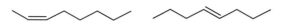

- **A.** Conformers
- **B.** Enantiomers
- **C.** Epimers
- **D.** Not stereoisomers

Question 249

How are the molecules shown below related?

- **A.** Conformers
- **B.** Enantiomers
- **C.** Structural isomers
- **D.** Geometric isomers

Question 250

Which of the following conformers has the highest energy?

- **A.**
- **B.**
- **C.**
- **D.**

Question 251

What is the conformer shown below called?

- **A.** Antistaggered
- **B.** Gauche
- **C.** Fully eclipsed
- **D.** Eclipsed

Question 252

What is the conformer shown below called?

- **A.** Antistaggered
- **B.** Gauche
- **C.** Fully eclipsed
- **D.** Eclipsed

Question 253

How many carbon-carbon bonds in the structure shown below have conformers?

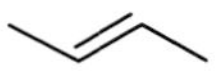

- ○ A. 1
- ○ B. 2
- ○ C. 3
- ○ D. 4

Question 254

How are the pair of molecules shown below related?

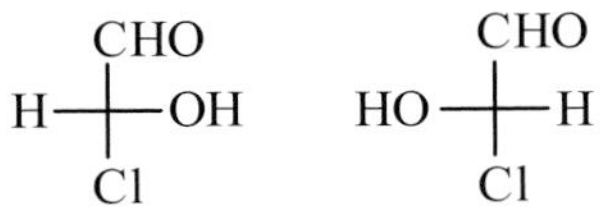

CHO
H——OH
Cl

CHO
HO——H
Cl

- ○ A. Conformers
- ○ B. Enantiomers
- ○ C. Structural isomers
- ○ D. Geometric isomers

▼

Only (L)-DOPA can react with the enzymes in the brain to form dopamine. The reaction is shown below. Refer to the reaction shown below to answers questions 255-256.

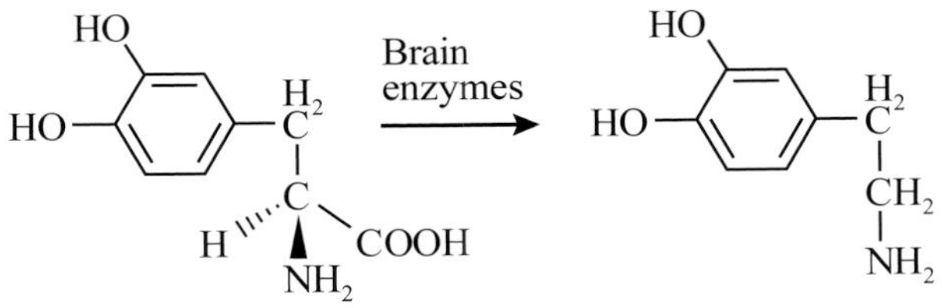

HO
HO——C²H₂
H——C——COOH
NH₂

(L)-DOPA

Brain enzymes →

HO
HO——C²H₂
CH₂
NH₂

dopamine

Question 255

Another name for (L)-DOPA is:

- ○ A. (+)-DOPA.
- ○ B. (−)-DOPA.
- ○ C. (D)-DOPA.
- ○ D. (R)-DOPA.

Question 256

The enantiomer of (L)-DOPA is toxic. Which of the following structures is the enantiomer of (L)-DOPA?

- ○ A.

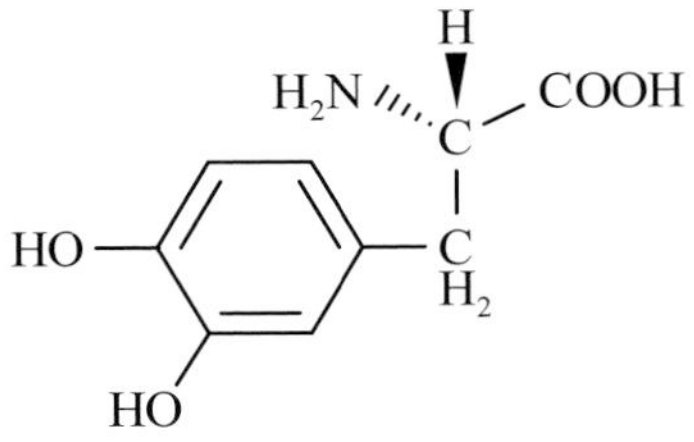

H_2N ,,,,C——COOH
H
C
H₂
HO
HO

- ○ B.

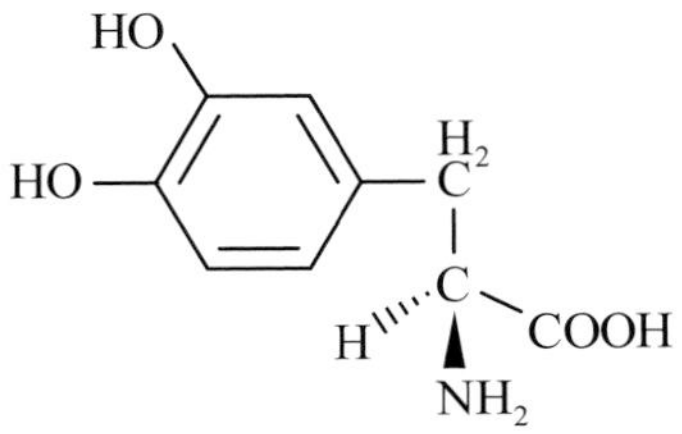

HO
HO
C²H₂
C
H,,,, COOH
NH₂

- ○ C.

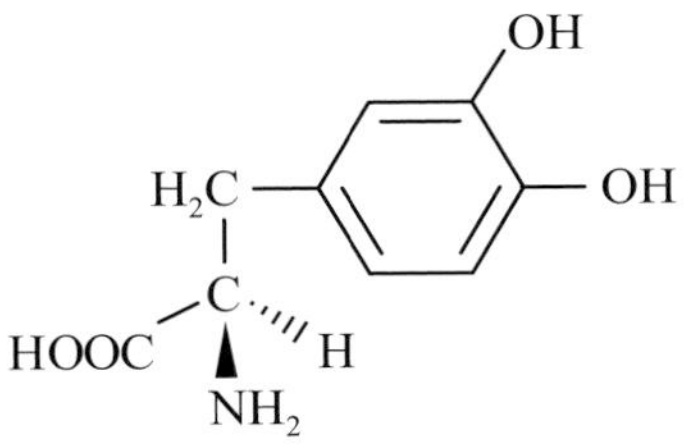

OH
OH
H₂C
C,,,,H
HOOC
NH₂

- ○ D.

OH
OH
H₂C
C,,,,NH₂
HOOC
H

▲

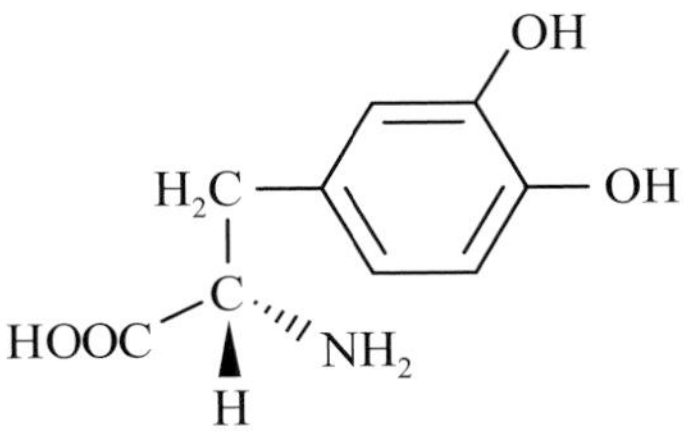

Question 257

How are the pair of molecules shown below related?

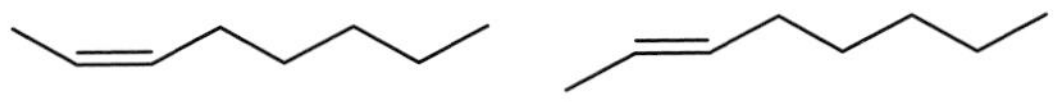

- ○ A. Diastereomers
- ○ B. Enantiomers
- ○ C. Epimers
- ○ D. Geometric isomers

Question 258

The equilibrium for glucose is shown below.

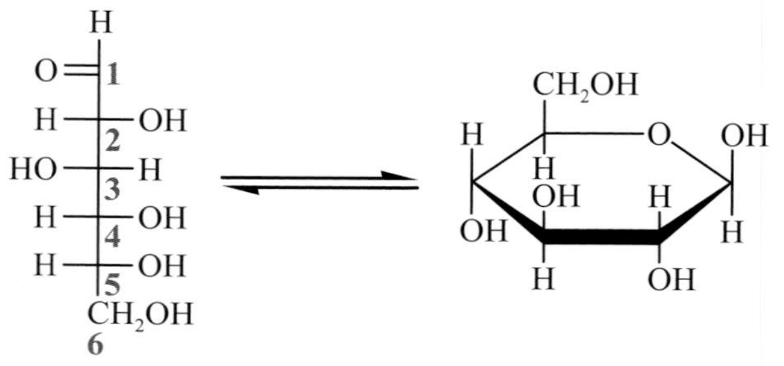

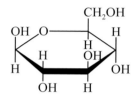

How is the structure shown below related to the pyranose structure in the equilibrium?

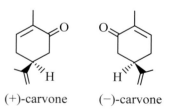

- ○ **A.** Enantiomer
- ○ **B.** Structural isomer
- ○ **C.** Epimer
- ○ **D.** Same molecule

Carvone has two stereoisomers that are shown below. (+)-carvone smells like caraway seed and (-)-carvone has a spearmint odor. Refer to the carvone structures to answer questions 259-260.

(+)-carvone   (−)-carvone

Question 259

What is the relationship between (+)-carvone and (−)-carvone?

- ○ **A.** Diastereomers
- ○ **B.** Enantiomers
- ○ **C.** Epimers
- ○ **D.** Geometric isomers

Question 260

What physical properties will be different for (+)-carvone and (−)-carvone?

- I.   Density
- II. Boiling point
- III. Rotation of plane polarized light

- ○ **A.** I only
- ○ **B.** III only
- ○ **C.** II and III only
- ○ **D.** I and III only

Question 261

Amino acids can be synthesized by reductive amination as shown below.

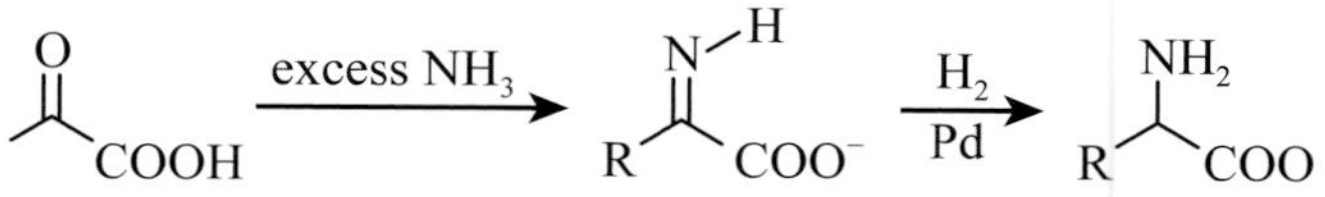

If valine is synthesized via reductive amination, what is true about the product?

- ○ **A.** The absolute configuration is R.
- ○ **B.** The absolute configuration is S.
- ○ **C.** The product is racemic.
- ○ **D.** The product is not chiral.

Question 262

In the assignment of absolute configuration, what priority does the ethyl group have in the structure shown below?

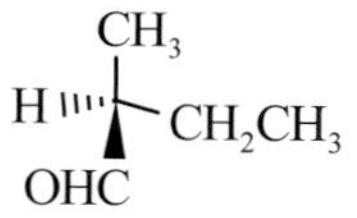

- ○ **A.** 1
- ○ **B.** 2
- ○ **C.** 3
- ○ **D.** 4

Question 263

The structures of D-aldoses synthesized from D-glyceraldehyde are displayed below.

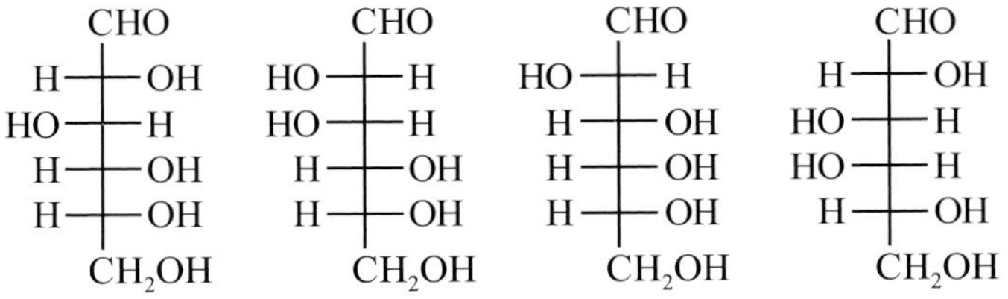

CHO
H OH
HO H
H OH
H OH
CH2OH
CHO
HO H
HO H
H OH
H OH
CH2OH
CHO
HO H
H OH
H OH
H OH
CH2OH
CHO
H OH
HO H
HO H
H OH
CH2OH

D-Glucose D-Mannose D-Altrose D-Galactose

What is the maximum number of optically active stereoisomers for the glucose molecule?

- A. 0
- B. 4
- C. 8
- D. 16

Question 264

The structure of naturally occurring epinephrine is shown below.

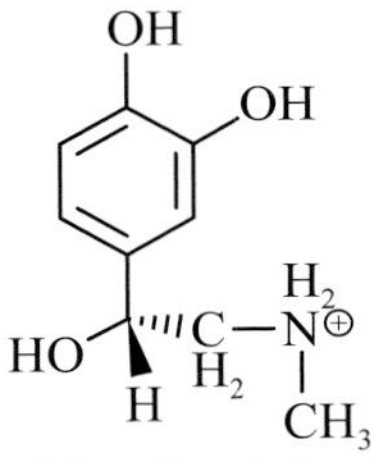

OH
OH
HO
H
C
H2
H2
N⊕
CH3

(L)-epinephrine

What is the absolute configuration of the chiral carbon in (L)-epinephrine?

- A. *R*
- B. *S*
- C. D
- D. L

Question 265

The structures of (+)-1-phenylethanol and (−)-1-phenylethanol are shown below. What is the absolute configuration of the (+) and (−) isomer, respectively?

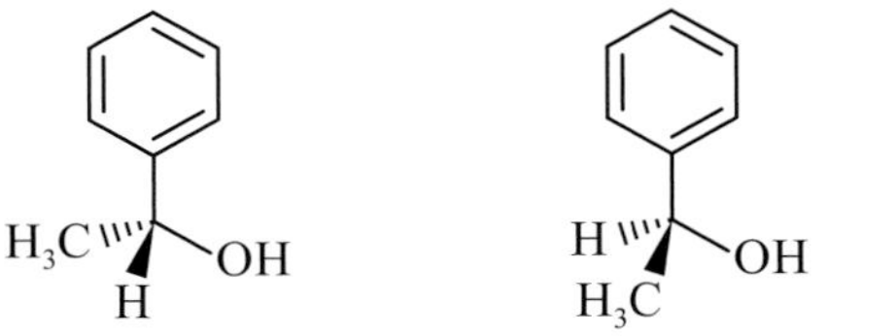

H3C
OH
H
H
OH
H3C

(+)-1-phenylethanol (−)-1-phenylethanol

- A. *R*, *R*
- B. *S*, *S*
- C. *S*, *R*
- D. *R*, *S*

Question 266

Given that a neat sample of (+)-1-phenylethanol rotates the sodium D line +42°, what can be determined from the observation that a pure neat sample of 1-phenylethanol rotates the sodium D line +12°?

- A. The sample contains a mixture of *R* and *S* isomers, with more *R* isomer present.
- B. The sample contains a mixture of *R* and *S* isomers, with more *S* isomer present.
- C. The sample contains pure *R* isomer.
- D. The sample contains pure *S* isomer.

Question 267

What is the absolute configuration of the malic acid molecule shown below?

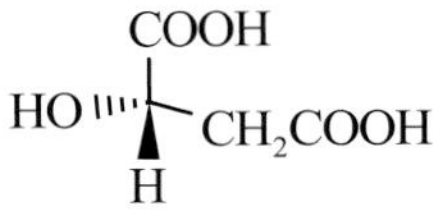

COOH
HO
CH2COOH
H

- A. *R*
- B. *S*
- C. D
- D. L

LECTURE 2

Question 268

What is the absolute configuration of the lactic acid molecule shown below?

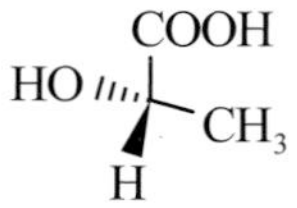

COOH
HO⟍ |
    C—CH₃
    |
    H

- A. R
- B. S
- C. D
- D. L

Question 269

What is the absolute configuration of the C2 and C5 carbons in D-glucose, respectively?

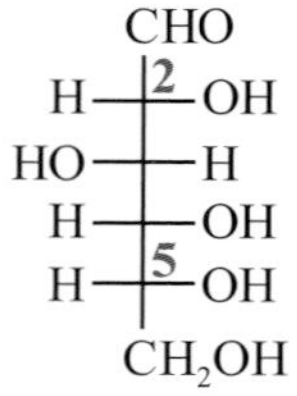

CHO
H——2—OH
HO——H
H——OH
H——5—OH
CH₂OH

D-Glucose

- A. R, R
- B. R, S
- C. S, R
- D. S, S

Tartaric acid was found to have distinctly different crystals. Two structures of tartaric acid are shown below. Refer to them to answer questions 270-272.

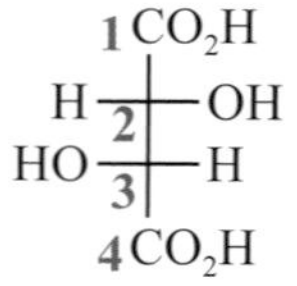

1 CO₂H   1 CO₂H
H——2—OH   HO——2—H
HO——3—H   H——3—OH
4 CO₂H   4 CO₂H

(+)-tartaric acid 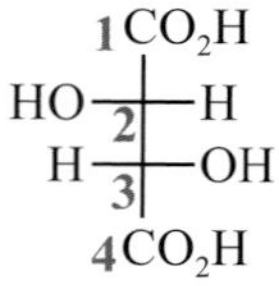   (−)-tartaric acid

Question 270

What is the absolute configuration of C2 and C3 of (+)-tartaric acid?

- A. R, R
- B. R, S
- C. S, R
- D. S, S

Question 271

What is the absolute configuration of C2 and C3 of (−)-tartaric acid, respectively?

- A. R, R
- B. R, S
- C. S, R
- D. S, S

Question 272

What is the name of the amino acid shown below?

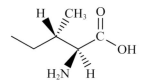

- A. (2S,3S)-2-Amino-3-methylpentanoic acid
- B. (3S,2S)-2-Amino-3-methylpentanoic acid
- C. (2S,3R)-2-Amino-3-methylpentanoic acid
- D. (3R,2S)-2-Amino-3-methylpentanoic acid

Refer to the structure below to answer questions 273-274.

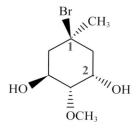

Question 273

What is the absolute configuration at labeled C1 and C2 carbons, respectively?

- A. R, R
- B. S, S
- C. S, R
- D. None of the above

Question 274

Assume the hydroxyl substituent at C2 carbon is changed to an ethyl group. What is the absolute configuration at the labeled C1 and C2 carbons, respectively?

- A. R, R
- B. S, S
- C. S, R
- D. None of the above

Question 275

X-Ray crystallographic analysis determined the absolute configurations about an unknown molecule's respective chiral centers. The analysis is displayed in the table.

Carbon	Absolute configuration
2	R
3	S
4	R

Which of the following compounds could be the unknown structure? Note that C1 is the aldehyde carbon.

A.

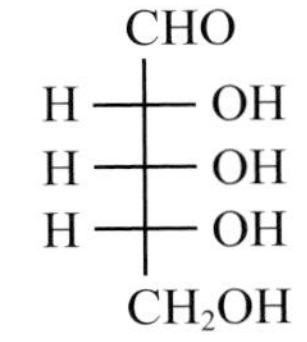

```
      CHO
  H ──┼── OH
  H ──┼── OH
  H ──┼── OH
     CH₂OH
```

B.

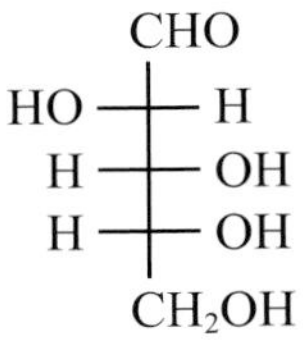

```
      CHO
 HO ──┼── H
  H ──┼── OH
  H ──┼── OH
     CH₂OH
```

C.

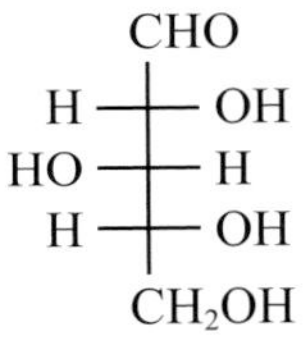

```
      CHO
  H ──┼── OH
 HO ──┼── H
  H ──┼── OH
     CH₂OH
```

D.

```
      CHO
 HO ──┼── H
 HO ──┼── H
  H ──┼── OH
     CH₂OH
```

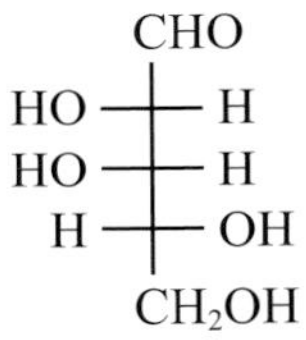

Question 276

A neat solution of 1-phenylethanol is optically active while 2-phenylethanol is not. The best explanation for this observation is:

○ **A.** 2-phenylethanol has a higher molecular weight than 1-phenylethanol.

○ **B.** 2-phenylethanol has a higher boiling point than 1- phenylethanol.

○ **C.** 1-phenylethanol is chiral while 2-phenylethanol is not.

○ **D.** 2-phenylethanol is chiral while 1-phenylethanol is not.

Question 277

What are possible explanations for molecules with chiral centers not rotating plane polarized light?

    I. There is a racemic mixture of the molecules.

    II. The molecule is a meso compound.

    III. Chiral molecules do not rotate light.

○ **A.** I only

○ **B.** III only

○ **C.** I and II only

○ **D.** I, II, and III

Question 278

The structure of cholesterol is shown below.

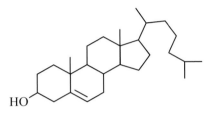

What geometric isomer is the cholesterol molecule?

○ **A.** *Trans*

○ **B.** *E*

○ **C.** *Z*

○ **D.** The geometric isomer cannot be determined.

Question 279

Polyunsaturated fats, such as the one shown below, are better for overall cardiovascular health than saturated fats. What is the name of the structure below?

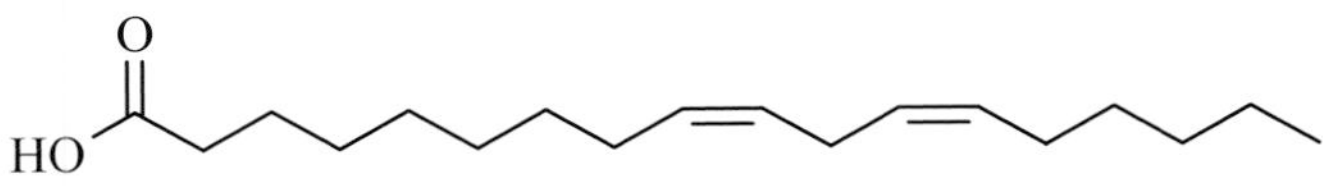

○ **A.** (9Z,12Z)-octadeca-9,12-dienoic acid

○ **B.** (9E,12Z)-octadeca-9,12-dienoic acid

○ **C.** (9Z,12E)-octadeca-9,12-dienoic acid

○ **D.** (9E,12E)-octadeca-9,12-dienoic acid

Substitution Reactions of Alkanes

Question 280

In an S_N2 reaction, what are the bond conversions?

- A. 2 sigma bonds are converted to 1 pi bond.
- B. 1 sigma bond is converted into 2 pi bonds.
- C. 1 pi bond is exchanged for 1 sigma bond.
- D. 1 sigma bond is exchanged for 1 sigma bond.

Question 281

What is true about an S_N1 reaction?

   I. A carbocation intermediate is formed.

   II. The rate determining step is bimolecular.

   III. The mechanism has two steps.

- A. I only
- B. II only
- C. I and III only
- D. I, II, and III

Question 282

The rate of an S_N2 reaction depends on:

- A. the concentration of the nucleophile only.
- B. the concentration of the electrophile only.
- C. the concentration of both the nucleophile and the electrophile.
- D. neither the concentration of the nucleophile nor the electrophile.

Question 283

How does the rate of step I in the mechanism shown below compare to the rate of step II?

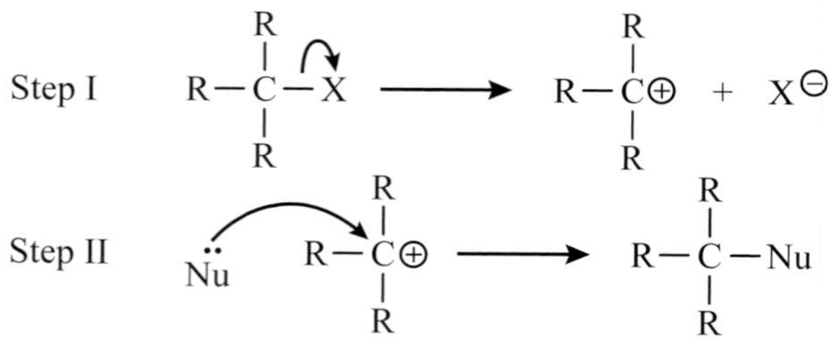

- A. Step I is faster than step II.
- B. Step II is faster than step I.
- C. Step I and step II happen at the same rate.
- D. The relationship cannot be determined.

The reaction of (2R)-iodobutane to form 2-methoxybutane proceeds by an S_N1 mechanism in methanol. However, in the presence of the methoxide ion (CH_3O^-), the mechanism is S_N2. Use this information to answer questions 284–285.

Question 284

Why does the mechanism change when methanol is replaced by methoxide?

- A. Iodide is a poor leaving group.
- B. Iodide is a good leaving group.
- C. Methanol is a weak nucleophile and methoxide is a strong nucleophile.
- D. Methanol is a strong nucleophile and methoxide is a weak nucleophile.

Question 285

Given the above information, what would be the product of the reaction of (2R)-iodobutane with methanol?

   I. (2R)-methoxybutane

   II. (2S)-methoxybutane

   III. Butane

- A. I only
- B. II only
- C. I and II only
- D. I, II, and III

Question 286

The rate of precipitate formation increases for the reaction of 1-bromobutane with NaI as the concentration of NaI is increased. When the concentration of NaI is increased in the reaction of 2-chloro-2-methylpropane, no rate change is observed. Why is there a change in rate in the first case and not in the second?

- A. Cl^- is a better leaving group than Br^-.
- B. Br^- is a better leaving group than Cl^-.
- C. 1-bromobutane proceeds via an S_N2 mechanism, while 2-chloro-2-methylpropane proceeds via an S_N1 mechanism.
- D. 1-bromobutane proceeds via an S_N1 mechanism, while 2-chloro-2-methylpropane proceeds via an S_N2 mechanism.

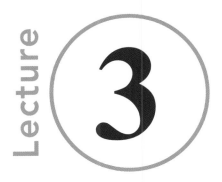

Lecture 3

Questions 287–429

Oxygen Containing Reactions

The Attackers: Nucleophiles

The Targets: Electrophiles

Substitution Reactions: Carboxylic Acids and their Derivatives

Addition Reactions: Aldehydes and Ketones

Oxidation and Reduction of Oxygen Containing Compounds

Carbonyls as Nucleophiles: Aldol Condensation

Bonding and Reactions of Biological Molecules

The Attackers: Nucleophiles

Question 287

Methyl mercaptan (CH_3SH) is similar to:

- ○ **A.** a primary alcohol.
- ○ **B.** a secondary alcohol.
- ○ **C.** a tertiary alcohol.
- ○ **D.** a quaternary alcohol.

Question 288

What is 2-methyl-2-butanol?

- ○ **A.** A primary alcohol
- ○ **B.** A secondary alcohol
- ○ **C.** A tertiary alcohol
- ○ **D.** A quaternary alcohol

Question 289

$KMnO_4$ forms a syn diol when reacted in a cold and dilute solution with an alkene. Oxidative cleavage results when it is reacted in a warm and concentrated solution. What would be the product if cold dilute $KMnO_4$ is reacted with 3-cyclohexene-1-ol?

○ **A.**

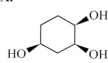

○ **B.**

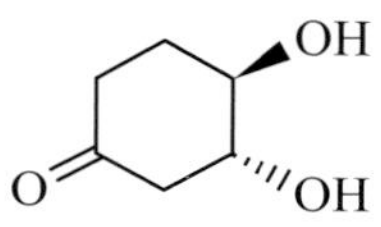

○ **C.**

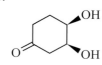

○ **D.**

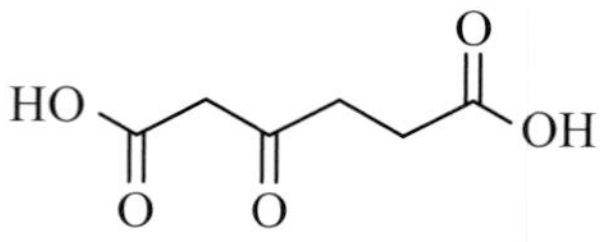

Question 290

What is the IUPAC name for the structure shown below?

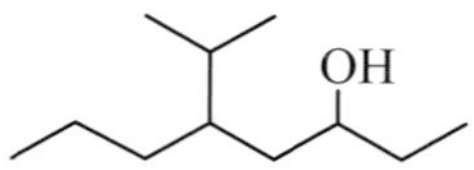

- ○ **A.** 4-Isopropyl-6-octanol
- ○ **B.** 5-Isopropyl-3-octanol
- ○ **C.** 5-Isopropyl-3-hexanol
- ○ **D.** 4-2-Butanol-5-methylhexane

Question 291

The Lucas test is used to determine whether an alcohol is primary, secondary, or tertiary based on the rate of reaction with HCl and $ZnCl_2$.

Class of alcohol	Approximate time of reaction	Mechanism
Primary	> 6 minutes	S_N2
Secondary	1-5 minutes	S_N1
Tertiary	< 1 minutes	S_N1

Which of the following alcohols will react the slowest?

- ○ **A.** 1-Pentanol
- ○ **B.** 2-Methyl-3-pentanol
- ○ **C.** 2-Methyl-2-pentanol
- ○ **D.** 2-Hexanol

Question 292

The word miscible means that one solvent forms a homogenous solution when mixed with another solvent in any amount. Which of the following would be miscible with water?

- ○ **A.** Ethanol
- ○ **B.** Cyclohexane
- ○ **C.** 2-Butene
- ○ **D.** Hexane

Question 293

Cyclohexanol is a solid in a cool room, while cyclohexane is a liquid. What is the best explanation for the different states?

- ○ **A.** Cyclohexanol has greater London dispersion forces than cyclohexane.
- ○ **B.** Cyclohexanol has weaker London dispersion forces than cyclohexane.
- ○ **C.** Cyclohexanol has hydrogen bonding and cyclohexane does not.
- ○ **D.** Cyclohexane has hydrogen bonding and cyclohexanol does not.

Question 294

Given that the boiling point for 1-propanol is 97°C and the boiling point of 1-pentanol is 138°C, what is the boiling point of 1-butanol?

- ○ **A.** 100°C
- ○ **B.** 118°C
- ○ **C.** 138°C
- ○ **D.** 150°C

LECTURE 3

Question 295

In the following reaction of ethanol with *para*-toluenesulfonyl chloride, ethanol is a(n):

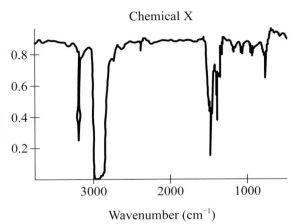

- ○ **A.** nucleophile.
- ○ **B.** electrophile.
- ○ **C.** radical.
- ○ **D.** reducing agent.

Question 296

Why does the presence of an acid facilitate the substitution of an alcohol?

- ○ **A.** The acid converts the OH group to a good nucleophile.
- ○ **B.** The acid converts the OH group to a good electrophile.
- ○ **C.** The acid converts the OH group to a good leaving group.
- ○ **D.** The acid neutralizes the bases in solution.

Question 297

Which of the following reagents will convert diethyl ether to ethanol and chloroethane?

- ○ **A.** HCl
- ○ **B.** Cl_2
- ○ **C.** $SOCl_2$
- ○ **D.** $AlCl_3$

Question 298

Chemical X was analyzed with IR spectroscopy prior to a reaction. Upon completion of the reaction, the product also underwent IR spectroscopy. How can the procedure be modified to maintain the functional group that was lost during the reaction?

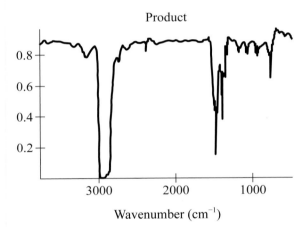

- ○ **A.** By reacting chemical X with two equivalents of an aldehyde to form a protecting group prior to the reaction
- ○ **B.** By reacting chemical X with two equivalents of a ketone to form a protecting group prior to the reaction
- ○ **C.** By reacting chemical X with HCl to form a protecting group prior to the reaction
- ○ **D.** By reacting chemical X with a tosylate to form a protecting group prior to the reaction

Question 299

Part of a multi-step synthesis to develop a cyanide-based pharmaceutical failed after an inadequate quantity of product was formed in the synthesis step below.

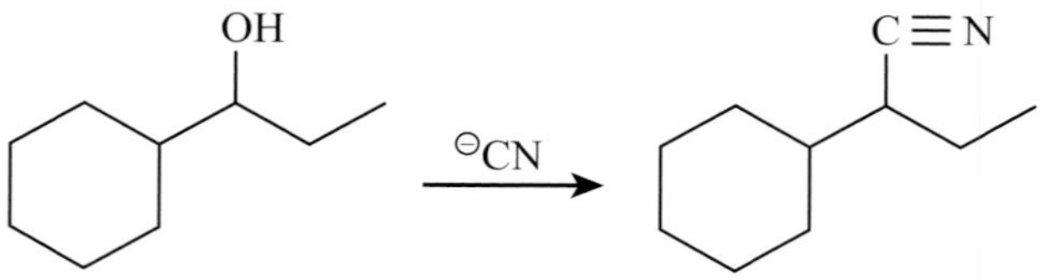

$$\text{OH} \xrightarrow{\ ^{\ominus}\text{CN}\ } \text{C} \equiv \text{N}$$

Which of the following reagents could be placed in the reaction vessel prior to this synthesis step in order to attain adequate product quantity?

○ **A.** NaOH

○ **B.**

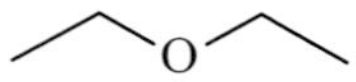

○ **C.**

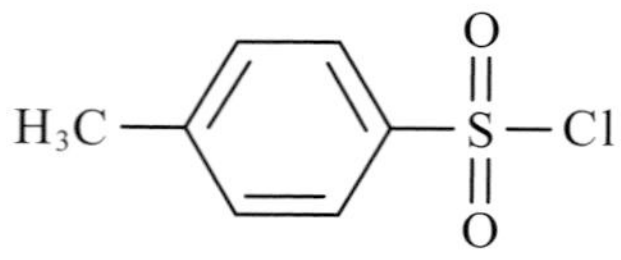

○ **D.**

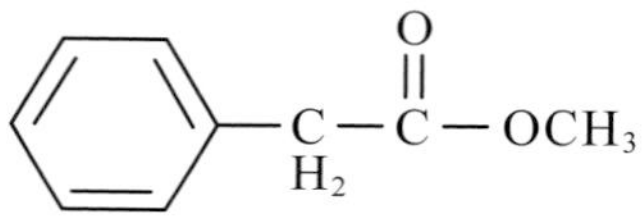

Question 300

Tetrahydrofuran (THF) is a common solvent for synthetic reactions because it is an ether. Ethers are relatively inert, so they do not participate in the reaction. Which of the following structures is THF?

○ **A.**

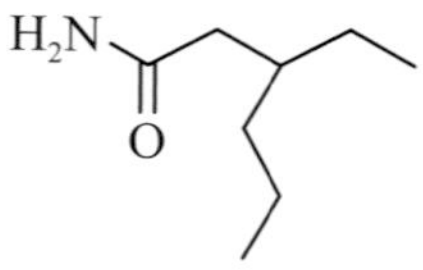

○ **B.**

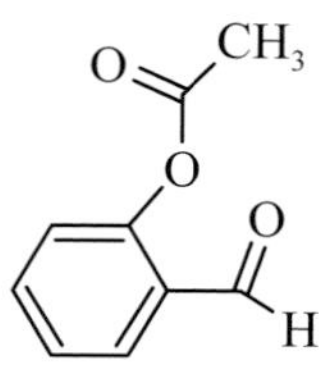

○ **C.**

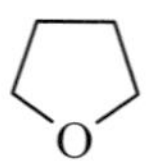

○ **D.**

$$CH_3CH_2OH$$

The Targets: Electrophiles

Question 301

Researchers reacted a particularly strong and bulky base with an aldehyde and a ketone and then measured the reaction rates. Results are displayed in the table. Compound identities were lost.

Compound	Reaction rate (mol/sec)
A	1×10^3
B	1×10^{14}

The identity of compound B is most likely:

○ **A.** an aldehyde, because the sp^2-hybridized geometry allows for quicker nucleophilic attack.

○ **B.** ketone, because the sp^2-hybridized geometry allows for quicker nucleophilic attack.

○ **C.** an aldehyde, because the reduced steric hindrance facilitates nucleophilic addition.

○ **D.** a ketone, because the reduced steric hindrance facilitates nucleophilic addition.

Question 302

A nucleophilic substitution reaction between $LiAlH_4$ and which of the following compounds would be least sterically hindered?

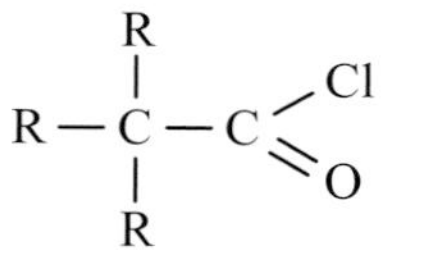

○ **A.**

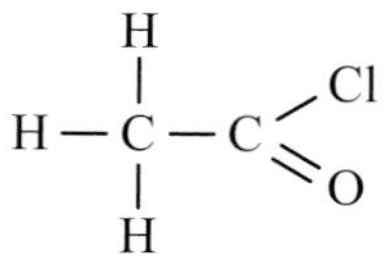

○ **B.**

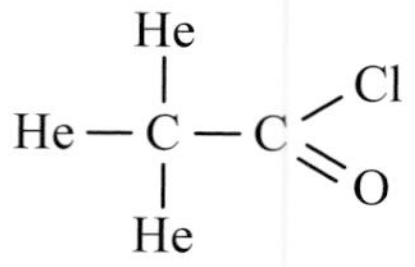

○ **C.**

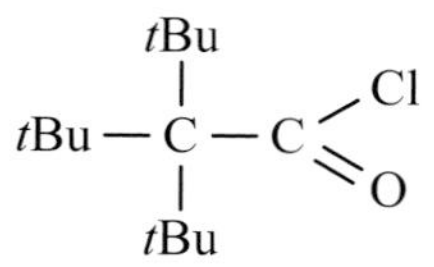

○ **D.**

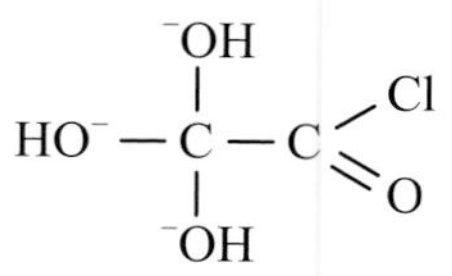

For questions 303-304, refer to the compounds provided below:

Compound A: $H_3C-C(=O)-CH_3$ Compound B: $H_3C-C(=O)-H$

Compound A   Compound B

Question 303

How can both compounds be rendered less reactive?

○ **A.** By reacting each compound with 1M of HCl.

○ **B.** By reacting each compound with 1M of acetic anhydride.

○ **C.** By reacting each compound with 1M of acetic acid.

○ **D.** By reacting each compound with 1M of N-ethylacetamide.

Question 304

Between compound A and compound B, which would be more useful in an experiment where high reactivity is essential?

○ **A.** Compound A, as it would be more electrophilic.

○ **B.** Compound A, as it would be less electrophilic.

○ **C.** Compound B, as it would be more electrophilic.

○ **D.** Compound B, as it would be less electrophilic.

Question 305

Which of the following compounds is the most reactive?

○ **A.** $(CH_3CO)_2O$

○ **B.** CH_3COCl

○ **C.** CH_3COOH

○ **D.** CH_3COCH_3

Question 306

A scientist is attempting to choose a reactant for a synthesis. An IR spectroscopy result of compound A indicates a broad stretch in the 3000 cm^{-1} range, and sharp peaks at 1750 cm^{-1}, 1272 cm^{-1}, and 1180 cm^{-1}. An IR spectroscopy result of compound B indicates a broad stretch in the 3000 cm^{-1} range, and sharp peaks at 2800 cm^{-1} and 1714 cm^{-1}. Which of the following is true based on this information?

○ **A.** Compound A is more vulnerable to nucleophilic attack than compound B.

○ **B.** Compound B is more vulnerable to nucleophilic attack than compound A.

○ **C.** Both compounds are equally susceptible to nucleophilic attack.

○ **D.** It is difficult to predict which compound is more susceptible to nucleophilic attack.

Question 307

Amide and esters are vulnerable to nucleophilic substitution due to their possession of:

○ **A.** planar stereochemistry, a partial negative charge on carbonyl oxygen, and a partial positive charge on the carbonyl carbon.

○ **B.** planar stereochemistry, a partial positive charge on the carbonyl oxygen, and a partial positive charge on the carbonyl carbon.

○ **C.** nonplanar stereochemistry, a partial negative charge on the carbonyl oxygen, and a partial positive charge on the carbonyl carbon.

○ **D.** nonplanar stereochemistry, a partial positive charge on the carbonyl oxygen, and a partial positive charge on the carbonyl carbon.

Question 308

Reacting acetyl chloride with which of the following reactants is most likely to occur the fastest?

○ **A.** H_3CCOOH

○ **B.** H_6C_2OH

○ **C.** H_3COH

○ **D.** H_3CNH_2

Question 309

Acyl chlorides are the most reactive acyl halide due to the electron-withdrawing nature of Cl and the stability of Cl$^-$ as a leaving group. Which of the following molecules CANNOT be used to form an acyl chloride?

- ○ **A.** HCl
- ○ **B.** SOCl$_2$
- ○ **C.** PCl$_3$
- ○ **D.** PCl$_5$

Question 310

The synthesis of methyl benzoate from benzoic acid and methanol requires an acid catalyst. However, methyl benzoate can be synthesized from benzoyl chloride and methanol without a catalyst. Why are different conditions required for these two reactions?

- ○ **A.** The product is more stable in the acid chloride reaction.
- ○ **B.** The product is more stable in the carboxylic acid reaction.
- ○ **C.** Acid chlorides are less reactive than carboxylic acids.
- ○ **D.** Acid chlorides are more reactive than carboxylic acids.

Question 311

Luminol is used in the detection of blood. The synthesis of luminol is shown below:

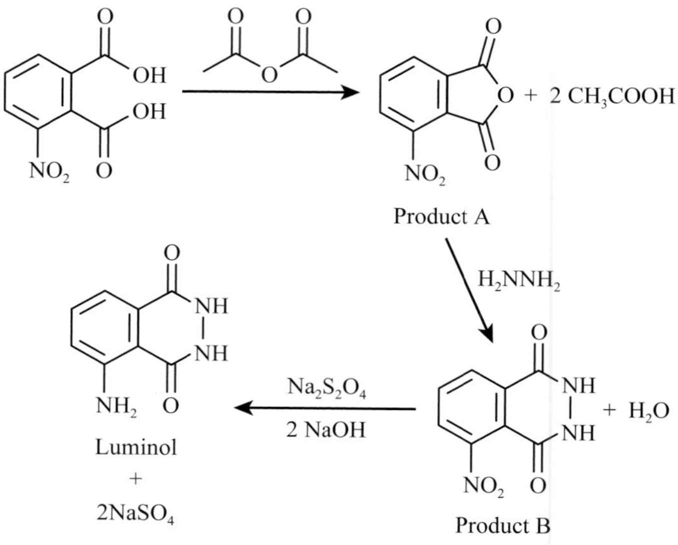

Why is product A used as an intermediate in the formation of product B?

- ○ **A.** Carboxylic acids are more reactive than anhydrides.
- ○ **B.** Anhydrides are more reactive than carboxylic acids.
- ○ **C.** Five membered rings are more reactive.
- ○ **D.** Five membered rings are less reactive.

Substitution Reactions: Carboxylic Acids and Their Derivatives

Question 312

Which of the following bonds are contained in the carboxyl terminus of 5Z,8Z,11Z,14Z-eicosatetraenoic acid?

   I. Polar covalent
   II. sp^2-hybridized
   III. sp^3-hybridized

- ○ **A.** I only
- ○ **B.** I and II only
- ○ **C.** II and III only
- ○ **D.** I, II, and III

Question 313

Which of the following statements LEAST describes carboxylic acids?

○ **A.** Carboxylic acids are more acidic than aldehydes.

○ **B.** Carboxylic acid functional groups are found on glutamate and aspartate.

○ **C.** Carboxylic acids cannot undergo nucleophilic substitution reactions.

○ **D.** Carboxylic acids have low boiling points.

Question 314

Which IUPAC definition best describes the following molecule?

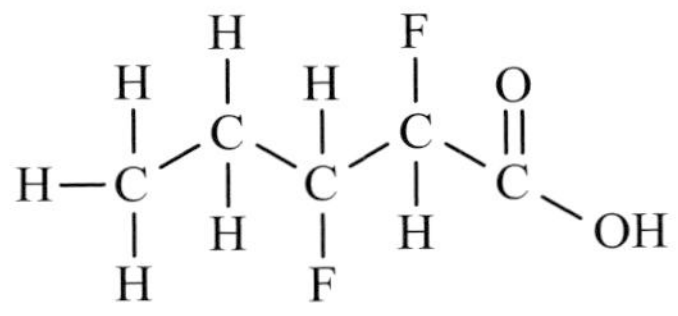

○ **A.** 2,3-difluropentaonic acid

○ **B.** 2,3-bifluropentanoic acid

○ **C.** 3,4-difluropenatonic acid

○ **D.** 3,4-bifluropenatonic acid

Question 315

Only (L)-DOPA can react with the enzymes in the brain to form dopamine. The reaction is shown below. The conversion that takes place in the brain when (L)-DOPA is converted to dopamine is a(n):

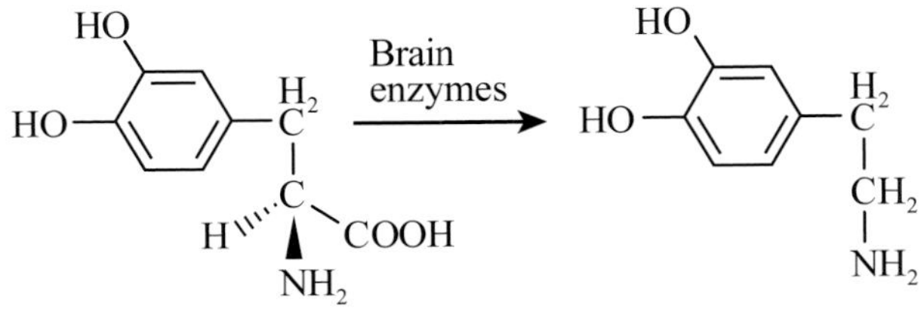

(L)-DOPA   dopamine

○ **A.** decarboxylation.

○ **B.** reduction of an amide to an amine.

○ **C.** oxidation of an amide to an amine.

○ **D.** carboxylation.

Use the table below to answer questions 316-317.

	Melting Point (°C)
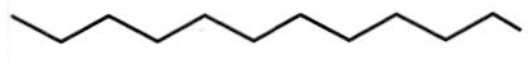 lauric acid	44
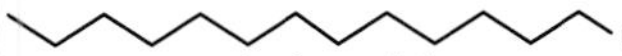 myristic acid	59
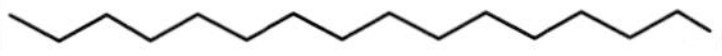 palmitic acid	64
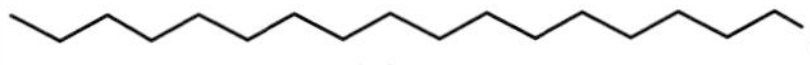 stearic acid	70
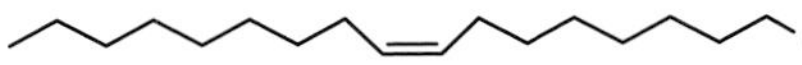 oleic acid	4
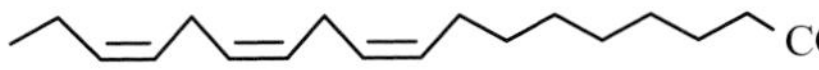 linolenic acid	−11

Question 316

The salt of which of the following would be most soluble in water?

○ **A.** Palmitic acid

○ **B.** Myristic acid

○ **C.** Lauric acid

○ **D.** Stearic acid

Question 317

A fatty acid that is a solid at room temperature is called a fat, while a fatty acid that is a liquid at room temperature is called an oil. Which of the following is an oil?

○ **A.** Oleic acid

○ **B.** Palmitic acid

○ **C.** Lauric acid

○ **D.** Stearic acid

Anthraquinone is synthesized from 2-benzoylbenzoic acid. Refer to the synthesis below to answer questions 318 - 319.

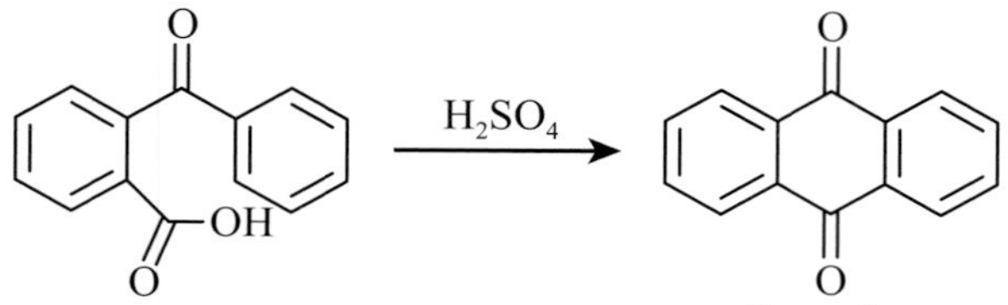

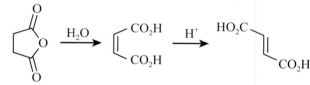

anthraquinone

Question 318

What is the structure of the benzoyl group in the starting material?

○ A.

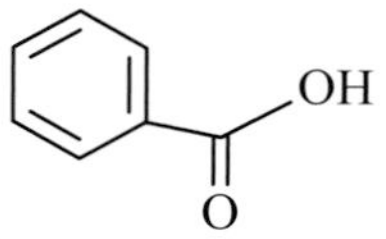

○ B.

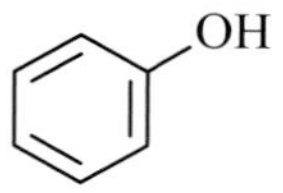

○ C.

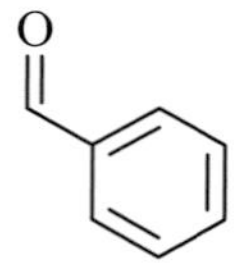

○ D.

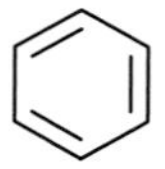

Question 319

In the synthesis of anthraquinone, the carboxylic acid group is:

○ A. the nucleophile.
○ B. the electrophile.
○ C. the catalyst.
○ D. the oxidant.

Question 320

Which of the following will lose CO_2 at room temperature?

○ A.

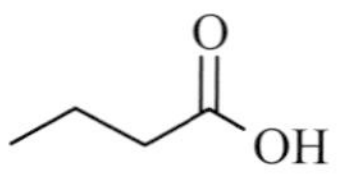

○ B.

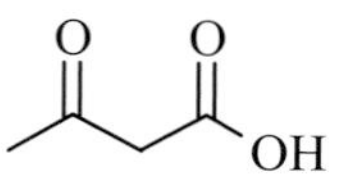

○ C.

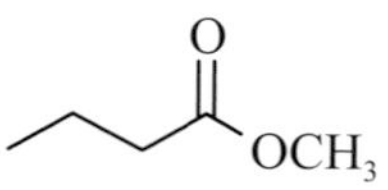

○ D.

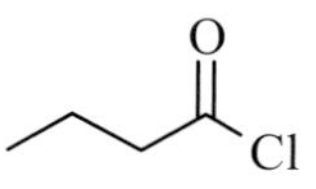

Question 321

If ethyl alcohol ferments in the presence of oxygen (an oxidant), vinegar is formed. What is vinegar?

○ A. Ethanoic acid
○ B. Diethyl ether
○ C. Ethanol
○ D. Ethane

Question 322

A scientist was synthesizing 3-oxo-pentaonic acid when bubbling was observed at room temperature. What is the cause of the bubbling?

○ A. Release of O_2
○ B. Release of H_2
○ C. Release of CO_2
○ D. Release of H_2O vapor

Use the reaction scheme below to answer questions 323 - 325.

maleic anhydride   maleic acid   fumaric acid

Question 323

The formation of maleic acid from maleic anhydride is a(n):

○ A. isomerization.
○ B. hydrolysis.
○ C. carboxylation.
○ D. decarboxylation.

Question 324

The carboxyl end of alanine can be reacted with the amino end of glycine to form which of the following bonds?

　I. Peptide
　II. Covalent
　III. Van der Waals

○ A. I only
○ B. II only
○ C. I and II only
○ D. I and III only

LECTURE 3

Question 325

In the formation of maleic acid from maleic anhydride, water is a(n):

○ **A.** catalyst.

○ **B.** acid.

○ **C.** nucleophile.

○ **D.** electrophile.

Question 326

What is the result of the reaction of an alcohol and an acid chloride?

○ **A.** An ester

○ **B.** An ether

○ **C.** An amide

○ **D.** An imide

Question 327

What is the result of the reaction of an amine and a carboxylic acid?

○ **A.** An ester

○ **B.** An ether

○ **C.** An amide

○ **D.** An imide

Bis(2,4,6-trichlorophenyl) oxalate is used in light sticks. When hydrogen peroxide and a fluorescer are added to this molecule, light is produced. Use the synthesis reaction for bis(2,4,6-trichlorophenyl) oxalate to answer questions 328-329.

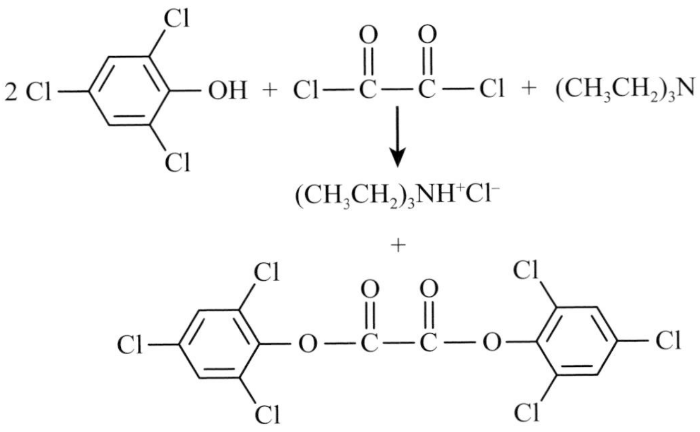

Bis(2,4,6-trichlorophenyl) oxalate

Question 328

Bis(2,4,6-trichlorophenyl) oxalate is a(n):

○ **A.** amide.

○ **B.** ester.

○ **C.** acid chloride.

○ **D.** carboxylic acid.

Question 329

In the synthesis of bis(2,4,6-trichlorophenyl) oxalate, 2,4,6-trichlorophenol is a(n):

○ **A.** nucleophile.

○ **B.** electrophile.

○ **C.** acid.

○ **D.** reductant.

Question 330

E-α-phenylcinnamic acid (shown below) undergoes decarboxylation to form *Z*-stilbene when reacted with a copper chromite catalyst and quinoline. What is the structure of *Z*-stilbene?

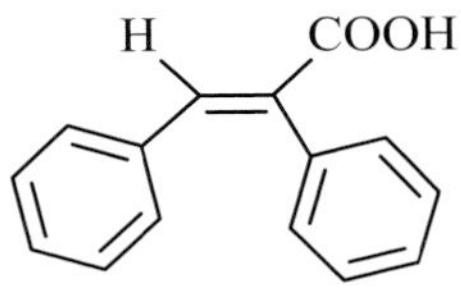

E-α-phenylcinnamic acid

○ **A.**

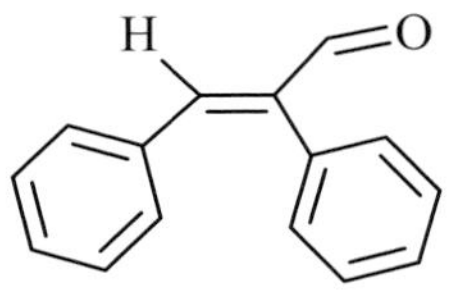

○ **B.**

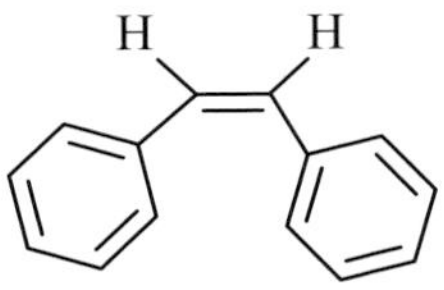

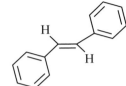

○ **C.**

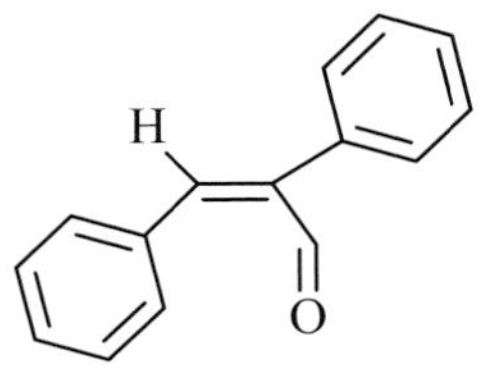

○ **D.**

Question 331

Which of the following will form acetic anhydride when reacted with the acetate ion?

- O **A.** Acetyl chloride
- O **B.** Acetic acid
- O **C.** Methyl acetate
- O **D.** *N*-ethylacetamide

Question 332

Which of the following reagents will convert butanoic acid into butyl chloride?

- O **A.** Cl_2
- O **B.** HCl
- O **C.** $SOCl_2$
- O **D.** $LiAlH_4$

Question 333

An enzyme intermediate to glycolysis and the citric acid cycle is called pyruvate decarboxylase. What is one expected product from this reaction?

- O **A.** Pyruvate
- O **B.** CO_2
- O **C.** HCO_3^-
- O **D.** H_2O

Question 334

Which rule dictates why decarboxylation reactions typically favor the product?

- O **A.** Le Châtelier's principle
- O **B.** The Bohr effect
- O **C.** Hund's rule
- O **D.** Michaelis-Menten kinetics

▼

A reaction for forming derivatives of unknown acids for the purpose of identification is shown below. Use this scheme to answer questions 335-336.

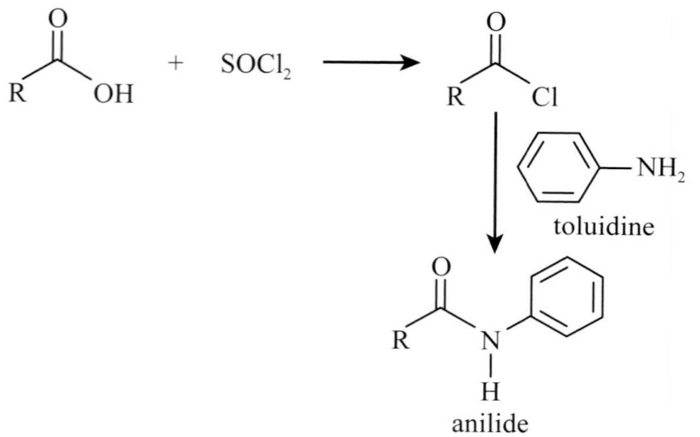

anilide

Question 335

The formation of the acid chloride is a(n):

- O **A.** elimination.
- O **B.** conjugate addition.
- O **C.** nucleophilic substitution.
- O **D.** nucleophilic addition.

Question 336

Why is the unknown acid reacted with $SOCl_2$ before reacting with toluidine?

- O **A.** Acid chlorides are more reactive than carboxylic acids.
- O **B.** Carboxylic acids are more reactive than acid chlorides.
- O **C.** The carbonyl of a carboxylic acid is more nucleophilic than the carbonyl of an acid chloride.
- O **D.** An acid chloride catalyzes the formation of an anilide.

▲

Question 337

Which of the following acids would be most reactive with the $SOCl_2$?

- O **A.** 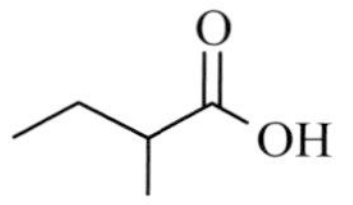
- O **B.** 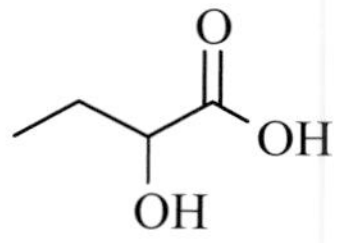
- O **C.** 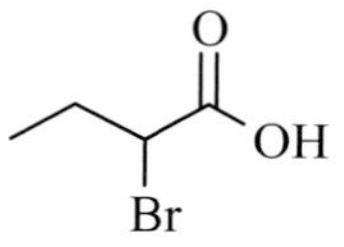
- O **D.**

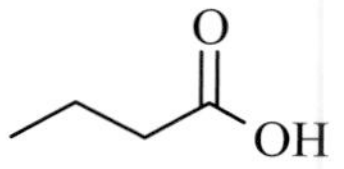

Question 338

Isoamylacetate is a honeybee pheromone that is released on the skin when a bee stings its victim. This pheromone has a sweet smell and attracts other bees to join the fight. The structure of isoamylacetate is shown below. What functional group does it contain?

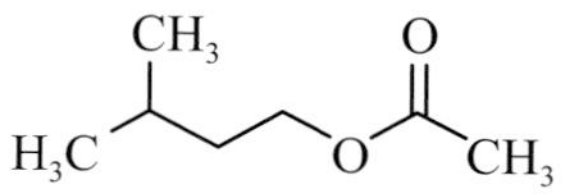

- O **A.** Ether
- O **B.** Ester
- O **C.** Carboxylic acid
- O **D.** Alcohol

Question 339

Bilirubin is a bile pigment found in human gallstones. The structure of bilirubin is shown below. How many amide functional groups are present in this pigment?

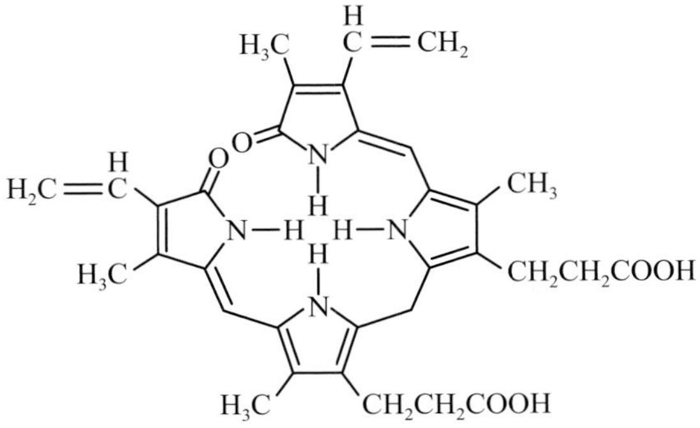

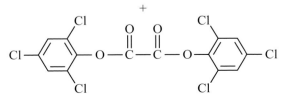

○ **A.** 1
○ **B.** 2
○ **C.** 3
○ **D.** 4

Question 340

Aspirin is the common name for acetylsalicylic acid. The structure is shown below, what three functional groups are present in this molecule?

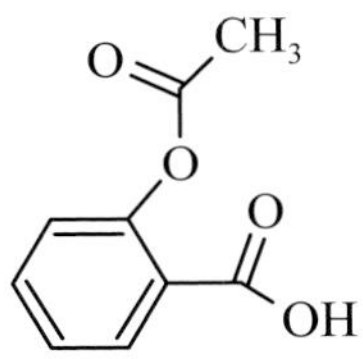

○ **A.** Ether, aromatic ring, carboxylic acid
○ **B.** Ester, phenyl, carboxylic acid
○ **C.** Alkene, aromatic ring, carboxylic acid
○ **D.** Alcohol, ether, carboxylic acid

Question 341

Bis(2,4,6-trichlorophenyl) oxalate is used in light sticks. When hydrogen peroxide and a fluorescer are added to this molecule, light is produced.

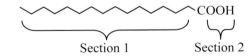

Bis(2,4,6-trichlorophenyl) oxalate

What does the prefix "bis" in bis(2,4,6 trichlorophenyl) oxalate indicate?

○ **A.** More than one chloride ion
○ **B.** Two 2,4,6-trichlorophenyl oxalate groups
○ **C.** Two moles of product
○ **D.** Two oxygens

Question 342

Which statement about the fatty acid below is true?

~~~~~~~COOH
Section 1   Section 2

○ **A.** Section 1 is polar and hydrophobic while section 2 is nonpolar and hydrophilic.
○ **B.** Section 1 is polar and hydrophilic while section 2 is nonpolar and hydrophobic.
○ **C.** Section 1 is nonpolar and hydrophobic while section 2 is polar and hydrophilic.
○ **D.** Section 1 is nonpolar and hydrophilic while section 2 is polar and hydrophobic.

Question 343

S(+)-Ethyl-3-hydroxybutanoate is the product of ethyl acetoacetate's reaction with yeast. This product can be further reacted with 3,5-dinitrobenzoyl chloride in the presence of pyridine to give 3,5-dinitrobenzoate (shown below).

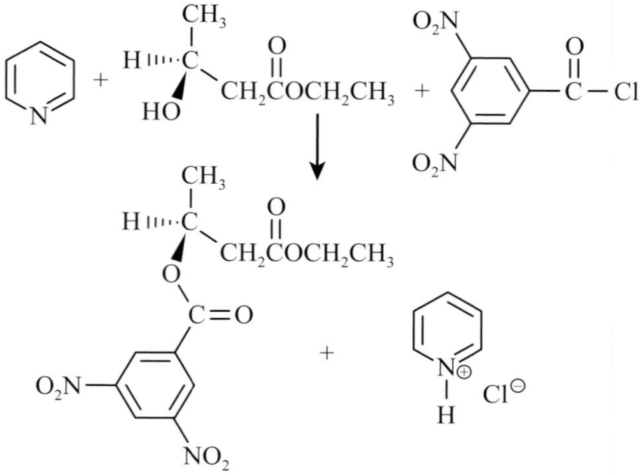

How do the nitro groups on the benzene ring in 3,5-dinitrobenzoyl chloride affect the reaction?

- **A.** They inhibit the reaction because they are deactivating.
- **B.** They inhibit the reaction because they are electron withdrawing.
- **C.** They enhance the reaction because they activate the nucleophile.
- **D.** They enhance the reaction because they activate the electrophile.

Question 344

Isoamyl propionate is one of the primary components in the pineapple odor. The reaction is shown below.

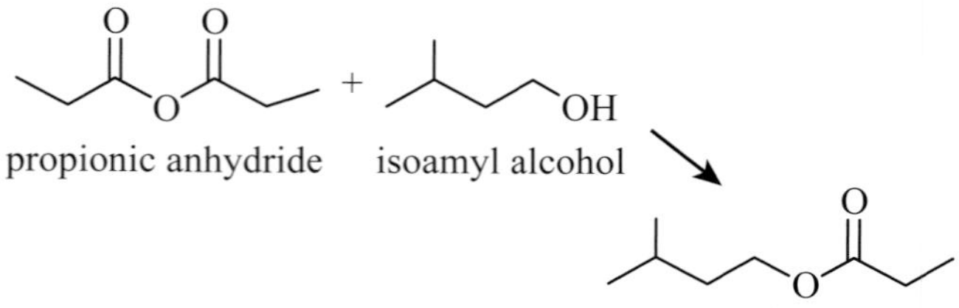

The synthesis is catalyzed by an acid. What does the acid do in the first step of the synthesis?

- **A.** Activate the electrophile by protonating the propionic anhydride
- **B.** Activate the nucleophile by protonating the propionic anhydride
- **C.** Activate the electrophile by protonating the isoamyl alcohol
- **D.** Activate the nucleophile by protonating the isoamyl alcohol

Use the following table to answer questions 345-347.

Name	Side Chain	pI
glycine	H	6.0
valine	$CH(CH_3)_2$	6.0
serine	CH_2OH	5.7
tyrosine	$CH_2C_6H_4OH$	5.7
asparagine	CH_2CONH_2	5.4
aspartic acid	CH_2COOH	2.8
lysine	$(CH_2)_4NH_2$	9.7
arginine	$(CH_2)_3NHC(NH)NH_2$	10.8

Question 345

Given the information in the table, the reductive amination of the α-ketoacid shown below results in the amino acid:

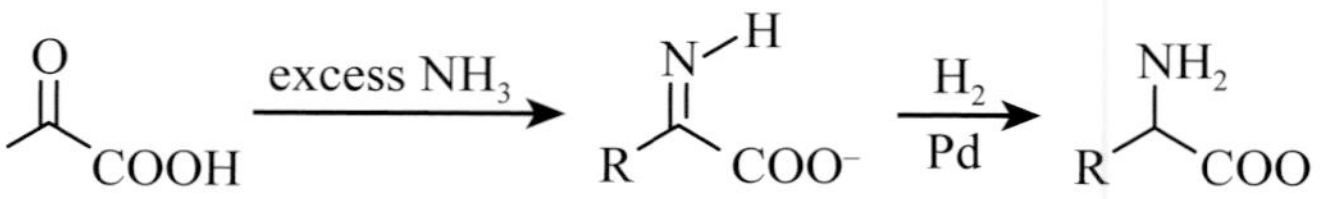

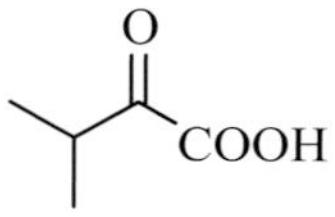

- **A.** glycine.
- **B.** valine.
- **C.** aspartic acid.
- **D.** lysine.

Question 346

Given the information in the table, the reductive amination of the α-ketoacid shown below results in the amino acid:

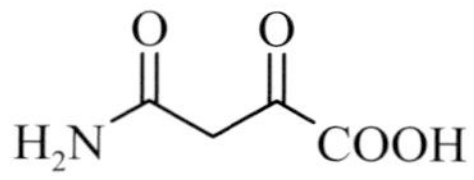

- **A.** glycine.
- **B.** serine.
- **C.** aspartic acid.
- **D.** asparagine.

LECTURE 3

Question 347

The structure of *N,N*-diethyl-*meta*-toluamide (DEET) is shown below. DEET is one of the best insect repellents. What two reagents would be best to use in order to synthesize DEET?

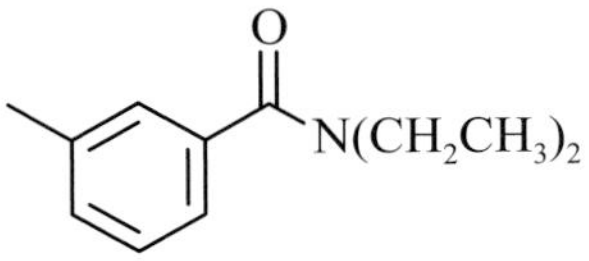

- ○ **A.** *meta*-methylbenzoyl chloride and ammonia
- ○ **B.** *meta*-methylbenzoyl chloride and diethyl amine
- ○ **C.** *meta*-methylbenzoic acid and diethyl amine
- ○ **D.** *meta*-methylbenzoic acid and ammonia

Question 348

Which of the following products would be expected in the reaction below?

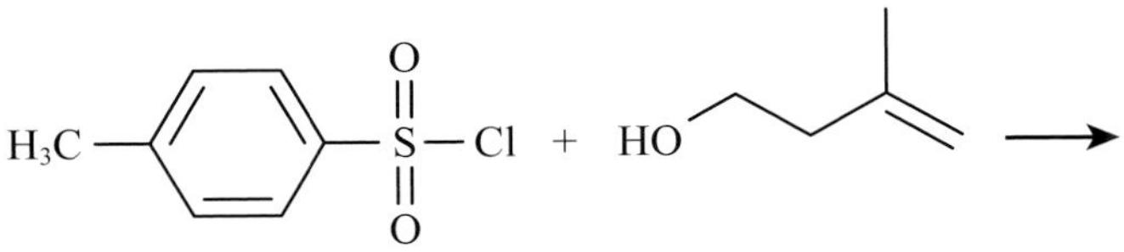

- ○ **A.** An aldehyde
- ○ **B.** A protected alcohol
- ○ **C.** A carboxylic acid
- ○ **D.** An alkyne

Question 349

Biotin is a vitamin that is popular for its supposed effects on skin and hair. Below is the structure of biotin, which is used as a cofactor in carboxylation reactions. Which of the following atoms likely serves as the nucleophile?

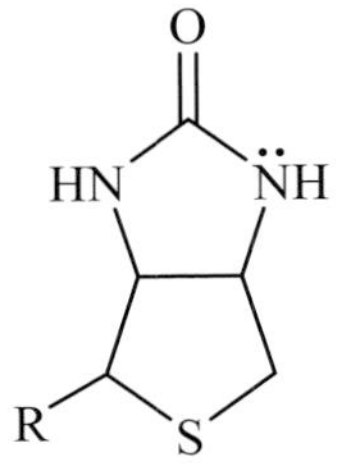

- ○ **A.** Carbon
- ○ **B.** Nitrogen
- ○ **C.** Oxygen
- ○ **D.** Sulfur

Question 350

Which of the following energy-storing molecules is NOT an electrophile in metabolism?

- ○ **A.** ATP
- ○ **B.** NAD^+
- ○ **C.** NADH
- ○ **D.** FAD

Question 351

One mole of (*R*)-3-methyl-3-bromohexane was added to water. Which of the following product yields is expected?

- ○ **A.**

Product	% of total
(*R*)-3-methyl-3-hexanol	25%
(*S*)-3-methyl-3-hexanol	25%
3-methyl-3-hexene	25%
3-methyl-2-hexene	25%

- ○ **B.**

Product	% of total
(*R*)-3-methyl-3-hexanol	0%
(*S*)-3-methyl-3-hexanol	50%
3-methyl-3-hexene	25%
3-methyl-2-hexene	25%

- ○ **C.**

Product	% of total
(*R*)-3-methyl-3-hexanol	0%
(*S*)-3-methyl-3-hexanol	50%
3-methyl-3-hexene	50%
3-methyl-2-hexene	0%

- ○ **D.**

Product	% of total
(*R*)-3-methyl-3-hexanol	30%
(*S*)-3-methyl-3-hexanol	30%
3-methyl-3-hexene	20%
3-methyl-2-hexene	20%

Use the synthesis below to answer questions 352-353.

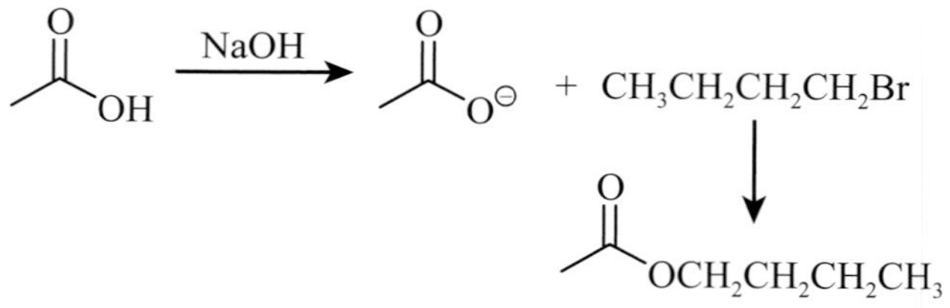

Question 352

In the synthesis of butyl acetate, the acetate ion is a(n):

- O **A.** nucleophile.
- O **B.** electrophile.
- O **C.** catalyst.
- O **D.** solvent.

Question 353

If (*S*)-2-bromobutane is used in place of the 1-bromobutane, what is true about the ester that is formed?

- O **A.** The ester will be optically active.
- O **B.** The ester will be optically inactive.
- O **C.** No product will form.
- O **D.** It will form faster than the butyl acetate.

Question 354

The formation of an ester by the reaction of a carboxylic acid and an alcohol is reversible. How can the yield of the ester be increased?

I. Increase the concentration of alcohol.
II. Substitute the appropriate anhydride for the carboxylic acid.
III. Add an acid catalyst.

- O **A.** I only
- O **B.** III only
- O **C.** I and III only
- O **D.** I, II, and III

Question 355

What does the acid catalyst do in the synthesis of an ester from a carboxylic acid and alcohol?

I. Creates a better leaving group
II. Activates the nucleophile
III. Activates the electrophile

- O **A.** I only
- O **B.** III only
- O **C.** I and III only
- O **D.** I, II, and III

Solid derivatives of tertiary amines can be formed from the two reactions shown below. Use these reactions to answer questions 356-357.

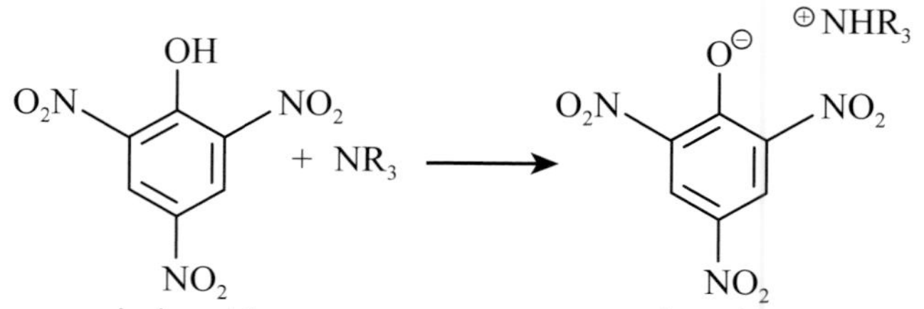

picric acid — amine picrate

$$NR_3 + CH_3I \longrightarrow R_3\overset{\oplus}{N}CH_3\ I^{\ominus}$$

methiodides

Question 356

The formation of methiodides is a(n):

- O **A.** dehydration.
- O **B.** hydration.
- O **C.** alkylation.
- O **D.** dehydrohalogenation.

Question 357

Which of the following would readily form an amine picrate?

O **A.**

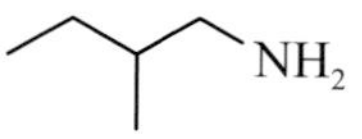

O **B.**

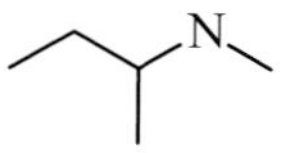

O **C.**

O **D.**

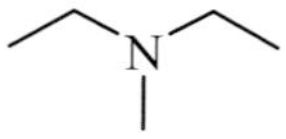

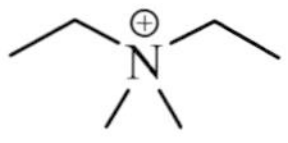

Question 358

Protein primary structure remains particularly intact in healthy individuals. Which statement best describes a reason for this?

○ **A.** Hydrolysis of an amide bond is only possible in a suboptimal pH environment.

○ **B.** Peptide bond breakage requires a strongly acidic and low temperature environment.

○ **C.** The lack of urea build-up in healthy individuals allows for favorable electronic interactions.

○ **D.** Primary structure disruption is only possible via genetic mutation.

Question 359

In the reaction that produces the energy needed for light emission (shown below), the intermediate is:

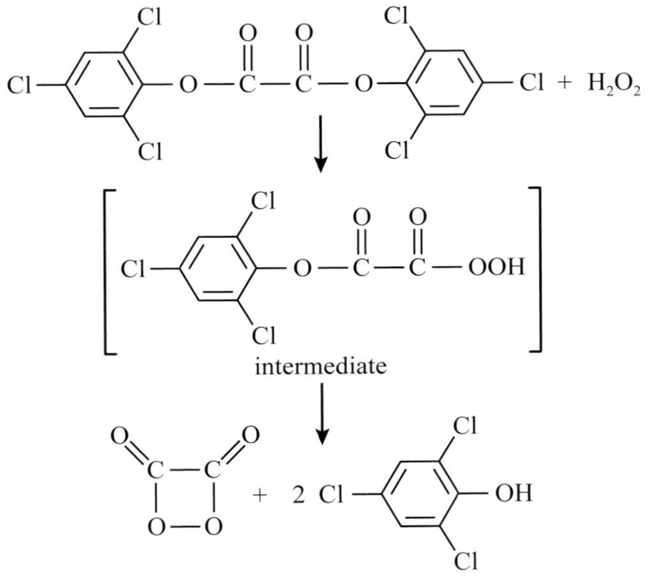

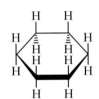

○ **A.** a stable molecule that is easy to isolate.

○ **B.** at a higher oxidation state than bis(2,4,6-trichlorophenyl) oxalate.

○ **C.** at a lower oxidation state than bis(2,4,6-trichlorophenyl) oxalate.

○ **D.** the same as a transition state.

Question 360

In an attempt to maximize reaction rate in the presence of sodium hydroxide, researchers are manipulating the compound below at the substituent labeled "X."

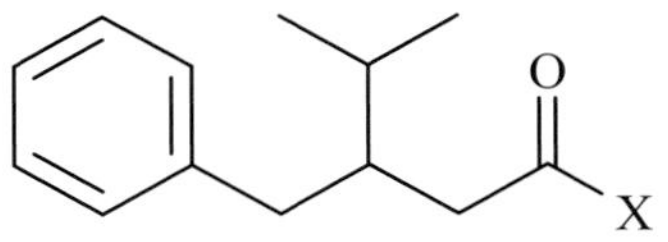

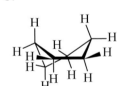

Which of the following substituents would maximize the reaction rate if placed at position "X"?

○ **A.** $-CH_3$

○ **B.** $-CCl_3$

○ **C.** $-OCH_3$

○ **D.** $-Br$

Question 361

Which of the following configurations of glucose experiences the least amount of ring strain?

○ **A.**   ○ **B.**

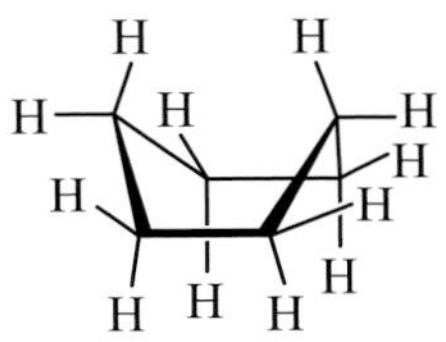

○ **C.**   ○ **D.**

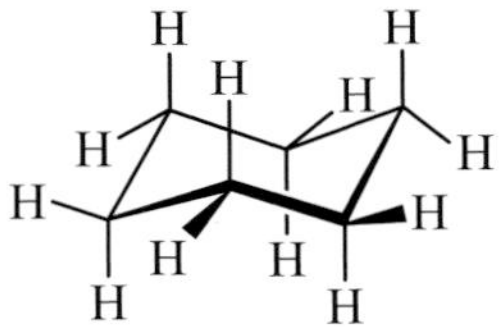

Question 362

Which of the following structures has the most ring strain?

○ **A.**

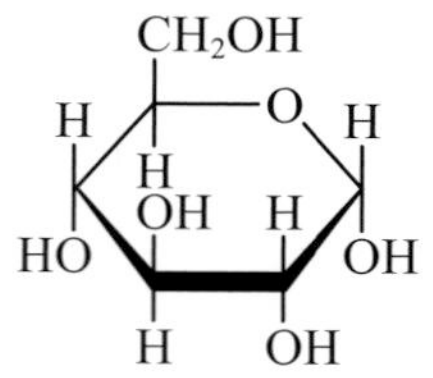

○ **B.**

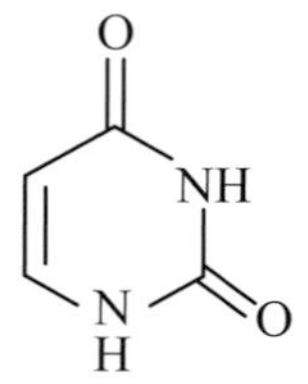

○ **C.**

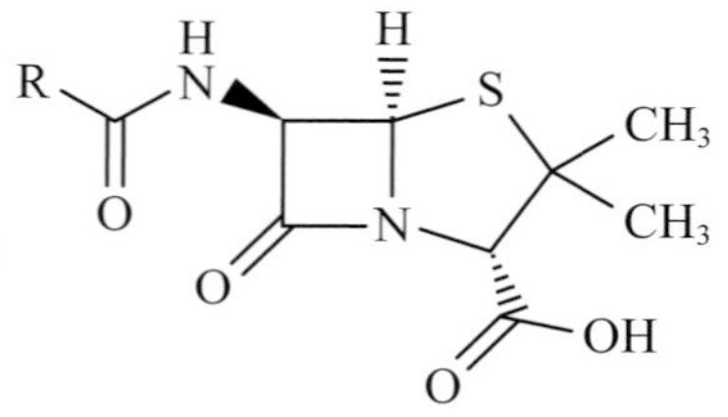

○ **D.**

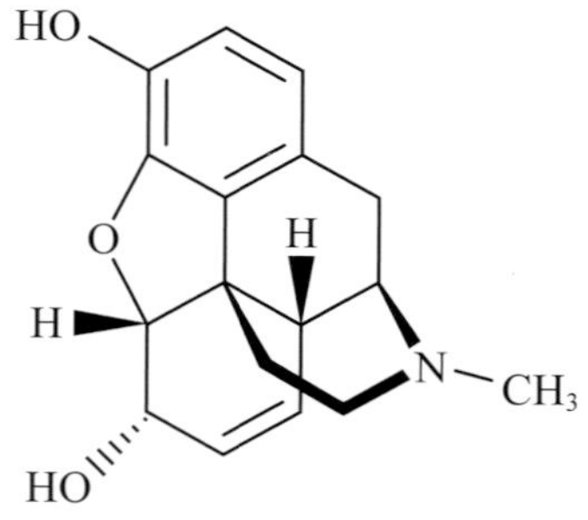

Question 363

Researchers hoped to test the efficacy of a modified penicillin (penicillin is shown below) but were worried about side reactions invalidating their results. Which of the following sites on penicillin is most at risk for side reactions?

○ **A.**

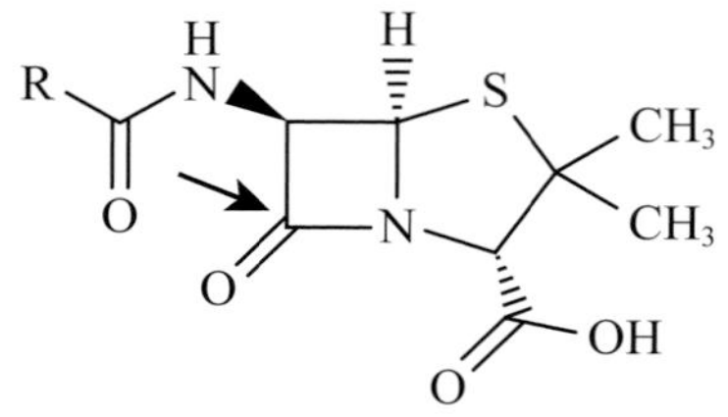

○ **B.**

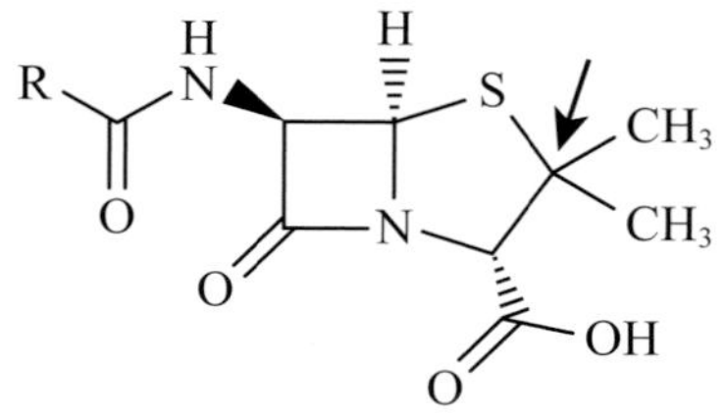

○ **C.**

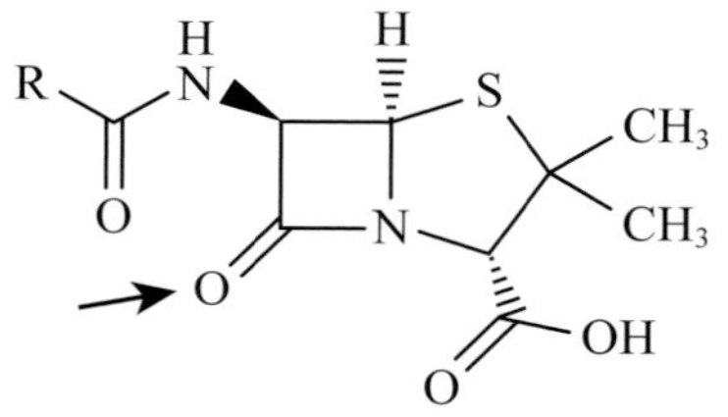

○ **D.**

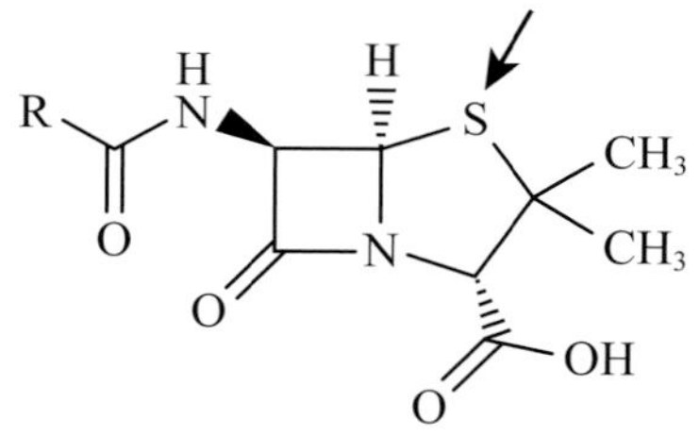

Addition Reactions: Aldehydes and Ketones

Question 364

Which of the following structures is a ketone?

○ **A.**

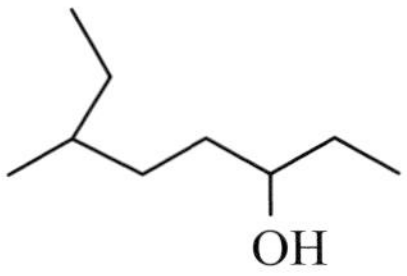

○ **B.**

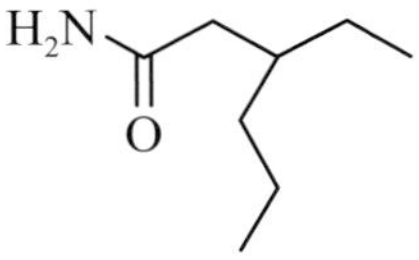

○ **C.**

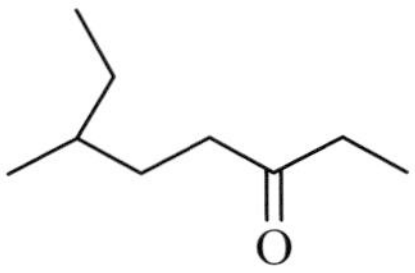

○ **D.**

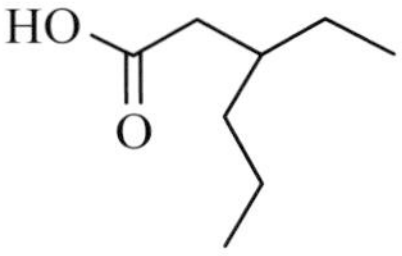

Question 365

In the reaction shown below, what is the functional group conversion that takes place?

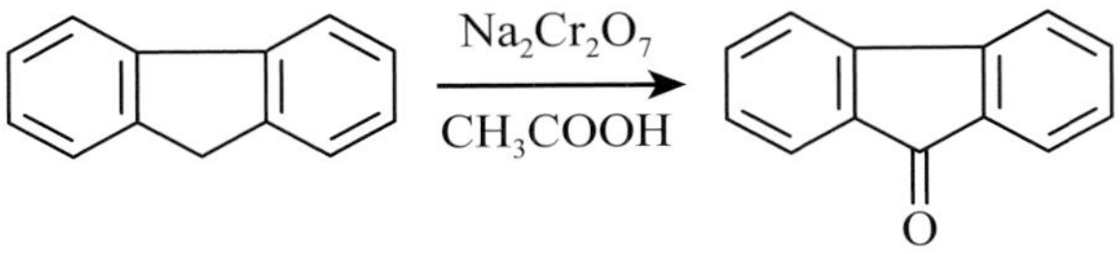

$$\xrightarrow[\text{CH}_3\text{COOH}]{\text{Na}_2\text{Cr}_2\text{O}_7}$$

○ **A.** Alkane to aldehyde

○ **B.** Cycloalkane to cycloketone

○ **C.** Alkane to cycloalkane

○ **D.** Cycloalkane to cycloether

Question 366

Which of the following hydrogen atoms is a beta hydrogen?

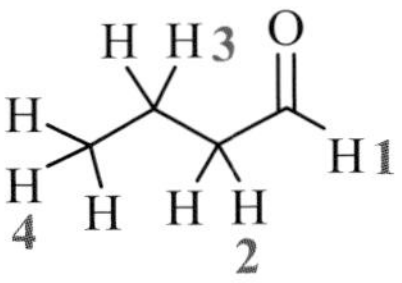

○ **A.** The hydrogen atom labeled 1.

○ **B.** The hydrogen atom labeled 2.

○ **C.** The hydrogen atom labeled 3.

○ **D.** The hydrogen atom labeled 4.

Question 367

The basic carbohydrate portion of the structure for a ribonucleoside is shown below.

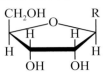

Given that R is a pyrimidine base, the carbohydrate portion of the ribonucleoside is a:

○ **A.** pyranose of a ketose.

○ **B.** pyranose of an aldose.

○ **C.** furanose of a ketose.

○ **D.** furanose of an aldose.

Question 368

Which of the following will have the greatest water solubility?

○ **A.** 1-Heptanol

○ **B.** Heptane

○ **C.** 2-Hepanone

○ **D.** Heptanal

Question 369

In the structure shown below, which carbon is the most electrophilic?

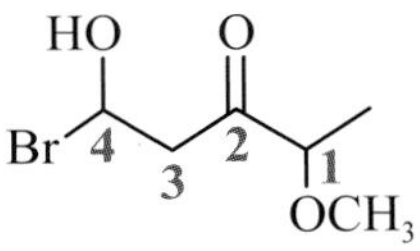

○ **A.** The carbon atom labeled 1.

○ **B.** The carbon atom labeled 2.

○ **C.** The carbon atom labeled 3.

○ **D.** The carbon atom labeled 4.

Question 370

Which of the following will have the highest boiling point?

○ **A.** 1-Heptanol

○ **B.** Heptane

○ **C.** 2-Hepanone

○ **D.** Heptanal

Use the scheme below to answer questions 371-374.

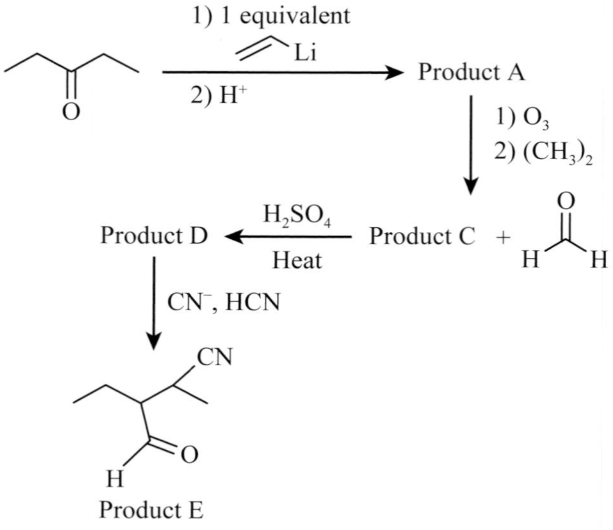

Question 371

How many carbonyls are present in product C?

- O **A.** 0
- O **B.** 1
- O **C.** 2
- O **D.** 3

Question 372

An excess of vinyl lithium was added to the 3-pentanone, producing product B. If product B was then reacted under the same conditions as product A, how many carbonyls are present in the final product?

- O **A.** 0
- O **B.** 1
- O **C.** 2
- O **D.** 3

Question 373

The transformation from product C to product D is a(n):

- O **A.** hydration.
- O **B.** dehydration.
- O **C.** aldol condensation.
- O **D.** hydrogenation.

Question 374

Where does the oxygen atom in product E come from?

- O **A.** The oxygen atom in 3-pentanone
- O **B.** An oxygen atom from O_3
- O **C.** An oxygen atom from H_2O
- O **D.** An oxygen atom from OH^-

Terminal alkynes can be used to synthesize methyl ketones. Refer to the example of this reaction below to answer questions 375-377.

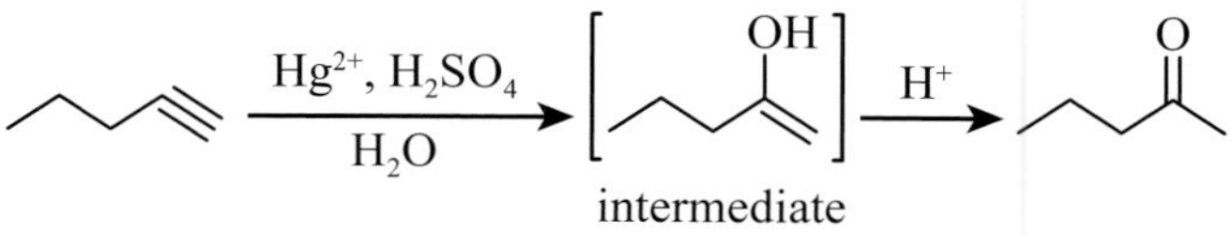

Question 375

Step one in the formation of 2-pentanone from 1-pentyne is a(n):

- O **A.** hydration.
- O **B.** dehydration.
- O **C.** hydrogenation.
- O **D.** nucleophilic substitution.

Question 376

Step two in the formation of 2-pentanone from 1-pentyne is a(n):

- O **A.** oxidation.
- O **B.** reduction.
- O **C.** tautomerization.
- O **D.** nucleophilic substitution.

Question 377

Why does the reaction shown for the synthesis of 2-pentanone only form a methyl ketone and not an aldehyde?

- O **A.** Only the Markovnikov alcohol product forms.
- O **B.** Only the anti-Markovnikov alcohol product forms.
- O **C.** Aldehydes are more unstable than ketones.
- O **D.** Aldehydes are more acidic than ketones.

LECTURE 3

Question 378

Butyraldehyde has a buttery odor and is used in margarine. What reagent could be used to synthesize butyraldehyde from 1-butanol?

○ **A.** $K_2Cr_2O_7$

○ **B.** PCC (mild oxidant)

○ **C.** $LiAlH_4$

○ **D.** O_3, Zn

▼

Dibezalacetone can be used as sunscreen because it has a large absorption band in the UV region. Use the synthesis shown below to answer questions 379-380.

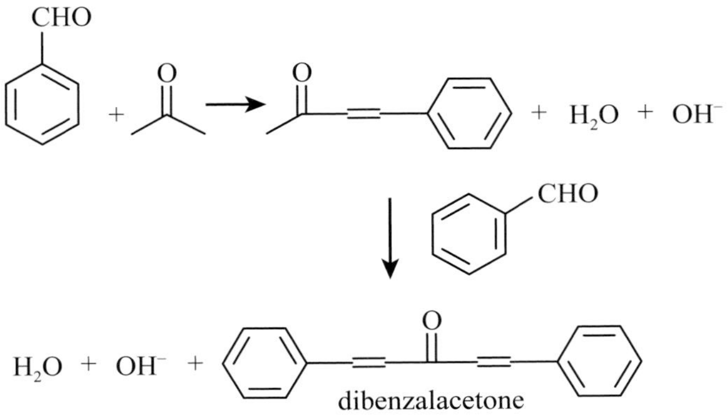

Question 379

In the formation of benzalacetone, acetone is the:

○ **A.** nucleophile.

○ **B.** electrophile.

○ **C.** acid.

○ **D.** oxidant.

Question 380

In the formation of dibenzalacetone from benzalacetone, benzaldehyde is the:

○ **A.** nucleophile.

○ **B.** electrophile.

○ **C.** base.

○ **D.** oxidant.

▲

Question 381

If a strong nucleophile is added to the compound shown below, which carbons are possible electrophiles?

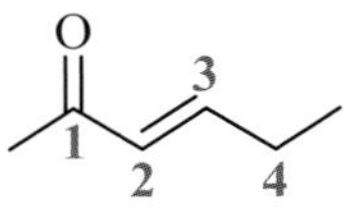

○ **A.** Only C1

○ **B.** C1 and C2

○ **C.** C1 and C3

○ **D.** C2 and C2

Question 382

Adipic acid is a monomer used in the formation of Nylon 6.6. The synthesis of adipic acid is shown below.

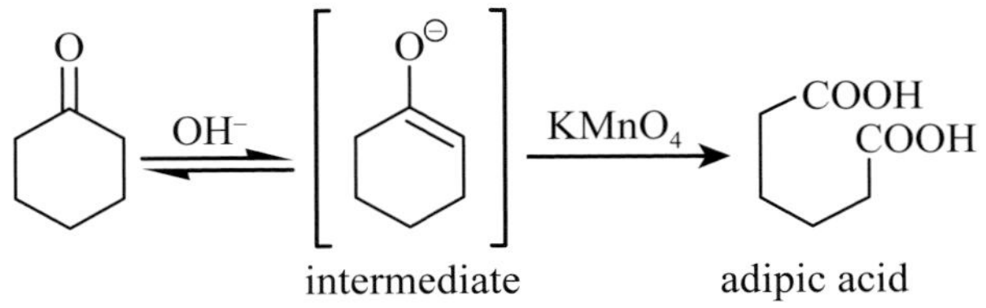

The formation of the intermediate from cyclohexanone is:

○ **A.** a nucleophilic substitution.

○ **B.** an electrophilic addition.

○ **C.** a tautomerization.

○ **D.** resonance stabilization.

Question 383

What reagents could be used to synthesize the acetal shown below?

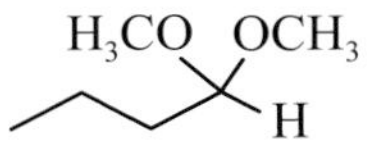

○ **A.** 1-Butanol with methanal

○ **B.** Butanal with methanol

○ **C.** 1,1-Dibutanol and water

○ **D.** Propanal with methanol

When reacted with water, formaldehyde forms formalin, which is used to preserve biological specimens. Use the reaction shown below to answer questions 384-386.

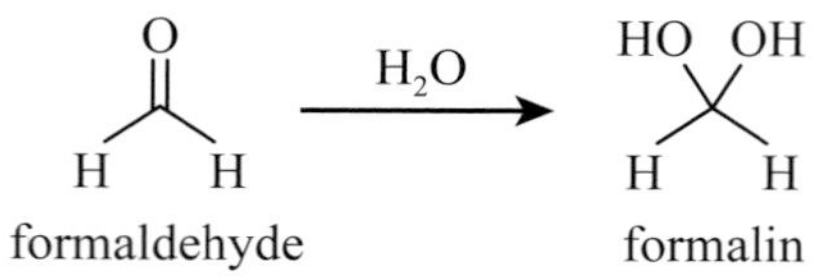

formaldehyde → formalin

Question 384

In a base catalyzed formation of formalin from formaldehyde, the nucleophile is:

○ **A.** the carbonyl carbon in formaldehyde.

○ **B.** the carbonyl oxygen in formaldehyde.

○ **C.** OH^-.

○ **D.** H_2O.

Question 385

In the acid catalyzed formation of formalin from formaldehyde, what does the acid catalyst do?

○ **A.** It activates the electrophile by protonating the oxygen of the carbonyl.

○ **B.** It activates the nucleophile by protonating the oxygen of the carbonyl.

○ **C.** It activates the electrophile by protonating the oxygen of water.

○ **D.** It activates the nucleophile by protonating the oxygen of water.

Question 386

In the acid catalyzed formation of formalin from formaldehyde, the nucleophile is:

○ **A.** the carbonyl carbon in formaldehyde.

○ **B.** the carbonyl oxygen in formaldehyde.

○ **C.** OH^-.

○ **D.** H_2O.

Question 387

The equilibrium of glucose is shown below.

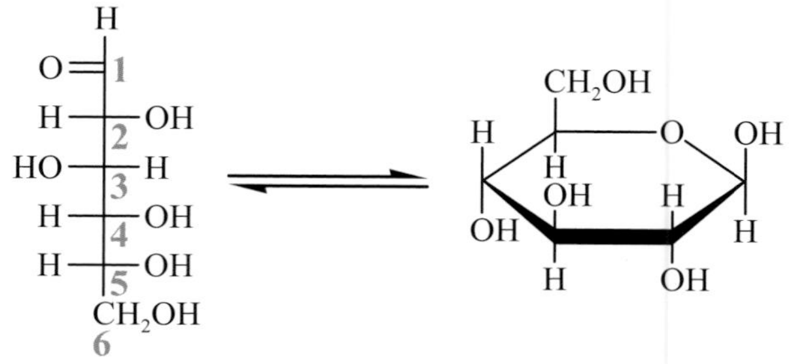

The pyranose form of glucose is a(n):

○ **A.** acetal.

○ **B.** hemiacetal.

○ **C.** ester.

○ **D.** ether.

Question 388

Which carbon shown below is the anomeric carbon?

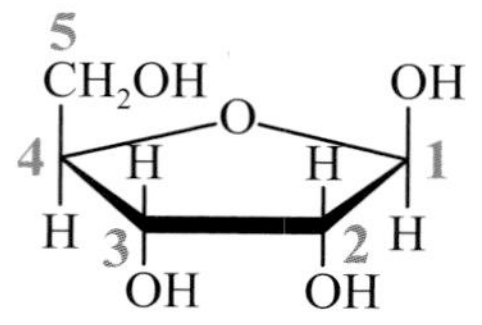

○ **A.** C1

○ **B.** C2

○ **C.** C4

○ **D.** C5

Question 389

The structure of cellulose is shown below.

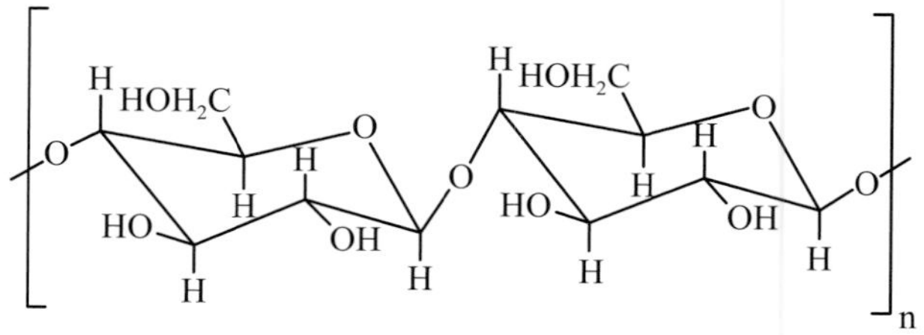

The anomeric carbon is a(n):

○ **A.** acetal.

○ **B.** hemiacetal.

○ **C.** ester.

○ **D.** ether.

Question 390

A patient visits the emergency room with a sweet odor on his breath. The molecules in this odor are taken to a laboratory and reacted with CH_3NH_2 and the result is an imine and an enamine. What could the original molecules have been?

○ **A.** Acetone and acetoacetic acid

○ **B.** Methane and sulfur dioxide

○ **C.** Hydrogen sulfide and dimethyl sulfide

○ **D.** Phenol and benzenes

Question 391

The reaction shown below is a(n):

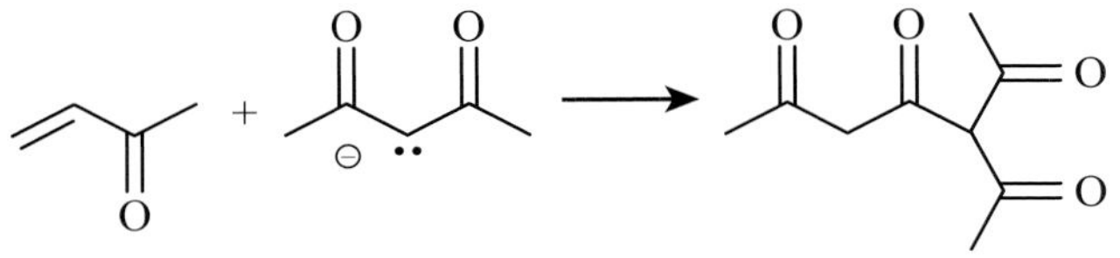

○ **A.** 1,2-conjugate addition.

○ **B.** 1,4-conjugate addition.

○ **C.** electrophilic addition.

○ **D.** nucleophilic substitution.

Question 392

cis-jasmone is a perfume that can be synthesized from *cis*-8-undecene-2,5-dione as shown below.

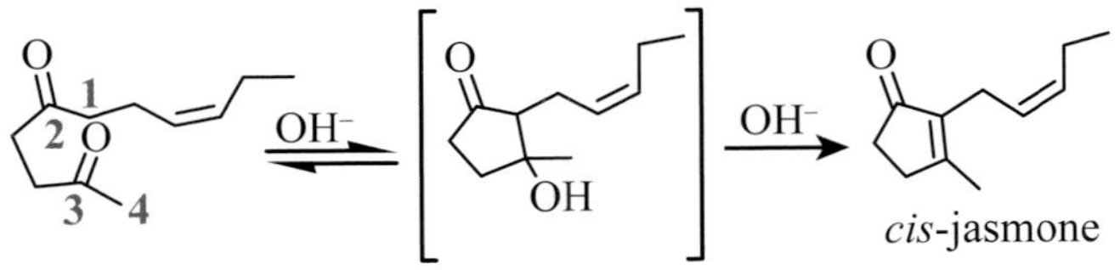

Which hydrogen is removed in the first step of the *cis*-jasmone synthesis to create the enolate ion?

○ **A.** The carbon labeled 1

○ **B.** The carbon labeled 2

○ **C.** The carbon labeled 3

○ **D.** The carbon labeled 4

Question 393

Tautomerization can racemize optically active ketones and aldehydes. Which of the following would no longer rotate plane polarized light after reacting with an acid?

○ **A.** (*S*)-3-methyl-2-heptanone

○ **B.** (*R*)-4-methyl-2-heptanone

○ **C.** (*S*)-3-*t*-butylpentanal

○ **D.** (*R*)-3-methylcyclopentanone

Question 394

In the structure shown below, which hydrogen is the most acidic?

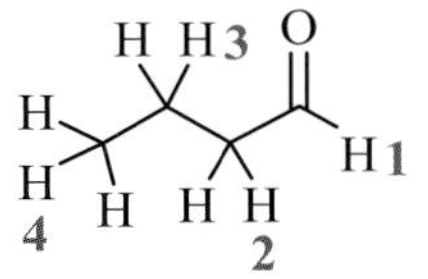

○ **A.** The hydrogen atom labeled 1

○ **B.** The hydrogen atom labeled 2

○ **C.** The hydrogen atom labeled 3

○ **D.** The hydrogen atom labeled 4

Question 395

Which of the following compounds is the most acidic?

○ **A.** Pentane

○ **B.** 1-Pentene

○ **C.** 2-Pentanone

○ **D.** Pentanal

Question 396

In the structure shown below, which hydrogen is the most acidic?

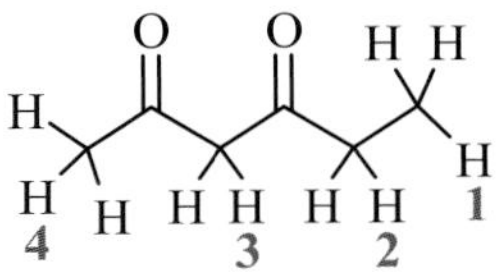

○ **A.** The hydrogen atom labeled 1

○ **B.** The hydrogen atom labeled 2

○ **C.** The hydrogen atom labeled 3

○ **D.** The hydrogen atom labeled 4

Question 397

Why are the alpha hydrogens of ketones more acidic than the hydrogens of alkanes?

○ **A.** The oxygen of the ketone promotes hydrogen bonding.

○ **B.** The oxygen of the ketone donates electrons to the base.

○ **C.** The ketone can resonance stabilize the anions generated when the proton is removed.

○ **D.** The ketone can resonance destabilize the anions generated when the proton is removed.

Question 398

What reagent could convert camphor to borneol?

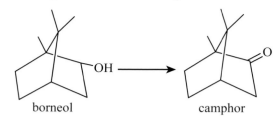

borneol → camphor

- ○ **A.** NaBH$_4$
- ○ **B.** PBr$_3$
- ○ **C.** Na$_2$Cr$_2$O$_7$
- ○ **D.** O$_3$

Use the scheme below to answer questions 399-400.

Product D ⟶ (HOCH$_2$CH$_2$CH$_2$OH / H$^+$) ⟶ Product A

Product A ⟶ (CH$_2$=CH–Li) ⟶ Product B

Product B ⟶ (H$_2$SO$_4$ / H$_2$O) ⟶ Product C

Question 399

If product D is reacted with LiAlH$_4$, then reacted with the 1-bromo-3-butanone and an acid catalyst, what is the product?

- ○ **A.**
- ○ **B.**
- ○ **C.**
- ○ **D.**

Question 400

If the first step of the scheme were skipped, what would be the result?

- ○ **A.** The vinyl lithium will not react with the 1-bromo-3-propanone.
- ○ **B.** The vinyl lithium would add to the carbonyl.
- ○ **C.** The same product would be obtained.
- ○ **D.** The reaction would proceed at a slower rate.

Question 401

What nucleophile could be used to form cyanohydrin (shown below) when reacted with 2-hexanone?

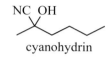

cyanohydrin

- ○ **A.** HCN
- ○ **B.** CN$^-$
- ○ **C.** H$_2$O
- ○ **D.** OH$^-$

Question 402

When HBr is reacted with an alkene in the presence of a peroxide, the anti-Markovnikov product results. What would be the product if 2-isopropyl-2-butene is reacted with HBr in the presence of hydrogen peroxide?

- ○ **A.** 2-Bromo-3-isopropylbutane
- ○ **B.** 2-Bromo-2-isopropylbutane
- ○ **C.** 2-Bromo-2-isopropylbutene
- ○ **D.** 2-Isopropylbutane

Oxidation and Reduction of Oxygen Containing Compounds

Question 403

Citronellol is converted to citronellal by PCC (pyridinium chlorochromate) according the reaction shown below. PCC is a(n):

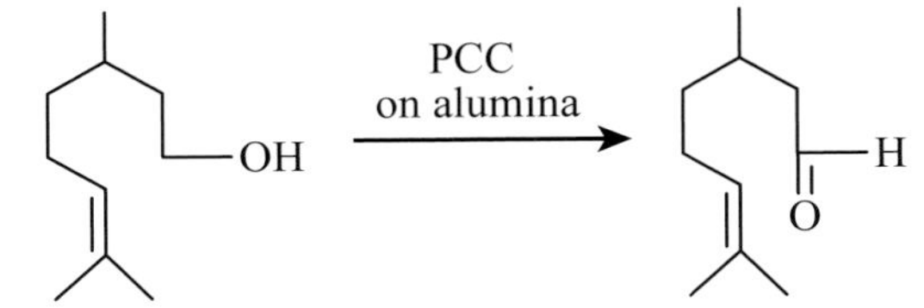

citronellol   cintronellal

- ○ **A.** oxidizing agent.
- ○ **B.** reducing agent.
- ○ **C.** acid.
- ○ **D.** base.

Question 404

Which of the following reagents will convert 3-hexanone to 3-hexanol?

- ○ **A.** $NaBH_4$
- ○ **B.** H_2CrO_4
- ○ **C.** $KMnO_4$
- ○ **D.** $AlCl_3$

Question 405

Which of the following will convert a primary alcohol to an aldehyde?

- ○ **A.** $LiAlH_4$
- ○ **B.** Dilute cold $KMnO_4$
- ○ **C.** K_2CrO_4
- ○ **D.** O_3 and $(CH_3)_2S$

Question 406

Which of the following will convert a primary alcohol to a carboxylic acid?

- ○ **A.** $LiAlH_4$
- ○ **B.** Dilute cold $KMnO_4$
- ○ **C.** K_2CrO_4
- ○ **D.** O_3 and $(CH_3)_2S$

Question 407

Phenolphthalein is an indicator for pH. In solutions of pH greater than 8, phenolphthalein is pink. This reaction is shown below.

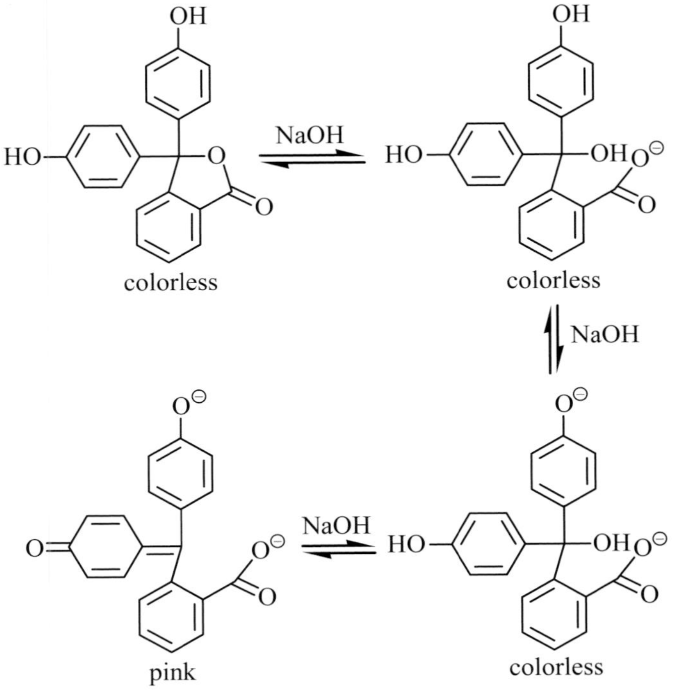

colorless   colorless

pink   colorless

The reaction with the first addition of an equivalent of NaOH to phenolphthalein is a(n):

- ○ **A.** hydrolysis.
- ○ **B.** dehydration.
- ○ **C.** hydrogenation.
- ○ **D.** decarboxylation.

Question 408

Which of the following will react with acetic acid to form ethyl acetate?

- ○ **A.** Acetic anhydride
- ○ **B.** Acetic acid
- ○ **C.** Ethanol
- ○ **D.** Ethyl chloride

Question 409

During an experiment, an investigator adds $LiAlH_4$ to pentatonic acid due to a mislabeling error. This would result in the formation of:

- ○ **A.** an alcohol due to random error.
- ○ **B.** an alcohol due to systematic error.
- ○ **C.** a ketone due to random error.
- ○ **D.** a ketone due to systematic error.

Question 410

Bromine water selectively oxidizes the carbonyl of aldehydes in the presence of alcohols. Which of the following would react with bromine water?

○ **A.** D-glucose

○ **B.** α-D-glucopyranose

○ **C.** D-fructose

○ **D.** α-D-fructofuranose

When reacted with water, formaldehyde forms formalin, which is used to preserve biological specimens. Use the reaction shown below to answer questions 411-412.

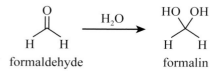

formaldehyde   formalin

Question 411

What would result if formaldehyde was dissolved in methanol rather than water?

○ **A.** The formation of hydrated formaldehyde

○ **B.** The formation of an acetal

○ **C.** The formation of a ketal

○ **D.** No reaction would occur.

Question 412

In the above reaction, the formation of the product (formalin) is favored over the starting compound (formaldehyde). However, when this reaction is conducted with 2-butanone as the reactant, the starting compound is favored over the hydrated product. What accounts for the difference in reactivity?

○ **A.** Alkyl groups are electron donating.

○ **B.** Alkyl groups are electron withdrawing.

○ **C.** Formaldehyde is sterically hindered.

○ **D.** Ketones are weaker nucleophiles.

Carbonyls as Nucleophiles: Aldol Condensation

Question 413

In an aldol reaction, the nucleophile is a(n):

○ **A.** carbonyl carbon.

○ **B.** carbonyl oxygen.

○ **C.** hydroxide ion.

○ **D.** enolate ion.

Question 414

In an aldol addition of 2-butanone and 3-pentanone, the product will have:

○ **A.** 2 carbonyl groups.

○ **B.** 2 hydroxyl groups.

○ **C.** 1 carbonyl group and 1 hydroxyl group.

○ **D.** 1 carbonyl group, 1 hydroxyl group, and one carbon-carbon double bond.

Question 415

What is the first step of a base catalyzed aldol condensation?

○ **A.** Protonation of the carbonyl oxygen to activate the nucleophile

○ **B.** Protonation of the enolate ion to activate the nucleophile

○ **C.** Deprotonation of the alpha hydrogen to activate the nucleophile

○ **D.** Deprotonation of the alpha hydrogen to activate the electrophile

Question 416

How does a base catalyzed aldol condensation compare with an acid catalyzed aldol condensation?

○ **A.** An acid catalyzed aldol condensation activates the electrophile, while the base catalyzed condensation activates the nucleophile.

○ **B.** An acid catalyzed aldol condensation activates the nucleophile, while the base catalyzed condensation activates the electrophile.

○ **C.** Both reactions activate the electrophile.

○ **D.** Both reactions activate the nucleophile.

Bonding and Reactions of Biological Molecules

Question 417

Hydrolysis of the glycosidic bonds in starch involves which of the following?

- ○ **A.** The addition of water and separation of the 1-6 carbon bond
- ○ **B.** The addition of water and separation of the 1-4 carbon bond
- ○ **C.** The removal of water and separation of the 1-6 carbon bond
- ○ **D.** The removal of water and separation of the 1-4 carbon bond

Question 418

All but which of the following may undergo hydrolysis of a glycosidic bond?

- ○ **A.** Hypoxanthine
- ○ **B.** Uridine
- ○ **C.** Lactose
- ○ **D.** Glycogen

Question 419

A mystery molecule is completely hydrolyzed in the presence of a strong acid. A student measures the molecular weight of the resulting molecules. The heaviest molecule in the mixture has a molecular weight of over 250 g/mol. Which of the following could be the mystery molecule?

- ○ **A.** DNA
- ○ **B.** ATP
- ○ **C.** Phospholipid
- ○ **D.** Glycogen

For questions 420-422, refer to the following reaction involving sucrose:

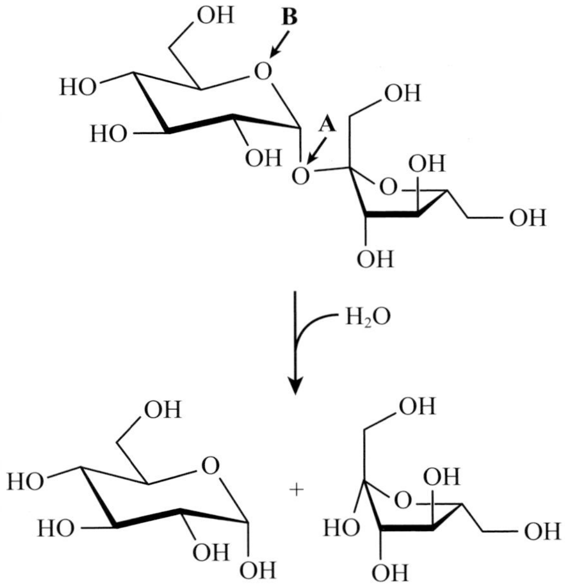

Question 420

Which of the following molecules most resembles the pyranose product?

- ○ **A.** Lactose
- ○ **B.** Mannose
- ○ **C.** Ribose
- ○ **D.** Xylose

Question 421

Prior to the formation of both products:

- ○ **A.** oxygen "A" will receive a proton from a hydronium ion.
- ○ **B.** oxygen "A" will receive a proton from a hydroxide ion.
- ○ **C.** oxygen "B" will receive a proton from a hydronium ion.
- ○ **D.** oxygen "B" will receive a proton from a hydroxide ion.

Question 422

Which of the following statements most accurately describes the bond that was broken during the reaction?

- **A.** The bond was a 1,1' glycosidic linkage. The linkage was alpha in respect to fructose but beta with respect to galactose.
- **B.** The bond was a 1,1' glycosidic linkage. The linkage was alpha in respect to fructose but beta with respect to glucose.
- **C.** The bond was a 1,1' glycosidic linkage. The linkage was alpha in respect to glucose but beta with respect to fructose.
- **D.** The bond was a 1,2' glycosidic linkage. The linkage was alpha in respect to glucose but beta with respect to fructose.

Question 423

Which of the following is likely to have a predominant enol, rather than keto, form at room temperature?

- **A.** Acetone
- **B.** Phenol
- **C.** Glucose
- **D.** Acetoacetic acid

Question 424

Fructose, a ketose sugar, is introduced into a test tube with lithium diisopropylamide, a strong base. Which of the following reaction conditions are most favorable to the tautomeric creation of glucose, an aldose sugar?

- **A.** High temperature and long reaction time
- **B.** High temperature and short reaction time
- **C.** Low temperature and long reaction time
- **D.** Low temperature and short reaction time

Question 425

Diacetyl, a simple dione, is introduced to a base. Which of the following reagents will inhibit keto-enol tautomerization?

- **A.** DCM
- **B.** THF
- **C.** Methanol
- **D.** Acetone

Question 426

Gelatin can be broken down to its constituent amino acids by refluxing in HCl, as shown below.

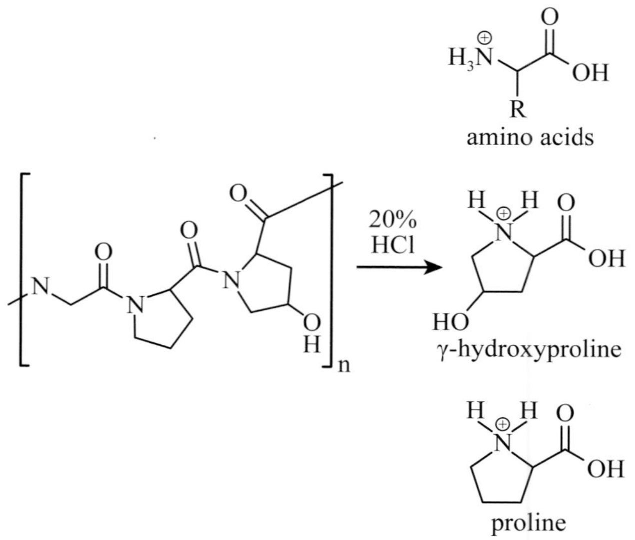

Gelatin is formed through the hydrolysis of collagen, a structural protein. In this reaction, water is a:

- **A.** catalyst.
- **B.** reactant.
- **C.** product.
- **D.** spectator ion.

Question 427

A dipeptide is hydrolyzed under acidic conditions. The resulting product is most likely:

- **A.** a denatured protein.
- **B.** a dipeptide.
- **C.** two amino acids and one H_2O.
- **D.** two amino acids.

Question 428

Which of the following bonds labeled in the protein segment below would be broken during acid-catalyzed hydrolysis?

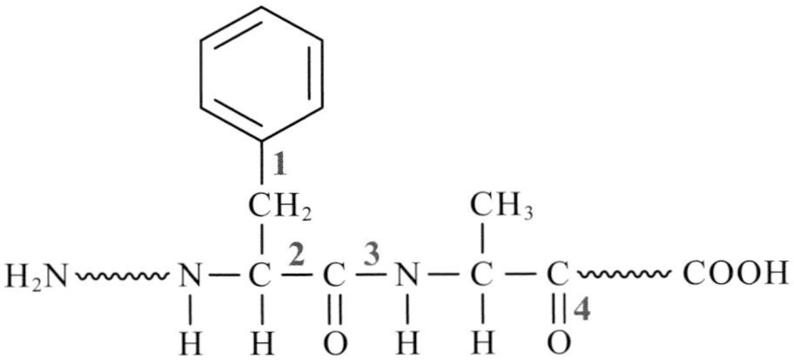

- ○ **A.** 1
- ○ **B.** 2
- ○ **C.** 3
- ○ **D.** 4

Question 429

What reagent is used to convert tristearin into stearate (pictured below), a soap?

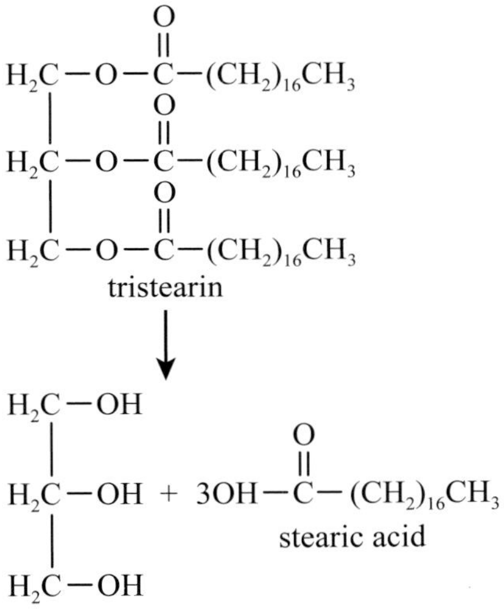

- ○ **A.** H_2O_2
- ○ **B.** HCl
- ○ **C.** NADH
- ○ **D.** NaOH

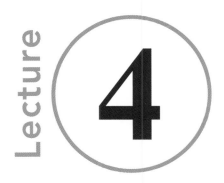

Lecture

Questions 430–572

Thermodynamics and Kinetics

Physical Properties of Systems and Surroundings
Chemical Kinetics
State and Path Functions: Internal Energy,
   Heat, and Work
Enthalpy and Entropy
Accounting for Energy: Gibbs Free Energy
   and Hess's Law
Equilibrium
Free Energy and Spontaneity

Physical Properties of Systems and Surroundings

Question 430

In an isolated system, which of the following can be exchanged between the system and its surroundings?

○ **A.** Energy only

○ **B.** Matter only

○ **C.** Both matter and energy

○ **D.** Neither matter nor energy

Question 431

In a closed system, what can be exchanged between the system and its surroundings?

○ **A.** Energy only

○ **B.** Matter only

○ **C.** Both matter and energy

○ **D.** Neither matter nor energy

Question 432

In an open system, what can be exchanged between the system and its surroundings?

○ **A.** Energy only

○ **B.** Matter only

○ **C.** Both matter and energy

○ **D.** Neither matter nor energy

Question 433

After running a reaction multiple times at varying temperatures, researchers determined that doubling the absolute temperature from the starting conditions results in the highest reaction rate. Assuming starting conditions of 23°C and 1 atm, at what temperature is reaction rate maximized?

○ **A.** 273 K

○ **B.** 310 K

○ **C.** 319 K

○ **D.** 592 K

Question 434

The Boltzmann constant best relates which of the following variables?

○ **A.** Kinetic energy and the temperature of a gas

○ **B.** Potential energy and the temperature of a gas

○ **C.** Kinetic energy and the intermolecular interactions of a gas

○ **D.** Potential energy and the intermolecular interactions of a gas

Question 435

What is the value of the Boltzmann constant of 1.7 moles of gas at 290 K that has an average kinetic energy of 1.4 MJ?

○ **A.** 7×10^{-24} J/K

○ **B.** 1.4×10^{-23} J/K

○ **C.** 6×10^{-3} J/K

○ **D.** 7×10^{-3} J/K

Question 436

Which of the following experimental designs would allow a scientist to measure the value of Boltzmann's constant?

  I. Determine the changes in rotational and translational energy as the temperature of a gas decreases.

  II. Determine the changes in rotational and translational energy as the temperature of a gas increases.

  III. Determine the changes in heat released from a gas as the temperature of a gas increases.

○ **A.** I only

○ **B.** III only

○ **C.** I and II only

○ **D.** II and III only

Chemical Kinetics

Question 437

Consider the complete combustion of ethanol (C_2H_6O) to form carbon dioxide and water. If the ethanol is consumed at a rate of 2.0 M s^{-1}, what is the rate at which carbon dioxide is produced?

○ **A.** 1.0 M s^{-1}

○ **B.** 2.0 M s^{-1}

○ **C.** 4.0 M s^{-1}

○ **D.** Cannot be determined from the information given

Question 438

The rate of a reaction between a solid and a liquid depends on:

   I. the temperature of the liquid.

   II. the surface area of the solid that is in contact with the liquid.

   III. the presence of a catalyst.

○ **A.** I only

○ **B.** III only

○ **C.** I and III only

○ **D.** I, II, and III

Question 439

Regarding chemical kinetics, which of the following is true?

○ **A.** The rate constant of a given reaction is independent of temperature.

○ **B.** Catalysts never change the mechanism of a reaction.

○ **C.** The rates of formation of different products in the same reaction under the same conditions are always the same.

○ **D.** Most collisions between reactants do not result in products being formed.

Question 440

According to the collision model, what three conditions are required for a reaction to occur?

○ **A.** A molecular collision, sufficient temperature and proper spatial orientation of the molecules

○ **B.** A molecular collision, sufficient temperature and sufficient duration of molecular contact

○ **C.** A molecular collision, sufficient energy of collision and proper spatial orientation of the molecules

○ **D.** A molecular collision, sufficient energy of collision and sufficient duration of molecular contact

Question 441

Based on the information shown in the graph below, what is the activation energy of the reaction?

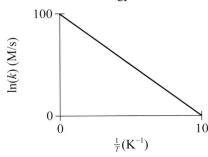

○ **A.** −83.1 J

○ **B.** 8.3 J

○ **C.** 83.1 J

○ **D.** 831.4 J

Question 442

The results from an experiment on an enzymatic reaction are shown below. Which of the following was/were decreased by using the enzyme?

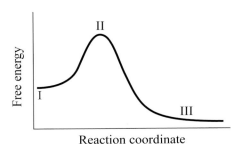

○ **A.** I only

○ **B.** II only

○ **C.** I and III only

○ **D.** I, II, and III

Question 443

A molecule is formed two different ways. In instance A, the kinetic product was formed. In instance B, the thermodynamic product was formed. Which reaction produced the most stable product?

○ **A.** Due to lower activation energy, the kinetic reaction will form the more stable product.

○ **B.** Due to higher activation energy, the kinetic reaction will form the more stable product.

○ **C.** Due to higher activation energy, the thermodynamic reaction will form the more stable product.

○ **D.** Due to lower activation energy, the thermodynamic reaction will form the more stable product.

Question 444

An asymmetric ketone is exposed to basic conditions and kept at a low temperature. Which of the following statements best describes the product that would form?

○ **A.** The most substituted enolate would form as it would require less activation energy.

○ **B.** The least substituted enolate would form as it would require less activation energy.

○ **C.** The most substituted enolate would form as it would require more activation energy.

○ **D.** The least substituted enolate would form as it would require more activation energy.

Question 445

Which of the following identifies the rate law for the following unbalanced elementary reaction?

$$\text{Glucose} + O_2 \leftrightarrow CO_2 + H_2O$$

○ **A.** Rate = $[\text{Glucose}][O_2]$

○ **B.** Rate = $k[\text{Glucose}][O_2]$

○ **C.** Rate = $[\text{Glucose}][O_2]^6$

○ **D.** Rate = $k[\text{Glucose}][O_2]^6$

Question 446

A chemist is studying the kinetics of a complex reaction. He obtains the following data. How many moles of A should be used if one mole of both B and C are used?

[A]	[B]	[C]	Rate
1	1	1	0.2 mol L^{-1} s^{-1}
2	1	3	2.4 mol L^{-1} s^{-1}
2	2	1	1.6 mol L^{-1} s^{-1}

○ **A.** 1 mol

○ **B.** 2 mol

○ **C.** 3 mol

○ **D.** 4 mol

Question 447

Consider the dissociation of hydrogen gas:

$$H_2(g) \rightarrow 2H(g)$$

Rates were measured for a number of different concentrations:

[H_2]	Rate/M s^{-1}
1.0 M	1.2×10^4
1.5 M	2.7×10^4
2.0 M	4.8×10^4

What is the rate law for this reaction?

○ **A.** Rate = $k[H_2]$

○ **B.** Rate = $k[H_2]^2$

○ **C.** Rate = $k[H]^2/[H_2]$

○ **D.** The rate law cannot be determined from the information given.

Question 448

Consider the reaction

$$2H_2 + 2NO \rightarrow N_2 + 2H_2O$$

Rates were measured for a number of different concentrations:

[H_2]	[NO]	Rate/M s^{-1}
0.1 M	0.3 M	230
0.2 M	0.3 M	460
0.3 M	0.1 M	80
0.4 M	0.1 M	50

What rate law is most consistent with this data?

○ **A.** Rate = $k[H_2][NO]$

○ **B.** Rate = $k[H_2][NO]^2$

○ **C.** Rate = $k[H_2]^2[NO]$

○ **D.** Rate = $k[H_2]^2[NO]^3$

Question 449

The reaction below proceeds very slowly at room temperature, but at a greater rate at higher temperatures. This is because:

$$N_2(g) + 3H_2(g) \rightarrow 2NH_3(g)$$

- ○ **A.** the reaction is exothermic.
- ○ **B.** the reaction is endothermic.
- ○ **C.** at higher temperatures, collisions occur more frequently and are more likely to have sufficient energy to initiate the reaction.
- ○ **D.** at higher temperatures, the equilibrium constant is greater.

Question 450

For all reactants at 1 M concentration, a certain reaction proceeds at an initial rate of 0.030 M s^{-1}. The reaction is then repeated under identical conditions, except that the temperature is doubled. What is the new initial rate?

- ○ **A.** 0.015 M s^{-1}
- ○ **B.** 0.030 M s^{-1}
- ○ **C.** 0.060 M s^{-1}
- ○ **D.** Cannot be determined from the information given

Question 451

Using calculus, the rate law for a first order reaction can be transformed to:

$$\log[A]_t = -kt/2.303 + \log[A]_0$$

where $[A]_t$ is the concentration of A at time t, $[A]_0$ is the initial concentration of A, and k is the rate constant of the reaction. Methyl isonitrile is converted to acetonitrile in a first order process as follows:

$$CH_3NC(g) \rightarrow CH_3CN(g)$$

The rate constant for the conversion of methyl isonitrile is 5×10^{-5} s^{-1}. A scientist has a container containing methyl isonitrile gas with a partial pressure of 100 torr. After 12.8 hours (approx. 46,000 seconds), what is the partial pressure of methyl isonitrile gas inside the container?

- ○ **A.** 1 torr
- ○ **B.** 10 torr
- ○ **C.** 25 torr
- ○ **D.** 50 torr

Question 452

The rate constant for a reaction depends on which of the following?

  I. Temperature
  II. Concentration of reactants
  III. Concentration of products

- ○ **A.** I only
- ○ **B.** I and II only
- ○ **C.** II and III only
- ○ **D.** I, II, and III

Question 453

Which of the following methods could be used to determine the rate law for a reaction?

  I. Measure the initial rate of the reaction for a variety of reactant concentrations.
  II. Graph the concentration of the reactants as a function of time.
  III. Find the mechanism of the reaction.

- ○ **A.** I only
- ○ **B.** III only
- ○ **C.** II and III only
- ○ **D.** I, II, and III

Question 454

Suppose a certain reaction has the rate law:

$$\text{Rate} = k[A]^{1/2}[B]$$

Which of the following can be concluded about the reaction?

- ○ **A.** Two molecules of B react for every molecule of A.
- ○ **B.** Two molecules of A react for every molecule of B.
- ○ **C.** B reacts at twice the rate of A.
- ○ **D.** This reaction does not take place in a single step.

Question 455

The mechanism for the conversion of 2-iodo-2-methylpropane into an alcohol is displayed below.

2-iodo-2-methylpropane →
        2-methylpropane cation + iodide

2-methylpropane cation + water →
        protonated 2-methylpropanol

protonated 2-methylpropanol + water →
        2-methylpropanol + hydronium

In the mechanism shown, iodide is a(n):

○ **A.** reactant.

○ **B.** product.

○ **C.** intermediate.

○ **D.** catalyst.

Question 456

Scientist A proposes a mechanism for a certain reaction, and uses that mechanism to derive a rate law for the reaction. Scientist B then determines the rate law for the reaction experimentally, using the method of initial rates. If the two rate laws are the same, what can be concluded?

○ **A.** Assuming that the mechanism proposed by scientist A is correct, scientist B determined the correct experimental rate law.

○ **B.** Assuming that scientist B determined the correct experimental rate law, then the mechanism proposed by scientist A is correct.

○ **C.** Both the mechanism proposed by scientist A and the experimental rate law determined by scientist B are correct.

○ **D.** Either scientist A or scientist B made a mistake: rate laws determined by different techniques should be different.

Question 457

The rate law for a reaction is shown below. What is the order of the reaction?

$$Rate = k[A][B]^2$$

○ **A.** 2

○ **B.** 3

○ **C.** 4

○ **D.** 6

Question 458

The rate law for a reaction is shown below. What is the order of A in this reaction?

$$Rate = k[A]^2[B]^4$$

○ **A.** 2

○ **B.** 3

○ **C.** 4

○ **D.** 6

Question 459

The rate law for a reaction is shown below. If B is also a reactant, what is the order of B in this reaction?

$$Rate = k[A]^2$$

○ **A.** 0

○ **B.** 1

○ **C.** 2

○ **D.** Cannot be determined from the information given.

The following information is used for questions 460-461.

The following are the elementary steps of a reaction. The k's represent the rate constants for the respective reactions.

Step 1: $NO(g) + Br_2(g) \underset{k_{-1}}{\overset{k_1}{\rightleftharpoons}} NOBr_2(g)$ (fast)

Step 2: $NOBr_2(g) + NO(g) \overset{k_2}{\longrightarrow} 2NOBr_2(g)$ (slow)

Question 460

What is the overall reaction?

○ **A.** $2NO(g) + Br_2(g) \rightarrow 2NOBr(g)$

○ **B.** $NO(g) + Br(g) \rightarrow NOBr(g)$

○ **C.** $NO(g) + Br_2(g) \rightarrow NOBr_2(g)$

○ **D.** $NOBr_2(g) + Br_2(g) \rightarrow 2NOBr(g)$

Question 461

Which of the following is true concerning the reaction?

○ **A.** Step 1 is the rate determining step. The reaction will proceed at the rate of Step 1.

○ **B.** Step 2 is the rate determining step. The reaction will proceed at the rate of Step 2.

○ **C.** Step 1 is the rate determining step. The reaction will proceed at the rate of Step 1 plus Step 2.

○ **D.** Step 2 is the rate determining step. The reaction will proceed at the rate of Step 1 plus Step 2.

Question 462

Because $NOBr_2$ is a product of the fast step and a reactant of the slow step, and because the fast step precedes the slow step, which of the following concentrations of $NOBr_2$ should be used in the rate law for Step 2?

- **A.** Zero moles per liter
- **B.** The concentration of $NOBr_2$ that exists when Step 1 has run to completion
- **C.** The equilibrium concentration of $NOBr_2$
- **D.** The concentration for $NOBr_2$ in Step 2 cannot be predicted because Step 1 is the fast step.

Question 463

Consider the following mechanism:

$$Br_2 + H_2O_2 \rightarrow 2Br^- + 2H^+ + O_2$$
$$2Br^- + H_2O_2 + 2H^+ \rightarrow Br_2 + 2H_2O$$

Which substance is a catalyst?

- **A.** Br_2
- **B.** H_2O_2
- **C.** H^+
- **D.** O_2

Question 464

Ammonia produced from molecular nitrogen and hydrogen can be used to synthesize amino acids *in vitro*. However, this process often requires a metal oxide catalyst. Which of the following is accomplished by use of the metal oxide catalyst?

- I. The rate of production of ammonia increased.
- II. The energy of activation was raised.
- III. The equilibrium shifted to the products.

- **A.** I only
- **B.** II only
- **C.** I and II only
- **D.** I, II, and III

Question 465

Which of the following can be changed by a catalyst?

- I. The rate constant of a reaction
- II. The rate law of a reaction
- III. The equilibrium constant of a reaction

- **A.** I only
- **B.** I and II only
- **C.** I and III only
- **D.** I, II, and III

Question 466

The energy diagram below compares the kinetic energy of molecules in a reaction with the fraction of molecules colliding in that reaction.

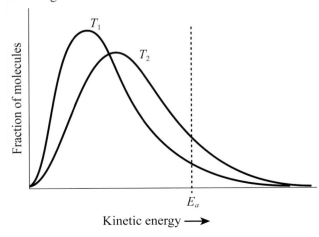

What changes to the diagram would reflect the addition of a catalyst to the reaction?

- **A.** The curves would be flattened and spread over a broader kinetic energy range.
- **B.** The curves would be heightened and narrowed.
- **C.** The curves would be shifted to the right.
- **D.** The vertical line marking the energy of activation would be shifted to the left.

Question 467

Angiotensin converting enzyme converts the hormone angiotensin I to the active vasoconstrictor angiotensin II. Which of the following thermodynamic values is angiotensin converting enzyme likely to change?

- **A.** $G°_{reactants}$
- **B.** $G°_{products}$
- **C.** $\Delta G^{\ddagger}$
- **D.** $\Delta G°$

Question 468

When heat is added to potassium chlorate, it generally disproportionates into potassium perchlorate and potassium chloride. If manganese dioxide is present during the process, however, the products are potassium chloride and oxygen gas. Which of the following is a possible explanation for these observations?

- ○ **A.** In the absence of manganese dioxide, the first set of products is more stable than the second. Manganese dioxide is a catalyst that stabilizes the second set of products.
- ○ **B.** Although the second set of products are more stable than the first, in the absence of manganese dioxide the second reaction occurs at a negligible rate. Manganese dioxide is a catalyst that increases the rate of the second reaction.
- ○ **C.** Manganese dioxide cannot be a catalyst, since it changes the products of the reaction; it must be actively involved with the second reaction.
- ○ **D.** Manganese dioxide cannot be a catalyst, since the presence of a catalyst would affect the reverse reaction as well; it must be a kinetic promoter of the second reaction.

State and Path Functions: Internal Energy, Heat, and Work

Question 469

Which of the following properties of a gas are state functions?

- I. Temperature
- II. Heat
- III. Work

- ○ **A.** I only
- ○ **B.** I and II only
- ○ **C.** II and III only
- ○ **D.** I, II, and III

Question 470

When the enthalpy of a system decreases, the surroundings:

- ○ **A.** experience an increase in entropy and an increase in enthalpy.
- ○ **B.** experience an increase in entropy and a decrease in enthalpy.
- ○ **C.** experience a decrease in entropy and an increase in enthalpy.
- ○ **D.** experience a decrease in entropy and a decrease in enthalpy.

Question 471

The Helmholz function, F, is a state function. From this alone, what can be concluded about F?

- ○ **A.** In a closed system, it is conserved.
- ○ **B.** In an open system, it is not conserved.
- ○ **C.** It must be a function of pressure, volume, and temperature only.
- ○ **D.** If the system is taken from one state to another, the change in F will be independent of the process used.

Question 472

Two objects of differing temperatures are put in direct contact of one another. Which statement best describes the final temperature?

- ○ **A.** The equilibrium temperature would directly match the original temperature of the larger object.
- ○ **B.** The equilibrium temperature would directly match the original temperature of the smaller object.
- ○ **C.** The equilibrium temperature would fall somewhere between the two original temperatures.
- ○ **D.** The equilibrium temperature would first rise towards the larger object's temperature, and then eventually fall to the temperature of the smaller object.

Question 473

What is the zeroth law of thermodynamics?

- ○ **A.** Energy cannot be created or destroyed.
- ○ **B.** The entropy of the system and surroundings must increase in a spontaneous process.
- ○ **C.** If two systems are in thermodynamic equilibrium with a third, then they are in equilibrium with each others.
- ○ **D.** The entropy of a crystal cooled to 0 K is 0.

Question 474

The system shown below contains three chambers, separated by a wall permeable only to heat. If no net heat exchange occurs between C_1 and C_2 or C_2 and C_3, what is the temperature of chamber 2?

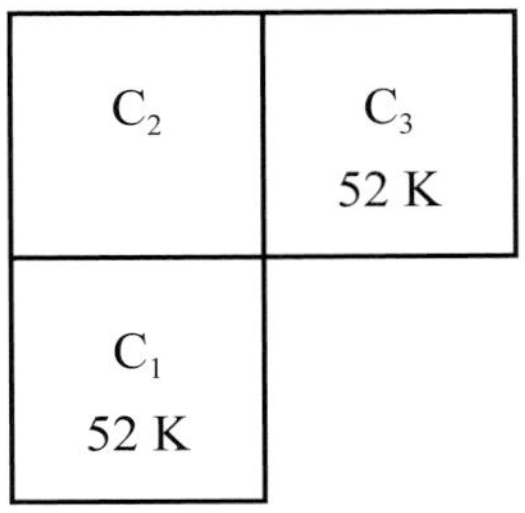

C_2	C_3 52 K
C_1 52 K	

- ○ **A.** 0 K
- ○ **B.** 52 K
- ○ **C.** 104 K
- ○ **D.** 156 K

Question 475

A sealed container with hollow walls is quite effective at maintaining its inside temperature. What is the purpose of the hollow walls?

- ○ **A.** The air in the hollow walls is an excellent insulator, cutting down on conduction.
- ○ **B.** The air in the hollow walls provides an additional source of heat for the container.
- ○ **C.** The hollow walls trap air trying to escape from the box, reducing convection.
- ○ **D.** Reactions can take place within the walls, helping to maintain the temperature of the container.

Question 476

Considering that all objects radiate heat, which of the following statements must be true?

- ○ **A.** All objects are continually getting colder.
- ○ **B.** Any object that gets warmer must be experiencing conduction or convection.
- ○ **C.** No object can reach a temperature of absolute zero.
- ○ **D.** The First Law of Thermodynamics does not apply when radiation is considered.

Question 477

Which of the following phases of a substance typically has the greatest resistance to conduction?

- ○ **A.** Solid
- ○ **B.** Liquid
- ○ **C.** Gas
- ○ **D.** It depends upon the substance.

Use the following information to answer questions 478–480.

The rate of heat transfer through a slab is given by the equation:

$$\frac{Q}{t} = \kappa A \frac{T_h - T_c}{L}$$

where Q is heat, t is time, κ is the thermal conductivity constant, A is the cross-sectional area of each slab face, L is the length of the slab, and T_h and T_c are the hot and cold ends of the slab respectively.

Six contiguous slabs at six temperatures, T_1, T_2, etc.., are placed in a row as shown. Heat flows from left to right through the slabs. The cross-section of each slab face is square. (Unless otherwise stated assume that each slab is made from the same material and the temperature of the slabs do not change over time.)

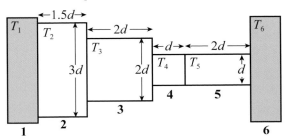

Question 478

Through which slab is the rate of heat flow, Q/t, the greatest?

- ○ **A.** Slab 2
- ○ **B.** Slab 3
- ○ **C.** Slab 4
- ○ **D.** The rate of heat flow is the same through all slabs.

Question 479

Consider only slabs 2, 3, and 4. Which slab experiences the greatest temperature difference between its left and right sides?

- ○ **A.** Slab 2
- ○ **B.** Slab 3
- ○ **C.** Slab 4
- ○ **D.** The temperature difference across each of these slabs is the same.

Question 480

If each slab is made of a different material and the temperature difference is the same across each slab, which slab has the greatest thermal conductivity constant, k?

- A. Slab 2
- B. Slab 3
- C. Slab 4
- D. Slab 5

Question 481

By how much would the length of a 50 cm stainless steel instrument ($\alpha = 17 \times 10^{-6}$ °C^{-1}) used in a laparoscopic surgery change upon entering the body? Room temperature is 20°C, while the body temperature is 37°C.

- A. 8.5×10^{-6} m
- B. 1.4×10^{-4} m
- C. 8.5 m
- D. 17 m

Question 482

Maximizing oxygen delivery lends a particular competitive advantage for highly-trained endurance athletes. In an attempt to develop an artificial hemoglobin-like molecule for intra-workout utilization, researchers recorded the molecule's cubic expansion in varying temperatures. Results are displayed in the table below.

Dimension	25°C	30°C
X (m)	2.05×10^{-9}	2.97×10^{-9}
Y (m)	3.89×10^{-9}	4.01×10^{-9}
Z (m)	5.09×10^{-9}	1.00×10^{-8}

Based on the results, which of the following values is most likely the volumetric coefficient of expansion?

- A. 6.4×10^{-25}
- B. 3.9×10^{-1}
- C. 1.0×10^{-1}
- D. 1.2

Refer to the diagram below to answer questions 483-486.

The diagram below displays the pressure and volume of a sample of ideal gas as it is taken very slowly through six states: A, B, C, D, E, and F, along the pathway shown. ($R = 8.314$ J K^{-1} mol^{-1})

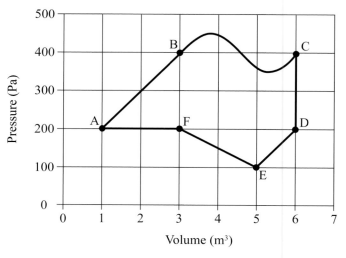

Question 483

What is the approximate net work done on the gas as it goes directly from state F to state A?

- A. −400 J
- B. 0 J
- C. 400 J
- D. 600 J

Question 484

What is the approximate net work done on the gas as it goes directly from state C to state D?

- A. −1200 J
- B. 0 J
- C. 1200 J
- D. 2400 J

Question 485

What is the approximate net work done on the gas as it goes directly from state A to state B?

- A. −1000 J
- B. −600 J
- C. −400 J
- D. 1000 J

LECTURE 4

Question 486

What is the approximate net work done on the gas as it goes from state A, through states B, C, D, E, and F, and back to state A?

- ○ **A.** −1600 J
- ○ **B.** −950 J
- ○ **C.** 0 J
- ○ **D.** 950 J

Question 487

The net work done on a gas is 55 J, and the net heat flow into the gas is −23 J. What is the net work done by the gas?

- ○ **A.** −55 J
- ○ **B.** 0 J
- ○ **C.** 32 J
- ○ **D.** 78 J

Question 488

The net work done on a gas is 55 J, and the net heat flow into the gas is –23 J. What is the change in energy of the gas?

- ○ **A.** −55 J
- ○ **B.** 0 J
- ○ **C.** 32 J
- ○ **D.** 78 J

Question 489

Which of these systems violate(s) the first law of thermodynamics?

- I. A pendulum, perfectly isolated from its environment, which swings forever
- II. A battery that never "dies" or needs recharging
- III. A refrigerator that uses all of the heat it removes from its interior to provide electricity to an apartment

- ○ **A.** I only
- ○ **B.** II only
- ○ **C.** I and III only
- ○ **D.** I, II, and III

Use the diagram below to answer questions 490-492.

The diagram below shows a cross-section of an insulated cylinder-piston apparatus filled with gas and connected to a heat reservoir. The volume of the cylinder can be expanded via the piston at constant pressure or constant temperature.

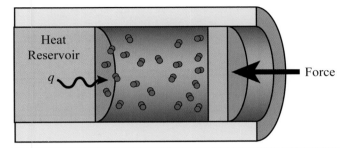

Question 490

Which of the following is true concerning the gas molecules in the cylinder?

- I. If no heat is added to the gas, it will cool as it expands.
- II. The average kinetic energy of the molecules is proportional to the temperature of the gas.
- III. The gas does work on the surroundings as it expands.

- ○ **A.** I only
- ○ **B.** I and II only
- ○ **C.** II and III only
- ○ **D.** I, II, and III

Question 491

If the cylinder is held at constant volume and heat is added, what will become of the added energy?

- ○ **A.** The energy does work on the surroundings.
- ○ **B.** If heat is added, the gas must expand.
- ○ **C.** All the energy becomes kinetic energy of the gas molecules, raising the temperature and pressure of the gas.
- ○ **D.** All the energy becomes kinetic energy of the gas molecules, raising the temperature but not the pressure of the gas.

Question 492

If the cylinder is allowed to expand while heat is added so that the pressure stays constant, what will become of the added heat energy?

○ **A.** All the energy does work on the surroundings.

○ **B.** All the energy becomes kinetic energy of the gas molecules raising the temperature of the gas.

○ **C.** Some of the energy does work on the surroundings and some of the energy becomes the kinetic energy of the gas molecules, raising the temperature of the gas.

○ **D.** The cylinder cannot be expanded at constant pressure because the added heat energy becomes molecular kinetic energy which must raise the temperature and the pressure.

Enthalpy and Entropy

Question 493

Which of the following expressions defines enthalpy? (q is heat; U is internal energy; P is pressure, V is volume)

○ **A.** q

○ **B.** ΔU

○ **C.** $U + PV$

○ **D.** $U + q$

Questions 494-495 refer to the following reaction:

$$P_4(s) + 6Cl_2(g) \rightarrow 4PCl_3(l) \qquad \Delta H° = -1279 \text{ kJ/mol}$$

Question 494

What is the standard enthalpy change for the following reaction?

$$3P_4(s) + 18Cl_2(g) \rightarrow 12PCl_3(l)$$

○ **A.** −3837 kJ/mol

○ **B.** −1279 kJ/mol

○ **C.** −426 kJ/ mol

○ **D.** 1279 kJ/mol

Question 495

What is the standard enthalpy change for the following reaction?

$$4PCl_3(l) \rightarrow P_4(s) + 6Cl_2(g)$$

○ **A.** −3837 kJ/mol

○ **B.** −1279 kJ/mol

○ **C.** −426 kJ/ mol

○ **D.** 1279 kJ/mol

Question 496

Given that the bond energy of hydrogen-hydrogen bonds is 436 kJ/mol, that of hydrogen-oxygen bonds is 464 kJ/mol, and those in oxygen molecules 496 kJ/mol, what is the approximate heat of reaction for $2H_2 + O_2 \rightarrow 2H_2O$?

○ **A.** −488 kJ/mol

○ **B.** −440 kJ/mol

○ **C.** 440 kJ/mol

○ **D.** 488 kJ/mol

Use the information below to answer questions 497-498.

The heat of hydration for NaCl is −783 kJ/mol. The change in enthalpy for the formation of solid NaCl from its ions in gaseous state is −786 kJ/mol.

Question 497

What is the heat of solution when NaCl is dissolved in water?

○ **A.** −3 kJ/mol

○ **B.** +3 kJ/mol

○ **C.** −1569 kJ/mol

○ **D.** +1586 kJ/mol

Question 498

Based on the heat of hydration of NaCl, what can be said about the hydrogen bonds of water compared to the bonds between the water molecules and the ions of NaCl?

○ **A.** The hydrogen bonds are stronger because hydrogen bonds are the strongest dipole-dipole forces.

○ **B.** The hydrogen bonds are stronger because the heat of hydration is negative.

○ **C.** The water-ion bonds are stronger because they are ionic bonds.

○ **D.** The water-ion bonds are stronger because the heat of hydration is negative.

Question 499

Which of the following reactions is likely to give off the most heat per gram of reactants?

○ **A.** $2H \rightarrow H_2$

○ **B.** $2O \rightarrow O_2$

○ **C.** $3O \rightarrow O_3$

○ **D.** $Xe + 3F_2 \rightarrow XeF_6$

Question 500

In order to measure the energy contained in the covalent bonds of taxane, a chemotherapeutic that inhibits depolymerization of microtubules, researchers should measure:

   I. the heat added to the synthesis reaction of taxane from its precursors.

   II. the heat released from the synthesis reaction of taxane from its precursors.

   III. the change in entropy of the reactants of the synthesis reaction of taxane from its precursors.

○ **A.** I only

○ **B.** III only

○ **C.** I and II only

○ **D.** II and III only

Question 501

Which of the following would be most helpful in determining the heat of formation of a non-flammable compound?

○ **A.** Bomb calorimeter

○ **B.** Mass spectrometer

○ **C.** Chromatograph

○ **D.** Coffee-cup calorimeter

Question 502

Which of the following statements best describes the relationship between the bond dissociation energy (BDE) and the heat of formation (HF) for a compound used to treat high blood pressure?

○ **A.** BDE > HF

○ **B.** BDE < HF

○ **C.** BDE = HF

○ **D.** BDE ≠ HF

Question 503

Which calculation would provide an estimate of the bond energy of an oxygen-oxygen double bond?

○ **A.** Finding the heat of formation of $O_2(g)$

○ **B.** Doubling the heat of formation of $O(g)$

○ **C.** Dividing the heat of formation of $CO_2(g)$ by two

○ **D.** Doubling the bond energy of an oxygen-oxygen single bond

Question 504

Which of the following statements best explains why biological reactions often utilize ATP or GTP as co-reactants?

○ **A.** The energy released when the γ phosphate is cleaved drives the exothermic reaction.

○ **B.** The energy released when the γ phosphate is cleaved drives the endothermic reaction.

○ **C.** The energy released when the β phosphate is cleaved drives the exothermic reaction.

○ **D.** The energy released when the β phosphate is cleaved drives the endothermic reaction.

Question 505

In order to prepare a solution of 10 g/mL dextrose, the dextrorotatory form of glucose, a scientist must cool a solution by 7°C. This reaction is most likely to be:

   I. exothermic.

   II. endergonic.

   III. exergonic.

○ **A.** I only

○ **B.** II only

○ **C.** I and II only

○ **D.** I and III only

Question 506

Which of the following correctly identifies the thermodynamic properties of the reaction below ?

$$AB \rightarrow A + B + heat$$

○ **A.**

Property	Sign
ΔH	$-$
ΔS	$-$
ΔG	$-$

○ **B.**

Property	Sign
ΔH	$-$
ΔS	$+$
ΔG	$-$

○ **C.**

Property	Sign
ΔH	$+$
ΔS	$+$
ΔG	$-$

○ **D.**

Property	Sign
ΔH	$-$
ΔS	$+$
ΔG	$+$

Question 507

Under constant pressure conditions, enthalpy can be described using two variables. These are:

○ **A.** the change in internal energy and the change in volume.

○ **B.** the change in internal energy and the change in heat.

○ **C.** the change in potential energy and the change in pressure.

○ **D.** the change in potential energy and the change in heat.

Question 508

If a reaction is endothermic, the system:

○ **A.** can do positive work.

○ **B.** feels cold.

○ **C.** produces heat.

○ **D.** may be dangerous.

Question 509

For the reaction shown below, what are the signs of the enthalpy and entropy changes?

$$2O(g) \rightarrow O_2(g)$$

○ **A.** Both are negative.

○ **B.** The enthalpy change is negative, while the entropy change is positive.

○ **C.** The enthalpy change is positive, while the entropy change is negative.

○ **D.** Both are positive.

Question 510

The standard molar entropy of O_2 gas is 0 J mol^{-1} K^{-1} at:

○ **A.** 0 K.

○ **B.** 273 K.

○ **C.** 298 K.

○ **D.** the standard molar entropy of a substance does not depend upon temperature.

Use the following information to answer questions 511–512.

A man finds one hundred blocks scattered across the floor of an empty room. He neatly stacks the blocks in the center of the room.

Question 511

Which of the following increases in entropy as a result of the man's actions?

    I. The blocks

    II. The man

    III. The universe

○ **A.** II only

○ **B.** III only

○ **C.** II and III only

○ **D.** I, II, and III

Question 512

Whenever entropy of the universe increases, some energy permanently loses some of its potential to do work. Which energy best represents this lost potential when the man stacks the blocks?

○ **A.** The potential energy of the blocks

○ **B.** The heat energy created by the man

○ **C.** The chemical energy of the nutrients in the man's body

○ **D.** The kinetic energy of the air molecules in the room

Question 513

The diagrams below represent glass tubes with black and white marbles. Which system has the greatest entropy?

○ **A.**

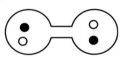

○ **B.**

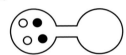

○ **C.**

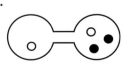

○ **D.**

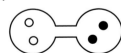

Question 514

Which of the following systems violate(s) the second law of thermodynamics?

I. A pendulum, perfectly isolated from its environment, which swings forever

II. A battery that never "dies" or needs recharging

III. A refrigerator that uses all of the heat it removes from its interior to provide electricity to an apartment

○ **A.** I only

○ **B.** III only

○ **C.** I and II only

○ **D.** I, II, and III

Question 515

Is it possible for the entropy of the universe to decrease when the system undergoes a spontaneous reaction?

○ **A.** Yes, but only if the entropy gain of the environment is smaller in magnitude than the magnitude of the entropy loss in the system.

○ **B.** Yes, but only if the reaction is exothermic.

○ **C.** No, because this would violate the first law of thermodynamics.

○ **D.** No, because this would violate the second law of thermodynamics.

Question 516

When 100 mL of a 2 M NaCl solution and 100 mL of a 2 M $AgNO_3$ solution are mixed, a precipitate is formed. Considering the two solutions to be the system:

○ **A.** the entropy of the system and the entropy of the surroundings both increase.

○ **B.** the entropy of the system increases but the entropy of the surroundings decreases.

○ **C.** the entropy of the system decreases but the entropy of the surroundings increases.

○ **D.** the entropy of the system and the entropy of the surroundings both decrease.

Question 517

Which of the following 5 g samples of CO_2 has the highest entropy?

○ **A.** $CO_2(s)$

○ **B.** $CO_2(l)$

○ **C.** $CO_2(g)$

○ **D.** $CO_2(aq)$

Question 518

Which choice is ranked correctly from lowest to highest entropy per gram of NaCl?

○ **A.** NaCl(g), NaCl(aq), NaCl(l), NaCl(s)

○ **B.** NaCl(s), NaCl(aq), NaCl(l), NaCl(g)

○ **C.** NaCl(s), NaCl(l), NaCl(aq), NaCl(g)

○ **D.** NaCl(s), NaCl(l), NaCl(g), NaCl(aq)

Question 519

Which of the following compounds has the smallest entropy per mole?

○ **A.** $O_2(g)$

○ **B.** $CH_4(s)$

○ **C.** $C_5H_{12}(s)$

○ **D.** NaCl(aq)

Question 520

Entropy will generally increase during:

I. sublimation.

II. condensation.

III. combustion reactions.

○ **A.** I only

○ **B.** II only

○ **C.** I and III only

○ **D.** I, II, and III

Accounting for Energy: Gibbs Free Energy and Hess's Law

Question 521

Which of the following conditions are required for the formula: $\Delta G = \Delta H - T\Delta S$?

   I. Constant pressure

   II. Constant temperature

   III. Constant volume

○ **A.** I only

○ **B.** II only

○ **C.** I and II only

○ **D.** I, II, and III

Question 522

Which of the following is/are true concerning Gibbs free energy?

   I. The Gibbs free energy of the universe is conserved.

   II. Gibbs free energy of a system is conserved.

   III. Gibbs free energy does not obey the first law of thermodynamics.

○ **A.** I only

○ **B.** II only

○ **C.** III only

○ **D.** I and II only

Question 523

Given the fact that the standard free energies of formation of water vapor and liquid water are –229 kJ/mol and –237 kJ/mol respectively, what is the free energy of the vaporization of water? Assume all measurements were performed at 25°C.

○ **A.** –466 kJ/mol

○ **B.** –8 kJ/mol

○ **C.** +8 kJ/mol

○ **D.** +466 kJ/mol

Question 524

The standard free energies of formation (at 25°C) of the gas phase of several compounds are given below. If samples of the gases were placed in separate containers at 25°C and 1 atm and allowed to reach equilibrium, which container would end up with the greatest proportion of nonpolar gases?

Container	Gas	$\Delta G°$
1	HF	174 kJ/mol
2	HCl	187 kJ/mol
3	NO	211 kJ/mol

○ **A.** 1

○ **B.** 2

○ **C.** 3

○ **D.** More information is needed.

Question 525

A reaction is spontaneous at all temperatures. The reaction is:

○ **A.** exothermic and decreases the entropy of the system.

○ **B.** exothermic and increases the entropy of the system.

○ **C.** endothermic and decreases the entropy of the system.

○ **D.** endothermic and increases the entropy of the system.

Question 526

Is the dissolution of NaCl in water a spontaneous process at all temperatures?

○ **A.** Yes, because the change in enthalpy is positive.

○ **B.** No, because it is an endothermic reaction.

○ **C.** It depends upon the temperature because the change in entropy is positive.

○ **D.** It depends upon the temperature because the change in enthalpy depends upon temperature.

Use the following information to answer questions 527-528.

Under constant pressure conditions, the enthalpy change of a reaction represents the heat transferred into the system. If the enthalpy change is negative, heat is transferred to the surroundings. When heat is transferred to the surroundings, the entropy of the surroundings increases. The entropy change of the universe equals the negative of the Gibbs energy change of the system divided by the temperature. Putting this together gives:

$$\Delta G = \Delta H - T\Delta S$$

Question 527

Under which of the following conditions must a reaction be spontaneous?

- ○ **A.** Both enthalpy change and entropy change are negative.
- ○ **B.** Both enthalpy change and entropy change are positive.
- ○ **C.** Enthalpy change is negative and entropy change is positive.
- ○ **D.** Enthalpy change is positive and entropy change is negative.

Question 528

If a reaction is exothermic but experiences a decrease in entropy of the system, under what conditions is the reaction most likely to be spontaneous?

- ○ **A.** Low temperature
- ○ **B.** High temperature
- ○ **C.** Low pressure
- ○ **D.** High pressure

Question 529

A particular endothermic reaction causes a decrease in the entropy of the system. This reaction:

- ○ **A.** can never occur, since it decreases system entropy.
- ○ **B.** can never occur, since the free energy change will be positive.
- ○ **C.** can only occur at low temperatures, where entropy is a smaller factor.
- ○ **D.** can occur if coupled to another reaction.

Question 530

Is it possible for the entropy of a system to decrease when the system undergoes a spontaneous reaction?

- ○ **A.** Yes, but only if the entropy gain of the environment is greater in magnitude than the magnitude of the entropy loss in the system.
- ○ **B.** Yes, but only if the reaction is endothermic.
- ○ **C.** No, because this would violate the first law of thermodynamics.
- ○ **D.** No, because this would violate the second law of thermodynamics.

Question 531

In order for this reaction below to be spontaneous under standard conditions, the reaction:

$$A(g) + 2B(g) \rightarrow C(l)$$

- ○ **A.** must result in an increase in entropy of the system.
- ○ **B.** must take place in the presence of a catalyst.
- ○ **C.** must be exothermic.
- ○ **D.** could not be spontaneous under standard conditions.

Question 532

Suppose a scientist made the claim that all spontaneous reactions were exothermic. Which of the following would provide the strongest challenge to this claim?

- ○ **A.** An endothermic reaction that only proceeds when coupled to an exothermic reaction
- ○ **B.** An endothermic reaction that only proceeds at a reasonable rate when a catalyst is present
- ○ **C.** An endothermic reaction which is not spontaneous
- ○ **D.** An exothermic reaction which is not spontaneous

Question 533

$$2NO(g) \rightarrow N_2O_2(g)$$
$$2N_2O_2(g) + O_2(g) \rightarrow 2NO_2(g)$$

Which substance serves as an intermediate in the mechanism shown above?

- ○ **A.** $NO(g)$
- ○ **B.** $N_2O_2(g)$
- ○ **C.** $O_2(g)$
- ○ **D.** $NO_2(g)$

Question 534

Methanol can be used as antifreeze within solar water heaters to prevent bursting due to expansion as a result of water freezing. The first step in a synthesis of methanol is listed below:

$$CH_4(g) + H_2O(g) \rightarrow CO(g) + 3H_2(g)$$

Use the enthalpy changes below to determine the total enthalpy change in this first synthesis step.

1. $CO(g) + \frac{1}{2}O_2(g) \rightarrow CO_2(g)$ $\Delta H_1 = -283$ kJ

2. $H_2(g) + \frac{1}{2}O_2(g) \rightarrow H_2O(g)$ $\Delta H_2 = -242$ kJ

3. $CH_4(g) + 2O_2(g) \rightarrow CO_2(g) + 2H_2O(g)$ $\Delta H_3 = -803$ kJ

The total enthalpy change is:

O **A.** −1330 kJ

O **B.** −844 kJ

O **C.** 206 kJ

O **D.** 608 kJ

Question 535

Cyanide acts as a lethal poison by binding to complex IV of the electron transport chain and rendering it inactive. Gaseous cyanide smells like almonds, and it can be synthesized from methane and ammonia via the following reaction:

$$CH_4(g) + NH_3(g) \rightarrow HCN(g) + H_2(g)$$

Using the enthalpy changes listed below, calculate the total enthalpy change of HCN production from methane and ammonia.

1. $N_2(g) + 3H_2(g) \rightarrow 2NH_3(g)$ $\Delta H_1 = -91.8$ kJ

2. $C(s) + 2H_2(g) \rightarrow CH_4(g)$ $\Delta H_2 = -74.9$ kJ

3. $H_2(g) + 2C(s) + N_2(g) \rightarrow 2HCN(g)$ $\Delta H_3 = +270.3$ kJ

The total enthalpy change is:

O **A.** −135 kJ

O **B.** −52.3 kJ

O **C.** 104 kJ

O **D.** 260 kJ

Question 536

The activated complex in the reaction catalyzed by glyceraldehyde 3-phosphate dehydrogenase is LEAST likely to have:

O **A.** higher energy than the reactant.

O **B.** higher energy than the product.

O **C.** higher energy than the reactant and the product.

O **D.** lower energy than the reactant and the product.

Question 537

Which of the following statements best describes the transition state of a reaction?

O **A.** The lowest energy molecule of a reaction

O **B.** The highest energy molecule of a reaction

O **C.** Can be isolated and characterized by mass spectrometry

O **D.** Can be isolated and characterized by nuclear magnetic resonance (NMR)

▼

Refer to the following information for questions 538-539.

A particular reaction proceeds via formation of an intermediate compound. The reaction coordinate is displayed below.

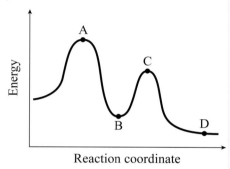

Question 538

Which of the labeled points on the reaction coordinate represents a transition state?

O **A.** A only

O **B.** B only

O **C.** C only

O **D.** A and C only

Question 539

At which point(s) of the reaction coordinate can researchers isolate a product for further analysis?

O **A.** D only

O **B.** B and C only

O **C.** B and D only

O **D.** A, B, C, and D

▲

Question 540

In second order nucleophilic substitution, there is a moment when five bonds are found on the electrophilic carbon. An example is shown below. This is known as:

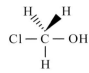

$$Cl - C - OH$$

- ○ **A.** the intermediate.
- ○ **B.** the reactant.
- ○ **C.** the product.
- ○ **D.** the transition state.

Question 541

Enzymes function to lower the activation energy of a reaction by:

- ○ **A.** changing the transition state.
- ○ **B.** stabilizing the transition state.
- ○ **C.** bringing the products in closer proximity.
- ○ **D.** keeping the reactants further apart.

Question 542

Which of the following locations on the curve represents the time point where the transition state is present?

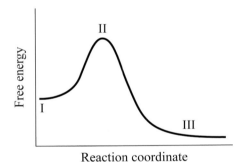

- ○ **A.** I only
- ○ **B.** II only
- ○ **C.** I and II only
- ○ **D.** I, II, and III

For questions 543–545, refer to the energy diagram for the reaction pathway of the isomerization of methyl isonitrile given below.

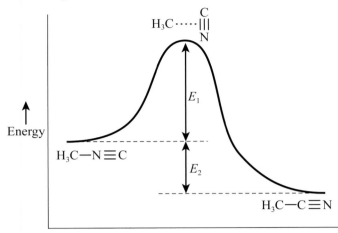

Reaction pathway

Question 543

In the reaction pathway shown above, which of the following represents the energy of activation for the forward reaction?

- ○ **A.** E_1
- ○ **B.** E_2
- ○ **C.** $E_1 + E_2$
- ○ **D.** $E_2 - E_1$

Question 544

In the reaction pathway shown above, which of the following represents the energy of activation for the reverse reaction?

- ○ **A.** E_1
- ○ **B.** E_2
- ○ **C.** $E_1 + E_2$
- ○ **D.** $E_2 - E_1$

Question 545

Which of the following is true concerning the isomerization of methyl isonitrile?

- ○ **A.** Energy is absorbed to begin the reaction, and energy is absorbed by the overall reaction.
- ○ **B.** Energy is absorbed to begin the reaction, but energy is released by the overall reaction.
- ○ **C.** Energy is released to begin the reaction, but energy is absorbed by the overall reaction.
- ○ **D.** Energy is released to begin the reaction, and energy is released by the overall reaction.

Question 546

A single-step reaction has an activation energy of 25 kJ/mol and a heat of reaction of −85 kJ/mol. What is the activation energy of the reverse reaction?

- ○ **A.** −25 kJ/mol
- ○ **B.** 25 kJ/mol
- ○ **C.** 60 kJ/mol
- ○ **D.** 110 kJ/mol

Equilibrium

Question 547

Suppose the first reaction below has an equilibrium constant of 530. What is the equilibrium constant of the second reaction?

$$CO(g) + Cl_2(g) \rightarrow COCl_2(g)$$
$$2CO(g) + 2Cl_2(g) \rightarrow 2COCl_2(g)$$

- ○ **A.** 530
- ○ **B.** 1060
- ○ **C.** 2120
- ○ **D.** 2.81×10^5

Question 548

At 740 K, the reaction below has an equilibrium constant of 50. If, at 740 K, the concentration of hydrogen gas is 0.2 M, iodine gas is 0.3 M, and hydrogen iodide gas is 5 M:

$$H_2(g) + I_2(g) \rightarrow 2HI(g)$$

- ○ **A.** the concentration of hydrogen iodide will increase over time.
- ○ **B.** the concentration of hydrogen iodide will decrease over time.
- ○ **C.** the system is at equilibrium.
- ○ **D.** there must be an error in measurement of concentration.

Question 549

In considering the reaction:

$$3NO_2(g) + H_2O(l) \rightarrow 2HNO_3(aq) + NO(g)$$

student A writes the equilibrium expression as:

$$K = \frac{[NO][HNO_3]^2}{[NO_2]^3}$$

while student B writes:

$$K = \frac{P_{NO}[HNO_3]^2}{[NO_2]^3}$$

Which of the following is a true statement?

- ○ **A.** Student B is incorrect; it is not permissible to mix concentrations and partial pressures in one equilibrium expression.
- ○ **B.** Student A is incorrect; gases should always appear as partial pressures in equilibrium expressions.
- ○ **C.** Both students are correct, and will arrive at the same value of K.
- ○ **D.** Both students are correct, but they will arrive at different values of K.

Question 550

The change in free energy of the reaction converting glucose to glucose-6-phosphate is −20 kJ/mol. The K_{eq} is most likely:

- ○ **A.** positive and favors the products.
- ○ **B.** positive and favors the reactants.
- ○ **C.** negative and favors the products.
- ○ **D.** negative and favors the reactants.

Question 551

Which of the following values of the equilibrium constant of the reaction catalyzed by carbonic anhydrase would release the most CO_2 in the lungs?

- ○ **A.** 1×10^{-7}
- ○ **B.** 2.5×10^{-6}
- ○ **C.** 3.1×10^{-6}
- ○ **D.** 1.1×10^{-5}

Refer to the information below for questions 552-553.

Gaseous nitric oxide, NO(g), is a potent vasodilator with a short half-life. Although NO(g) is endogenously synthesized from L-arginine, researchers performed the following reaction to yield product:

$$2N_2O(g) + O_2(g) \rightleftharpoons 4NO(g)$$

The researchers noted the values at which the reactants' and products' concentrations stopped significantly changing. The results are recorded below.

Species	Concentration (mol L^{-1})
$N_2O(g)$	2×10^{-2}
$O_2(g)$	5×10^1
$NO(g)$	1×10^3

Question 552

Which of the following conclusions can be most validated from the researchers' results?

○ **A.** $K = 5 \times 10^{22}$

○ **B.** The reaction has not yet reached equilibrium.

○ **C.** At $Q = 3.67 \times 10^{19}$, the concentration of $N_2O(g)$ will decrease.

○ **D.** At $Q = 2.13 \times 10^{22}$, the concentration of $NO(g)$ will increase.

Question 553

Which of the following, if true, would most likely invalidate the researchers' results?

○ **A.** After removing all compounds from the reaction vessel, the researchers' instrument reads 2.5×10^{-1} M.

○ **B.** The researchers only conducted the experiment once.

○ **C.** The researchers miscalculated the size of the reaction vessel.

○ **D.** The temperature was not recorded.

Question 554

Suppose a scientist claims when two reactions are in competition, the one that occurs at the greater rate always dominates. What criticism could be made of this scientist's claim?

○ **A.** The reaction that occurs at the greater rate also depletes its reactants faster, so the slower reaction will eventually surpass it.

○ **B.** A reaction that dominates at one temperature may not dominate at another temperature.

○ **C.** The scientist has ignored the role of the reverse reactions.

○ **D.** Reactions are never in competition.

Question 555

The reaction below is found to stop before the reactants are completely converted to products. What is a possible explanation?

$$NH_3(aq) + HC_2H_3O_2(aq) \rightarrow NH_4^+(aq) + C_2H_3O_2^-(aq)$$

○ **A.** As the quantity of reactants decreases, ammonia molecules and acetic acid molecules stop colliding.

○ **B.** As the quantity of products increases, the acetic acid begins to dissociate, stopping the reaction.

○ **C.** The reverse rate increases and the forward rate decreases until they exactly balance.

○ **D.** The catalyst is used up.

For Questions 556–558 refer to the Haber Process shown below:

$$N_2(g) + 3H_2(g) \rightleftharpoons 2NH_3(g)$$

In 1912 Fritz Haber developed the Haber process for making ammonia from nitrogen and hydrogen. His development was crucial for the German war effort of World War I, providing the Germans with ample fixed nitrogen for the manufacture of explosives.

The Haber process takes place at 500°C and 200 atm. It is an exothermic reaction. The graph below shows the change in concentrations of reactants and products as the reaction progresses.

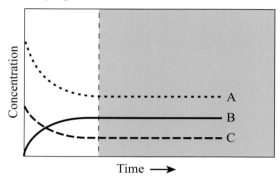

Question 556

In the diagram, the letters A, B, and C represent which of the following?

- ○ **A.** A = NH_3, B = H_2, and C = N_2
- ○ **B.** A = NH_3, B = N_2, and C = H_2
- ○ **C.** A = H_2, B = NH_3, and C = N_2
- ○ **D.** A = N_2, B = NH_3, and C = H_2

Question 557

Which of the following most accurately describes the shaded area of the graph?

- ○ **A.** A limiting reagent has been used up.
- ○ **B.** The catalyst has been used up.
- ○ **C.** The reaction has reached equilibrium.
- ○ **D.** The reaction has run to completion.

Question 558

Which of the following graphs could also accurately reflect the establishment of equilibrium between nitrogen, hydrogen, and ammonia?

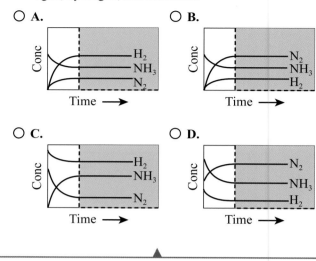

Question 559

Consider the following conversion

$$O_2(g) \rightarrow O_2(aq)$$

What is the equilibrium expression?

- ○ **A.** $[O_2(aq)]/[O_2(g)]$
- ○ **B.** $[O_2(aq)]$
- ○ **C.** $1/[O_2(g)]$
- ○ **D.** $[O_2(g)]$

Question 560

What is the equilibrium expression in the below reaction?

$$ZnO(s) + CO(g) \rightarrow Zn(s) + CO_2(g)$$

- ○ **A.** $K = \dfrac{[Zn][CO_2]}{[ZnO][CO]}$
- ○ **B.** $K = [Zn][CO_2]$
- ○ **C.** $K = \dfrac{[ZnO][CO]}{[Zn][CO_2]}$
- ○ **D.** $K = \dfrac{[CO_2]}{[CO]}$

Question 561

What is the equilibrium expression in the below reaction?

$$[Fe(H_2O)_6]^{2+}(aq) + Cl^-(aq) \rightarrow [FeCl(H_2O)_5]^+(aq) + H_2O(l)$$

○ **A.** $K = [FeCl(H_2O)_5^+][H_2O]/[Fe(H_2O)_6^{2+}][Cl^-]$

○ **B.** $K = [FeCl(H_2O)_5^+][H_2O]$

○ **C.** $K = [Fe(H_2O)_6^{2+}][Cl^-]/[FeCl(H_2O)_5^{2+}][H_2O]$

○ **D.** $K = [FeCl(H_2O)_5^+]/[Fe(H_2O)_6^{2+}][Cl^-]$

Question 562

A college student studying a reaction with colored reactants and products believes the reaction defies the law of mass action. His data are shown below. Which of the following statements are correct?

$$A + B \rightarrow C$$

Textbook data:

Wavelength	Absorptivity of A	Absorptivity of B	Absorptivity of C
450 nm	0 M^{-1}cm^{-1}	0 M^{-1}cm^{-1}	10 M^{-1}cm^{-1}
650 nm	0 M^{-1}cm^{-1}	20 M^{-1}cm^{-1}	0 M^{-1}cm^{-1}
850 nm	10 M^{-1}cm^{-1}	0 M^{-1}cm^{-1}	0 M^{-1}cm^{-1}
$K = 100$			

Initially:

Wavelength	Absorbance
450 nm	1
650 nm	20
850 nm	10

At equilibrium:

Wavelength	Absorbance
450 nm	10
650 nm	2
850 nm	1

○ **A.** Neither the data nor the conclusion is valid.

○ **B.** The data are valid, but the conclusion is not valid.

○ **C.** The data are not valid, but the conclusion is valid.

○ **D.** The data and the conclusion are valid.

Question 563

Which of the following would decrease the proportion of water vapor at equilibrium in the below reaction?

$$2H_2(g) + O_2(g) \rightarrow 2H_2O(g)$$

○ **A.** Increasing the partial pressure of oxygen gas

○ **B.** Decreasing the volume of the container

○ **C.** Reducing the amount of catalyst present

○ **D.** Raising the temperature

Question 564

When sulfur trioxide is heated, it produces sulfur dioxide and oxygen in the following endothermic reaction:

$$2SO_3(g) + heat \rightleftharpoons 2SO_2(g) + O_2(g)$$

In a container sealed by a piston, the reaction can be driven to the left by:

○ **A.** adding calcium sulfite ($CaSO_3(s)$).

○ **B.** burning the excess O_2 in the container in a combustion reaction.

○ **C.** placing the container in a colder environment.

○ **D.** increasing the volume of the container by moving the piston upward.

Refer to the following chemical equation for questions 565-566.

$$SnO_2(g) + 2C(s) \rightleftharpoons Sn(s) + 2CO(g)$$

Question 565

Researchers added heat to the reaction vessel and the concentration of $SnO_2(g)$ increased. Which of the following conclusions can be validated based on this information?

○ **A.** The reaction is exothermic.

○ **B.** The reaction is endothermic.

○ **C.** The addition of heat will increase entropy.

○ **D.** Lowering the temperature will increase $C(s)$.

Question 566

Researchers slowly decrease the size of the reaction vessel while concurrently adding $CO(g)$. At the end of the compression, what is most likely true of the reaction vessel?

○ **A.** The partial pressure of $CO(g)$ has decreased.

○ **B.** The number of moles of solids has increased.

○ **C.** The reaction vessel will weigh less.

○ **D.** The mass of $Sn(s)$ will increase.

Question 567

Instead of developing an aqueous catalyst for a novel chemical reaction, a scientist raised the temperature of the reaction only to observe that the reaction did not occur. Which of the following best explains why the reaction failed?

○ A. The reaction was exothermic, so raising the temperature would have decreased the rate of the reaction.

○ B. The reaction was exothermic, so raising the temperature would have reduced the yield of the reaction.

○ C. Higher temperatures would have caused an increase in pressure lowering the yield of the reaction.

○ D. Higher temperatures might have decomposed the hydrogen.

Question 568

Magnesium hydroxide ($Mg(OH)_2$) is a white solid commonly prepared in tablets or suspensions to be used in everyday antacids. $Mg(OH)_2$ can be precipitated from a reaction between magnesium and hydroxide.

$$Mg(OH)_2(s) \leftrightarrow Mg^{2+}(aq) + 2OH^-(aq)$$

With adjustments in the acidity or pressure of the environment, the chemistry of the equilibrium can change. Which pair of statements best describes the solution under the two independent conditions of added NaOH and added pressure?

○ A. For both conditions, relative mass will increase, entropy will decrease, and Mg^{2+} concentration will decrease.

○ B. For NaOH, relative mass will increase, entropy will decrease, and Mg^{2+} concentration will decrease; for added pressure, relative mass will decrease, entropy will increase, and Mg^{2+} concentration will increase.

○ C. For NaOH, relative mass will decrease, entropy will increase, and Mg^{2+} concentration will increase; for added pressure, relative mass will increase, entropy will increase, and Mg^{2+} will decrease.

○ D. For NaOH, relative mass will decrease, entropy will increase, and Mg^{2+} concentration will decrease; for added pressure, relative mass will decrease, entropy will increase, and Mg^{2+} concentration will increase.

Free Energy and Spontaneity

Refer to the following information for questions 569-570.

Atmospheric sulfur trioxide is the primary agent in acid rain. Its mode of synthesis is described below:

$$2SO_2(g) + O_2(g) \rightleftharpoons 2SO_3(g)$$

Researchers measured the concentrations of reactants and products over time and saw that the rate of concentration change reached zero when all compounds reached 1 mol L^{-1}. Recording was conducted at 298 K.

Question 569

Based on the given results, what conclusion can be drawn regarding $\Delta G°$?

○ A. $\Delta G°$ could be greater than one.

○ B. $\Delta G°$ must be below zero.

○ C. $\Delta G°$ equals zero.

○ D. The experiment must be run at multiple temperatures to determine $\Delta G°$.

Question 570

At a given point in the reaction, the concentrations of $SO_2(g)$, $O_2(g)$, and $SO_3(g)$ are 0.05 M, 0.01 M, and 0.05 M. At 298 K, which direction is the reaction likely to proceed? ($R = 8.312$ J K^{-1} mol^{-1})

○ A. The reaction will proceed leftward.

○ B. The reaction will proceed rightward.

○ C. The reaction will remain at equilibrium.

○ D. This cannot be determined.

Use the following information to answer questions 571-572.

Untreated liver cirrhosis could lead to increased levels of ammonia in the blood. Researchers interested in long-term cirrhosis treatment used the ammonia synthesis method below at 27°C.

$$N_2(g) + 3H_2(g) \rightleftharpoons 2NH_3(g) \; \Delta G° = -30 \text{ kJ}$$

Question 571

What is the expression for equilibrium constant K at 300 K and 1 bar? ($2.3\log(x) \approx \ln(x)$)

○ **A.** $10^{-30/690R}$

○ **B.** $10^{30/2.3R(300)}$

○ **C.** $e^{-(2.3)(30)/2.3R(300)}$

○ **D.** $-300^{R(-30)}$

Question 572

Which of the following statements must be true at 27°C? When the concentrations of $N_2(g)$, $H_2(g)$, and $NH_3(g)$ are all 1 mol L^{-1}, the concentration(s) of:

○ **A.** $H_2(g)$ only is expected to decrease.

○ **B.** $NH_3(g)$ is expected to increase.

○ **C.** $N_2(g)$ is expected to increase.

○ **D.** all gases in the reaction vessel will likely remain the same.

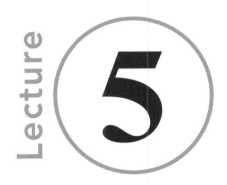

Lecture

5

Questions 573–715

Phases

Behavior of Gases
Real Gases
The Liquid and Solid Phases
Calorimetry
Phase Changes

Behavior of Gases

Question 573

Which of the following is NOT a feature of an ideal gas?

○ **A.** Elastic collisions

○ **B.** Atoms lack volume

○ **C.** Obeys $PV = nRT$

○ **D.** Nonexistent intramolecular forces

Question 574

Which of the following properties of the inhaled anesthetic isoflurane, shown below, causes it to behave as a real gas?

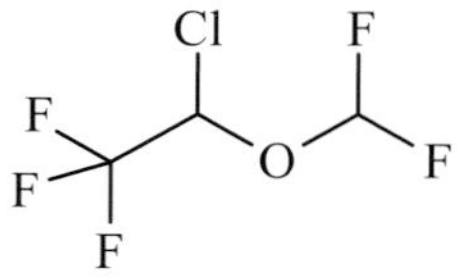

○ **A.** Presence of an ester functional group

○ **B.** Presence of fluorine atoms

○ **C.** Presence of sp^2 bonds

○ **D.** Presence of s orbital hybridized bonds

Question 575

During vaporization of liquid oxygen, gaseous oxygen molecules collide with each other, generating 0.00003 J/L of heat. The vaporizing O_2 most likely behaves as a(n):

○ **A.** ideal gas.

○ **B.** real gas.

○ **C.** noble gas.

○ **D.** halogen gas.

Question 576

Oxygen flowing through a nasal cannula, a tube used to deliver concentrated gas through the nose, can be approximated as an ideal fluid. Which of the following behaviors of the gas would NOT be observed?

   I. Irrotational flow

   II. Acceleration

   III. Turbulence

○ **A.** I only

○ **B.** III only

○ **C.** I and III only

○ **D.** I, II, and III

Question 577

At a temperature of 300 K, a mole of Kr has 30 J of kinetic energy. Assuming Kr behaves as an ideal gas, what is the kinetic energy of Kr at 600 K?

○ **A.** 15 J

○ **B.** 30 J

○ **C.** 45 J

○ **D.** 60 J

Question 578

Scientists found that they were only able to store 3.9 × 10^{16} molecules of N_2 in a rigid container, regardless of the applied pressure. Which of the following principles of an ideal gas does this NOT fulfill?

○ **A.** Gas molecules do not exert forces on one another.

○ **B.** Gas molecules have no molecular volume.

○ **C.** Gas molecules undergo completely elastic collisions.

○ **D.** Gas molecules have a velocity proportional to the temperature of the gas.

Question 579

Which of the following properties of a gas would promote behavior as an ideal gas?

○ **A.** Temperature at 0 K

○ **B.** No net dipole present

○ **C.** Large atomic radius

○ **D.** Ionized gas

Question 580

Real gases deviate from ideal behavior in a predictable manner based on the ideal gas law. The figure below depicts this deviation for four real gases. Which of the following correctly pairs the gas with the curve?

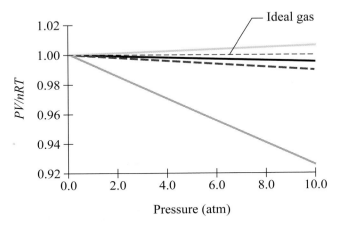

- **A.** Curve I: H_2, Curve II: N_2, Curve III: O_2, Curve IV: CO_2
- **B.** Curve I: O_2, Curve II: CO_2, Curve III: H_2, Curve IV: N_2
- **C.** Curve I: N_2, Curve II: H_2, Curve III: CO_2, Curve IV: O_2
- **D.** Curve I: CO_2, Curve II: O_2, Curve III: N_2, Curve IV: H_2

Question 581

For an ideal gas, internal energy depends upon:

   I. pressure.

   II. temperature.

   III. volume.

- **A.** I only
- **B.** II only
- **C.** I and III only
- **D.** I, II, and III

Question 582

Researchers interested in computationally modeling fluid dynamics must distinguish between properties of real liquids and gases. Compared to liquids, gases:

- **A.** have no intermolecular attractive or repulsive interactions.
- **B.** have greater intermolecular spacing.
- **C.** are more conducive to forming crystal lattice structures.
- **D.** tend to sort themselves due to differences in density.

Question 583

Researchers studying phase dynamics recorded the rates of four chemical reactions with reactants of varying phases. The researchers standardized the reaction such that each reaction generated the same number of moles of reactants and products. The standardized reactions and their results are displayed table below:

Reaction: $A + B \rightarrow C + D$

A	B	Reaction rate (mol $L^{-1} s^{-1}$)
Liquid	Liquid	7.3×10^{-3}
Liquid	Gas	3.2×10^{6}
Gas	Liquid	4.9×10^{3}
Gas	Gas	1.1×10^{11}

Which of the following explanations best explains the research results?

- **A.** Liquids tend to have smaller intermolecular collision frequencies than gases.
- **B.** Gaseous molecules tend to exist in larger quantities than liquid molecules.
- **C.** Gaseous reactants tend to form products faster than liquid reactants.
- **D.** Ideal gases exhibit no repulsive intermolecular forces to hinder product formation.

Question 584

Pulmonologists interested in modeling respiratory gas exchange assume that $CO_2(g)$ molecules exhibit no intermolecular attractions at the capillary-alveolus interface. Which statement best supports the validity of this assumption?

- ○ **A.** $CO_2(g)$ molecules are nonpolar and thus do not experience Van der Waals' forces.
- ○ **B.** The partial pressure of $O_2(g)$ is far greater than that of $CO_2(g)$, such that $CO_2(g)$ interactions are insignificant.
- ○ **C.** Gas movement is due to pressure gradients and not intermolecular interactions.
- ○ **D.** The average distance between $CO_2(g)$ nuclei is extremely large.

Question 585

Researchers are interested in how gas properties affect gaseous mixtures at STP. The gases will be injected concurrently into a 4.2 L vessel. The gases and their respective dipole moments are listed in the table below.

Gas	Dipole moment (Debyes)
CCl_4	0
H_2O	1.85
CO_2	0
CH_3Cl	1.87

Assuming ideal behavior, which of the following hypotheses is most likely to be validated following the experiment?

- ○ **A.** H_2O and CH_3Cl will form a gaseous layer above CCl_4 and CO_2.
- ○ **B.** CH_2O and CH_3Cl will form a gaseous layer below CCl_4 and CO_2.
- ○ **C.** The gases will form a single homogenous mixture.
- ○ **D.** Gas molecules may mix together irrespective of chemical composition.

Question 586

Reactions including real gaseous reactants tend to form product at a greater rate than reactions including aqueous reagents. Which of the following statements best explains this phenomenon?

- ○ **A.** The intermolecular mean free path is smaller for molecules in gaseous reagents.
- ○ **B.** Real gases exhibit intermolecular attractive/ repulsive forces to facilitate transition state formation.
- ○ **C.** A mixture of compounds in the gas phase tends to be homogenous, whereas liquids will sort by polarity.
- ○ **D.** Gases will occupy a greater volume in a given reaction vessel, allowing for a greater molecular collision frequency.

Question 587

A container appears to be marked "Ne, 3.5 moles," but has no pressure gauge. By measuring the temperature and checking the volume of the container, a scientist uses the ideal gas law to estimate the pressure inside the container. Unfortunately, the handwriting on the canister is difficult to read, and the container actually contains 3.5 moles of He, not Ne. How does this affect the scientist's estimate of the pressure inside the container?

- ○ **A.** The estimate is too low.
- ○ **B.** The estimate is too high.
- ○ **C.** The estimate is correct, but only because both gases are monatomic.
- ○ **D.** The estimate is correct, because the identity of the gas is irrelevant.

Question 588

In the ideal gas law, what does the variable V represent?

- ○ **A.** The average speed of a gas molecule
- ○ **B.** The average velocity of a gas molecule
- ○ **C.** The volume of a gas molecule
- ○ **D.** The volume of the container which holds the gas

Question 589

For an ideal gas, which of the following shows the relationship between pressure and temperature at constant volume?

A.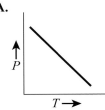

B.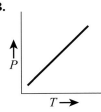

C.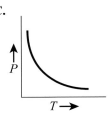

D.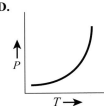

Question 590

A balloon has a volume of 500 mL when filled with gas at a pressure of 820 torr and a temperature of 300 K. How many moles of gas are inside the balloon? ($R = 0.08206$ L atm mol^{-1} K^{-1})

- **A.** 0.022 moles
- **B.** 0.22 moles
- **C.** 2.2 moles
- **D.** 22 moles

Question 591

Gas A exists in conditions of 25°C and 1 atmosphere. If the pressure is increased to 3 atmospheres without changing the volume, the new temperature will most likely be:

- **A.** −174°C.
- **B.** 8.3°C.
- **C.** 75°C.
- **D.** 621°C.

Question 592

A balloon initially contains 20 grams of helium at a pressure of 1000 torr. After some helium is let out of the balloon, the new pressure is 900 torr, and the volume is decreased by half. If the temperature has not changed, how much helium is now in the balloon?

- **A.** 9 grams
- **B.** 10 grams
- **C.** 11 grams
- **D.** Cannot be determined from the information given

Question 593

A researcher wishes to use two identical containers, one to store 5 moles of oxygen, and one to store 3 moles of nitrogen. Both are kept at 300 K and 5 atm. Is this possible?

- **A.** Yes, since oxygen and nitrogen have different molar masses.
- **B.** Yes, since these conditions are not STP.
- **C.** No, because once pressure, volume, and temperature of an ideal gas are known, the number of moles is determined.
- **D.** No, because number of moles and temperature are directly proportional.

Question 594

50.0 grams of oxygen are placed in an empty 10.0 liter container at 28°C. Compared to an equal mass of hydrogen placed in an identical container (also at 28°C), the pressure of the oxygen:

- **A.** is less than the pressure of hydrogen.
- **B.** is equal to the pressure of hydrogen.
- **C.** is greater than the pressure of hydrogen.
- **D.** has a relationship to the pressure of hydrogen that cannot be determined.

Question 595

If the partial pressure of carbon dioxide is 30 torr at STP, what is the mass of the carbon dioxide present?

- **A.** 0.04 grams
- **B.** 1.7 grams
- **C.** 44 grams
- **D.** Cannot be determined from the information given.

Question 596

In an 11.2 liter container, the partial pressure of nitrogen gas is 0.5 atmospheres at 25°C. What is the mass of nitrogen in the container?

- **A.** 3.5 g
- **B.** 7 g
- **C.** 14 g
- **D.** 28 g

Question 597

Why can pressure be used as a unit of concentration for a gas in the following reaction assuming constant temperature and volume?

$$CH_3NC(g) \rightarrow CH_3CN(g)$$

O **A.** The pressure is directly proportional to the number of moles per unit volume.

O **B.** The pressure is inversely proportional to the number of moles per unit volume.

O **C.** The pressure and concentration have the same value.

O **D.** The pressure of a gas is easier to measure than the concentration of a gas.

Question 598

An ideal gas with a pressure of 2 atm is expanded to twice its initial volume. What is the new pressure?

O **A.** 1 atm

O **B.** 2 atm

O **C.** 4 atm

O **D.** Cannot be determined from the information given.

Question 599

As a helium balloon rises through Earth's atmosphere, its volume:

O **A.** increases due to decreasing temperature.

O **B.** decreases due to increasing pressure.

O **C.** increases due to decreasing pressure.

O **D.** stays the same because it is impermeable to gases.

Question 600

A balloon containing 2 L of an ideal gas is at a pressure of 570 mmHg and a temperature of 273 K. When this balloon is at standard pressure, what is its new volume?

O **A.** 1 L

O **B.** 1.5 L

O **C.** 2 L

O **D.** 2.5 L

Question 601

A piston containing an ideal gas is pushed down to half of its maximum range of motion. If the final pressure in the piston is 4 atm, what was the initial pressure?

O **A.** 2 atm

O **B.** 4 atm

O **C.** 6 atm

O **D.** 8 atm

Question 602

A balloon is compressed to 4/5 of its initial volume at constant temperature. The ratio of the final pressure to the initial pressure is equal to:

O **A.** 0.2.

O **B.** 0.8.

O **C.** 1.25.

O **D.** 2.

Question 603

Which of the following gas laws explains why pressure decreases in the lungs as the thoracic cavity expands during inhalation?

O **A.** Charles' law

O **B.** Boyle's law

O **C.** Avogadro's law

O **D.** Dalton's law

Question 604

An ideal gas is placed in a 3.0 L container with a piston. The pressure of the gas is initially 850 torr. How much additional pressure must be exerted on the piston in order to lower the volume of the container to 1.0 L? Assume the temperature of the gas does not change.

O **A.** 283 torr

O **B.** 850 torr

O **C.** 1700 torr

O **D.** 2550 torr

Question 605

According to Charles' law, an increase in temperature at constant pressure causes:

O **A.** an increase in the number of moles of gas.

O **B.** a decrease in the number of moles of gas.

O **C.** an increase in volume.

O **D.** a decrease in volume.

Question 606

A researcher wishes to have two 20.0 L chambers containing equal moles of oxygen gas, one at 5 atm and the other at 3 atm. Is this possible?

O **A.** Yes, if the oxygen samples in the containers have different molecular weights.

O **B.** Yes, if the oxygen samples in the containers are at different temperatures.

O **C.** No, because once the volume and the number of moles of an ideal gas are known, all other parameters are determined.

O **D.** No, because volume and pressure are inversely proportional for an ideal gas.

Refer to the diagram below for questions 607-608.

The diagram below displays the pressure and volume of a sample of ideal gas as it is taken very slowly through six states: A, B, C, D, E, and F, along the pathway shown ($R = 8.314$ J K^{-1} mol^{-1}).

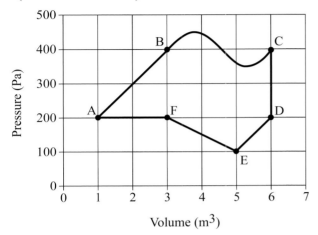

Question 607

As the gas is taken from A directly to F, the temperature of the gas:

○ **A.** increases.

○ **B.** decreases.

○ **C.** remains constant.

○ **D.** depends upon the heat transfer.

Question 608

If the sample contains one mole of gas, approximately what is the change in temperature of the gas as it goes directly from state A to state B?

○ **A.** 120 K decrease

○ **B.** 24 K decrease

○ **C.** 120 K increase

○ **D.** The temperature must be constant.

Question 609

A balloon is heated from 27°C to 77°C at constant pressure. The ratio of the final volume to the initial volume is closest to:

○ **A.** 1:3.

○ **B.** 3:1.

○ **C.** 6:7.

○ **D.** 7:6.

Question 610

A balloon containing an ideal gas at 25°C is heated at constant pressure until the volume of the balloon has doubled. What is the final temperature of the gas?

○ **A.** 50°C

○ **B.** 273°C

○ **C.** 300°C

○ **D.** 323°C

Question 611

Which of the following statements best explains Charles' law?

○ **A.** As more moles of gas are added to a flexible container, volume expands.

○ **B.** An increase in temperature leads to an increase in the volume of a flexible container.

○ **C.** The amount of a gas dissolved in a liquid is directly proportional to the partial pressure of that gas above the liquid.

○ **D.** As volume increases, gas molecules have more space to move, and pressure increases.

Question 612

An ideal gas inside a cylindrical piston is heated until the temperature is 300 K. If the height of the piston increases from 5 cm to 10 cm, what was the initial temperature of the gas? Assume constant pressure.

○ **A.** 75 K

○ **B.** 150 K

○ **C.** 600 K

○ **D.** 1500 K

Question 613

There are 0.3 moles of carbon dioxide in a balloon in a room that has a constant pressure and temperature. An additional 0.1 moles of oxygen are added to the balloon. What is the final volume of the balloon if the initial volume was 14 L?

○ **A.** 8.9 L

○ **B.** 12.4 L

○ **C.** 15 L

○ **D.** 18.7 L

Question 614

The volume occupied by 3 moles of an ideal gas at STP is approximately equal to:

- ○ **A.** 3 L.
- ○ **B.** 6.8 L.
- ○ **C.** 22.4 L.
- ○ **D.** 67.2 L.

Question 615

At standard temperature and pressure, a human can breathe in approximately 0.3 moles of air. On supplemental oxygen, the proportion of oxygen may increase from 21% to 32%. Assuming the remainder is nitrogen and the pressure inside the lungs remains the same, approximately how many moles are now in the lungs?

- ○ **A.** 0.5 mol
- ○ **B.** 0.4 mol
- ○ **C.** 0.3 mol
- ○ **D.** 0.2 mol

Question 616

A 5 L balloon at 3 atm contains 0.5 moles of He. If 2 moles of He are added to the balloon at constant temperature and pressure, what is the balloon's final volume?

- ○ **A.** 2.5 L
- ○ **B.** 5 L
- ○ **C.** 15 L
- ○ **D.** 25 L

Question 617

A flexible container holds 50,000 molecules of CO_2. If 30,000 molecules of CO_2 are added to the container at constant temperature and pressure, what is the percent change in volume of the container?

- ○ **A.** 6%
- ○ **B.** 30%
- ○ **C.** 40%
- ○ **D.** 60%

Question 618

$SO_2(g)$ and $O_2(g)$ react to form $SO_3(g)$ in a flexible container at constant temperature and pressure. If the initial volume of the container is 6 L, and the reactants are present in proportions to react fully, what is the final volume after the reaction is allowed to proceed to completion?

- ○ **A.** 2 L
- ○ **B.** 3 L
- ○ **C.** 4 L
- ○ **D.** 6 L

Question 619

A balloon containing an ideal gas is allowed to deflate from a volume of 1.8 L to 450 mL. If the balloon initially contained 1 mole of gas, how many moles of gas escaped from the balloon as it was deflated? Assume constant pressure and temperature.

- ○ **A.** 0.25 moles
- ○ **B.** 0.5 moles
- ○ **C.** 0.75 moles
- ○ **D.** 1 mole

Question 620

Which of the following is/are assumed in the kinetic-molecular theory of ideal gases?

    I. The molecules of gas all move at the same speed.

    II. The molecules of gas all have negligible volume.

    III. The molecules of gas exert no attractive forces on each other.

- ○ **A.** I only
- ○ **B.** I and III only
- ○ **C.** II and III only
- ○ **D.** I, II, and III

Question 621

Container A contains gas at 300°C. Container B contains the same gas, but at 150°C. Which of the following is a true statement?

- ○ **A.** All of the gas molecules in container A move faster than all of the gas molecules in container B.
- ○ **B.** All of the gas molecules in container A move slower than all of the gas molecules in container B.
- ○ **C.** Each of the gas molecules in container A has more mass than each of the gas molecules in container B.
- ○ **D.** None of the above statements are true.

Question 622

Which of the following formulas gives the kinetic energy of n moles of gas?

○ **A.** $\frac{1}{2}MV^2$, where M is the molar mass of the gas, and V is the volume of the container

○ **B.** $\frac{3}{2}nRT$, where n is the number of moles of gas, R is the ideal gas constant, and T is the absolute temperature

○ **C.** nPA, where n is the number of moles of gas, P is the total pressure, and A is the surface area of the container walls

○ **D.** $\frac{1}{2}nPA$, where n is the number of moles of gas, P is the total pressure, and A is the surface area of the container walls

Question 623

A polyatomic gas is held in a container with a piston and is heated in isobaric conditions. What is the molar heat capacity of the gas?

○ **A.** 8.31 J/mol K

○ **B.** 12.47 J/mol K

○ **C.** 37.41 J/mol K

○ **D.** 33.24 J/mol K

Question 624

After analyzing several hundred organic compounds, researchers discovered a direct correlation between the quantity of atoms within a compound and the constant pressure heat capacity, C_p. Which statement best explains this research finding? A greater number of atoms:

○ **A.** increases the chances that heat can be absorbed by atomic nuclei.

○ **B.** indicates that more energy can be diverted to intramolecular bond motion.

○ **C.** increases the amount of energy required to raise the temperature of the compound by 1 K.

○ **D.** indicates that the molecule has a greater molecular weight and thus possesses greater gravitational potential energy.

Question 625

A rigid container with 3 moles of oxygen inside is heated. What is the heat capacity?

○ **A.** 20.79 J/K

○ **B.** 12.47 J/K

○ **C.** 37.41 J/K

○ **D.** 62.35 J/K

Question 626

During vaporization, changes in the rotational axis of desflurane, an inhaled anesthetic, would be best characterized by:

○ **A.** constant gauge pressure calorimetry.

○ **B.** constant atmospheric pressure calorimetry.

○ **C.** constant gauge volume calorimetry.

○ **D.** constant atmospheric volume calorimetry.

Question 627

During an experiment, a scientist recorded that the heat released from a reaction increased with the addition of HCl. The scientist most likely used a:

○ **A.** coffee cup calorimeter.

○ **B.** bomb calorimeter.

○ **C.** both a coffee cup calorimeter and a bomb calorimeter.

○ **D.** neither a coffee cup calorimeter nor a bomb calorimeter.

Question 628

A scientist wants to measure the change in rotational energy of a reaction between warfarin and a clotting factor. He would most likely use:

○ **A.** a coffee cup calorimeter to measure the change in enthalpy.

○ **B.** a bomb calorimeter to measure the change in enthalpy.

○ **C.** a coffee cup calorimeter to measure the change in internal energy.

○ **D.** a bomb calorimeter to measure the change in internal energy.

Question 629

Heat capacities are typically provided at two conditions: constant pressure and constant volume. Why is the constant volume heat capacity typically smaller than the constant pressure heat capacity?

○ **A.** At a constant volume, compounds tend to require less energy to increase the temperature by 1 K.

○ **B.** The change in internal energy due to heat transfer is greater at a constant pressure.

○ **C.** Energy expended on the surroundings as work is minimized at a constant volume.

○ **D.** No energy is lost to PV work at a constant pressure.

Question 630

At which temperature is hemoglobin A most likely to exhibit reduced oxygen carrying capacity?

- ○ **A.** 37°C
- ○ **B.** 67°C
- ○ **C.** 310 K
- ○ **D.** 328 K

Question 631

Phosphodiester bond formation has a particularly high activation energy. Without the presence of a catalyst, at what temperature would this reaction proceed slowest?

- ○ **A.** 291 K
- ○ **B.** 301 K
- ○ **C.** 17°C
- ○ **D.** 23°C

Question 632

Which of the following could be used to estimate the value of absolute zero?

- ○ **A.** Plot pressure vs. temperature values for an ideal gas at constant volume and extrapolate the resulting line to low temperatures. The intercept with the temperature axis is an estimate of absolute zero.
- ○ **B.** Plot volume vs. temperature values for an ideal gas at constant pressure and extrapolate the resulting line to low temperatures. The intercept with the temperature axis is an estimate of absolute zero.
- ○ **C.** Allow both volume and pressure to vary and plot the product of pressure and volume vs. temperature. The intercept with the temperature axis is an estimate of absolute zero.
- ○ **D.** All of the above techniques would work.

Question 633

Which of the following is the lowest pressure?

- ○ **A.** 1 atm
- ○ **B.** 1 Pa
- ○ **C.** 1 torr
- ○ **D.** 1 mmHg

Question 634

Which of the following affects the average force (per unit area) exerted by a gas on the wall of its container?

   I. The average speed of a gas molecule
   II. The frequency of collisions between gas molecules and the wall
   III. The volume of a gas molecule

- ○ **A.** I only
- ○ **B.** II only
- ○ **C.** I and II only
- ○ **D.** I, II, and III

Question 635

Imagine that a cylinder was constructed with a cross-sectional area of 1 m^2 and spanning from the ground to the top of the atmosphere. Now imagine that the air inside the cylinder is weighed and the mass calculated. What would be the mass? (Note: Assume the acceleration due to gravity is 10 m/s^2.)

- ○ **A.** 101 kg
- ○ **B.** 1,010 kg
- ○ **C.** 10,100 kg
- ○ **D.** 101,000 kg

Question 636

Which of the following describes fluid pressure against a flat surface?

- ○ **A.** The pressure is equal to the change in momentum of the fluid molecules as they collide with the surface of the object divided by the time and the surface area.
- ○ **B.** The pressure is equal to the change in kinetic energy of the fluid molecules as they collide with the surface of the object divided by the time and the surface area.
- ○ **C.** The pressure is equal to the change in momentum of the fluid molecules as they collide with the surface of the object divided by the number of molecules and the surface area.
- ○ **D.** The pressure is equal to the temperature of the fluid molecules divided by the time and surface area.

LECTURE 5

Use the diagram below to answer questions 637–638.

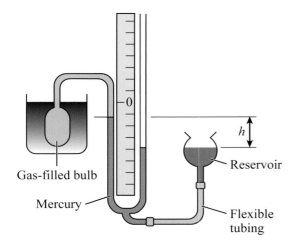

Gas-filled bulb

Mercury

Reservoir

Flexible tubing

h

The diagram shows a gas thermometer. A gas-filled bulb is connected to a mercury manometer. The reservoir can be raised or lowered so that the mercury level on the left is brought to the zero on the manometer. When this is done, the temperature T of any body in thermal equilibrium with the bulb is given as:

$$T = Cp$$

where p is the pressure of the gas and C is a constant. The pressure p is given by:

$$p = p_o - \rho g h$$

where p_o is atmospheric pressure and ρ is the density of mercury.

Question 637

Which of the following is true concerning the pressure of the gas in the diagram?

- O **A.** The gas is at atmospheric pressure.
- O **B.** The gas is below atmospheric pressure.
- O **C.** The gas is above atmospheric pressure.
- O **D.** The pressure of the gas relative to atmospheric pressure cannot be determined until the mercury level is brought to zero on the manometer.

Question 638

Why must the reservoir level match the level of the manometer in the diagram above?

- O **A.** Matching the level of the reservoir with the level of the manometer ensures that the gas remains at atmospheric pressure.
- O **B.** Matching the level of the reservoir with the level of the manometer ensures that the gas remains at constant temperature.
- O **C.** Matching the level of the reservoir with the level of the manometer ensures that the gas remains at constant pressure.
- O **D.** Matching the level of the reservoir with the level of the manometer ensures that the gas remains at constant volume.

Question 639

A 5 Newton weight is placed on a piston with an 8 centimeter radius. The piston compresses helium in a sealed container until the piston stops moving because of the increase in pressure inside the container. The pressure in the container is now recorded. Some helium is then removed from the container, causing the piston to fall so that the volume of the container drops by 25%, at which point the gas can again support the piston, and the pressure is again recorded. How do the two recorded pressures compare?

- O **A.** Since pressure and volume are directly proportional, the second pressure is lower.
- O **B.** Since pressure and volume are inversely proportional, the second pressure is higher.
- O **C.** Since the force on the piston is constant, the pressures are the same.
- O **D.** There is not enough information to answer this question.

Question 640

A large 60 L container of mustard gas ($C_4H_8Cl_2S$) is cooled to 0°C at 1 atm. Environmental chemists plan to deactivate the dangerous gas, which causes burns and cancer, with a reagent that must be equimolar to the gas. What is the minimum number of moles of reagent that can be used to react completely?

- O **A.** 0.4 moles
- O **B.** 2.7 moles
- O **C.** 20.1 moles
- O **D.** 22.4 moles

Question 641

1 mole of methane gas occupies 22.4 L at 1 atm and:

- ○ **A.** 0°C.
- ○ **B.** 25°C.
- ○ **C.** 37°C.
- ○ **D.** 100°C.

Question 642

The graph below represents work done to one mole of ideal gas. Assuming that one of the three energy changes is isovolumetric, what is the volume of the gas?

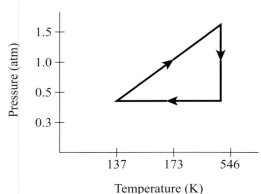

- ○ **A.** 22.4 L
- ○ **B.** 44.8 L
- ○ **C.** 11.2 L
- ○ **D.** 20.4 L

Question 643

One mole of nitric acid is reacted with a sufficient quantity of sodium carbonate to form sodium nitrate (solid), carbon dioxide (gaseous), and water (liquid). If the reaction is carried out at STP, what is the volume of gas produced?

- ○ **A.** 22.4 L
- ○ **B.** 44.8 L
- ○ **C.** 11.2 L
- ○ **D.** 20.4 L

Question 644

At 273 K and 1 atm of pressure, how many moles of gas are contained in a 38 L oxygen canister?

- ○ **A.** 1 mole
- ○ **B.** 1.7 moles
- ○ **C.** 2 moles
- ○ **D.** 2.7 moles

Question 645

Researchers hoped to record the properties of laughing gas (nitrous oxide) at 150 K. One researcher recalls that one mole of gas takes up 22.4 L of volume. Will this erroneous assumption affect the validity or reliability of the data?

- ○ **A.** Validity because at 100 K, 1 mole of gas does not occupy 22.4 L.
- ○ **B.** Reliability because at 100 K, 1 mole of gas does not occupy 22.4 L.
- ○ **C.** Validity because 1 mole of gas is not 6.022×10^{23} molecules.
- ○ **D.** Reliability because 1 mole of gas is not 6.022×10^{23} molecules.

Question 646

Hydrogen gas can react with oxygen to form water in a highly exothermic reaction. The reaction is displayed below:

$$2H_2(g) + O_2(g) \leftrightarrow 2H_2O(l)$$

60 liters of pure oxygen at STP are available to react. Assuming oxygen is the limiting reagent, what is the volume of water that will be created as product?

- ○ **A.** 0.096 L
- ○ **B.** 2.68 L
- ○ **C.** 5.3 L
- ○ **D.** 120 L

Question 647

A container contains only oxygen, nitrogen, carbon dioxide, and water vapor. If, at STP, the partial pressure of oxygen is 200 torr, the partial pressure of carbon dioxide is 10 torr, and the partial pressure of water vapor is 8 torr, what is the partial pressure of the nitrogen?

- ○ **A.** 218 torr
- ○ **B.** 542 torr
- ○ **C.** 760 torr
- ○ **D.** 978 torr

Question 648

The mole fraction of nitrogen in air is approximately 0.8. At STP, what is the partial pressure of nitrogen in air?

- ○ **A.** 608 torr
- ○ **B.** 760 torr
- ○ **C.** 800 torr
- ○ **D.** Cannot be determined from the information given

Question 649

A 10 L balloon at STP contains 0.3 atm oxygen and 0.45 atm nitrogen and the remainder helium. Approximately how many moles of helium are there in the balloon?

- **A.** 0.1 moles
- **B.** 2.4 moles
- **C.** 1 mole
- **D.** 0.25 moles

Question 650

Carbon monoxide is toxic at 1200 ppm by volume. What is the approximate mole fraction of CO, assuming that the remainder of the air is 20% oxygen and 80% nitrogen at STP?

- **A.** 0.1 moles
- **B.** 2.4 moles
- **C.** 1 mole
- **D.** 0.25 moles

Question 651

At sea level, air is 21% oxygen. What is the partial pressure of oxygen at sea level?

- **A.** 0.02 atm
- **B.** 0.2 atm
- **C.** 0.8 atm
- **D.** 1.0 atm

Question 652

In response to a heart attack, a patient is started on supplemental oxygen via a nasal cannula. Which of the following values is LEAST likely to increase?

- **A.** Mole fraction of oxygen
- **B.** Partial pressure of oxygen
- **C.** Mass of oxygen administered
- **D.** Volume of air inspired

Question 653

If the partial pressure of hydrogen in a container held at 5 atmospheres pressure is 35 torr, what is the mole fraction of hydrogen in the container?

- **A.** 0.009
- **B.** 0.046
- **C.** 0.23
- **D.** Cannot be determined from the information given

Question 654

Diving air tanks contain a lower partial pressure of oxygen to protect against free radical formation. If the pressure of gas at 30 feet in depth is double the surface pressure, and the ratio of nitrogen to oxygen is preserved, what is the mole fraction of the added helium needed to preserve the absolute partial pressure of oxygen at 30 feet?

- **A.** 1
- **B.** 2
- **C.** 0.5
- **D.** 0.05

Question 655

The atmosphere on Saturn's moon Titan is 1.45 atm. 95% of the pressure is nitrogen gas, 3.5% is methane gas, and 0.5% is hydrogen gas. Human life requires at least 19% oxygen on Earth. If enough nitrogen were replaced by oxygen to match the partial pressure of oxygen on Earth, which of the following would be the percent of nitrogen in the atmosphere?

- **A.** 13%
- **B.** 75%
- **C.** 82%
- **D.** 95%

Question 656

The partial pressures of carbon dioxide and oxygen in blood are 55 and 95 mmHg, respectively. If the alveolar partial pressures of oxygen and carbon dioxide are 36 and 105 mmHg, which of the following correctly explains the movement of gas across the alveolar membrane?

- **A.** The pressure of carbon dioxide in the alveoli is lower, resulting in movement of carbon dioxide into the alveoli.
- **B.** The pressure of carbon dioxide in the alveoli is lower, resulting in movement of carbon dioxide into the blood.
- **C.** The pressure of oxygen in the blood is lower, resulting in movement of oxygen into the alveoli.
- **D.** The pressure of carbon dioxide in the blood is lower, resulting in movement of oxygen into the blood.

Question 657

In which of the following scenarios would Dalton's law NOT apply?

○ **A.** The container is rigid.

○ **B.** The gases have high molecular weight.

○ **C.** The gases are at very high pressure.

○ **D.** There are many more moles of one gas than another.

Question 658

A graduated cylinder is inverted into a bowl of water such that there is a column of water inside the cylinder, with air trapped at the top. Inside the cylinder, a decomposition reaction that produces carbon dioxide occurs at STP, and all of the gas remains trapped inside the cylinder. Which of the following is required to experimentally determine the moles of CO_2 produced?

○ **A.** The identity of reactants

○ **B.** The moles of carbon in the reactants

○ **C.** Dalton's law

○ **D.** Bernoulli's law

Question 659

A scientist determined that the percentage of argon in the atmosphere is 1% at sea level. Which of the following additional results would most likely strengthen the scientist's finding?

○ **A.** Argon makes up 0.85% of the atmosphere at an elevation of 8,000 m.

○ **B.** Nitrogen has a partial pressure of 0.78 atm at sea level.

○ **C.** Oxygen makes up 21% of the atmosphere at an elevation of 8,000 m.

○ **D.** Argon has a partial pressure of 0.01 atm at sea level.

Question 660

If the partial pressure of carbon dioxide is 30 torr at STP, the gas is 10% carbon dioxide by mass, and there is only one other species of gas present, which of the following could be the other species of gas?

○ **A.** Hydrogen

○ **B.** Methane

○ **C.** Oxygen

○ **D.** Chlorine

Question 661

How would a scientist determine the partial pressure of nitrogen that a patient breathes out at sea level?

○ **A.** Measure the number of moles of nitrogen in one liter of a patient's expired air.

○ **B.** Measure the number of moles of nitrogen in one liter of a patient's inspired air.

○ **C.** Measure the number of moles of oxygen and argon in one liter of a patient's expired air.

○ **D.** Measure the number of moles of oxygen and argon in one liter of a patient's inspired air.

Question 662

Nitrogen narcosis occurs when the partial pressure of nitrogen in the alveoli exceeds 2400 mmHg. Assuming that the water pressure equals 1 atmosphere for every 30 feet under water, how deep can a diver go before experiencing narcosis while breathing tank air similar to atmospheric air?

○ **A.** 30 feet

○ **B.** 90 feet

○ **C.** 120 feet

○ **D.** 240 feet

Real Gases

Question 663

Which of the following is NOT a characteristic of a real gas?

○ **A.** Gas molecules have incompletely elastic collisions.

○ **B.** The average kinetic energy is directly proportional to the temperature of the gas.

○ **C.** Total gas volume is equal to that of its container.

○ **D.** The Van der Waals' equation quantifies gas behavior.

Question 664

Gases begin to deviate from ideal behavior when their:

○ **A.** molecules are close together under high pressure and low temperature.

○ **B.** molecules are far apart under high pressure and low temperature.

○ **C.** molecules are close together under low pressure and high temperature.

○ **D.** molecules are far apart under low pressure and high temperature.

Question 665

Two balloons were filled with similar gases. In balloon A, pressure was kept high while temperature was kept low. In balloon B, pressure was kept low while temperature was kept high. Assuming the same gas is present in both balloons, which balloon would exhibit more ideal behavior?

- ○ **A.** Balloon A
- ○ **B.** Balloon B
- ○ **C.** They will both behave ideally.
- ○ **D.** The answer cannot be determined.

Question 666

Octane gas most likely deviates from ideal gas behavior to a greater degree than methane because it:

- ○ **A.** generates less heat during collisions.
- ○ **B.** takes up less molecular space.
- ○ **C.** has fewer elastic collisions.
- ○ **D.** has fewer intermolecular interactions.

Question 667

Seeking to quantify the effects of a high pressure environment on gaseous compounds, researchers analyzed $N_2(g)$ in a compression chamber at 273 K. Results are displayed in the table below. Note that $R = 0.08206$ L atm K^{-1} mol^{-1}

Pressure	PV/RT
100	0.961
200	1.09
300	1.18
400	1.26

Which of the following statements could accurately explain the research findings? Increasing the pressure:

- ○ **A.** decreases electrostatic interactions.
- ○ **B.** increases intramolecular collision frequency.
- ○ **C.** generates significant intermolecular forces as predicted by Coulomb's law.
- ○ **D.** increases intermolecular attractions resulting from decreased gas volume.

Refer to the information below for questions 668-669.

Researchers used the Van der Waals' equation to quantitatively express the real gas behavior of the following gases: H_2, CO_2, and SO_2.

$$\left[P + \left(\frac{n^2 a}{V^2} \right) \right](V - nb) = nRT$$

Question 668

Which analyzed gas is most likely to have the greatest b variable?

- ○ **A.** H_2
- ○ **B.** CO_2
- ○ **C.** SO_2
- ○ **D.** Cannot be determined

Question 669

The researchers subsequently analyzed CCl_4 and were surprised to discover that it had smaller a and b variables than SO_2. Which statement best validates these findings?

- ○ **A.** Chlorine is more electronegative than oxygen.
- ○ **B.** SO_2 geometry permits greater intermolecular packing.
- ○ **C.** The greater number of p orbitals shields CCl_4 from non-ideal electrostatic interactions.
- ○ **D.** CCl_4 molecules are less likely to exert intermolecular attractive forces.

Refer to the graph below to answer questions 670–672.

The graph below shows PV/RT versus pressure for 1 mole of several gases at 300 K.

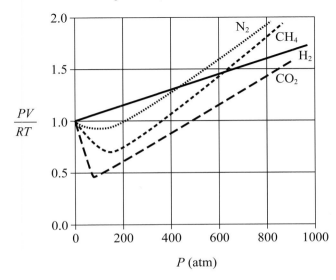

Question 670

At extremely high pressures, all gases deviate from the ideal gas law in the same direction. The greatest contributing factor to this deviation is:

- ○ **A.** molecular volume.
- ○ **B.** intermolecular attractions.
- ○ **C.** temperature.
- ○ **D.** molecular shape.

Question 671

Deviations from ideal behavior typically increase with which of the following molecular characteristics?

- ○ **A.** Molecular mass only
- ○ **B.** Molecular complexity only
- ○ **C.** Molecular mass and complexity
- ○ **D.** Deviations from ideal behavior depend upon temperature and pressure and are independent of molecular characteristics.

Question 672

At 100 atm, CO_2 deviates from ideal behavior. The direction of this deviation is best explained by:

- ○ **A.** molecular number.
- ○ **B.** molecular size.
- ○ **C.** temperature.
- ○ **D.** molecular shape.

Question 673

Under which set of conditions do gases most strongly deviate from ideal gas law behavior?

- ○ **A.** High pressures and low temperatures
- ○ **B.** High pressures and high temperatures
- ○ **C.** Low pressures and low temperatures
- ○ **D.** Low pressures and high temperatures

Question 674

In an attempt to model human ventilation, biomedical engineers developed an artificial lung and inflated it with gases mimicking atmospheric concentrations. The engineers used the ideal gas law to calculate the pressure at the peak of inspiration but were confused when the measured pressure was less than the calculated pressure. Which statement best explains this phenomenon?

- ○ **A.** Human inspiration primarily involves $O_2(g)$, not other atmospheric gases.
- ○ **B.** Real gases do not account for the volume of gas molecules.
- ○ **C.** Real $O_2(g)$ likely exhibits a decreased velocity prior to colliding with the artificial lung wall.
- ○ **D.** Ideal gas molecules have completely elastic collisions while real gases do not.

Question 675

Which of the following gases, when compared under identical conditions, is LEAST likely to behave ideally?

- ○ **A.** O_2
- ○ **B.** O_3
- ○ **C.** CO_2
- ○ **D.** CH_3OH

Question 676

As the volume of a container is decreased at constant temperature, the gas inside begins to behave less ideally. Compared to the pressure predicted by the ideal gas law, the actual pressure is most likely to be:

- ○ **A.** lower, due to the volume of the gas molecules.
- ○ **B.** lower, due to intermolecular attractions among gas molecules.
- ○ **C.** higher, due to the volume of the gas molecules.
- ○ **D.** higher, due to intermolecular attractions between gas molecules.

Question 677

As the temperature of a sample of gas is decreased at constant volume, the gas inside begins to behave less ideally. Compared to the pressure predicted by the ideal gas law, the actual pressure is most likely to be:

- ○ **A.** lower, due to the volume of the gas molecules.
- ○ **B.** lower, due to intermolecular attractions among gas molecules.
- ○ **C.** higher, due to the volume of the gas molecules.
- ○ **D.** higher, due to intermolecular attractions between gas molecules.

LECTURE 5

Question 678

Which of the following explains the pressure and volume deviations in a real gas compared to an ideal gas?

I. Ideal gas molecules do not have volume and real gas molecules do.

II. Ideal gas molecules do not exert forces on one another and real gas molecules do.

III. Ideal gas molecules all move at the same speed for a given temperature, whereas the speed of real gas molecules varies within a sample of gas at a given temperature.

- ○ A. I only
- ○ B. II only
- ○ C. I and II only
- ○ D. I, II, and III

Question 679

Which of the following experiments would help a scientist describe the principles of an ideal gas?

I. Compress a gas in a rigid container at constant pressure and temperature.

II. Use a colored gas and monitor the stream of gas as it moves through a pipe of varying widths.

III. Measure the pressure of a gas at a fixed volume and temperature.

- ○ A. I only
- ○ B. II only
- ○ C. I and III only
- ○ D. I, II, and III

Question 680

Some researchers have suggested that the use of a gas-filled, thin tube connected to an external liquid gauge more accurately reports body temperature during surgery. The thermometer is most accurate when the gas behaves like an ideal gas. Which of the following is most likely to increase the accuracy of the thermometer?

- ○ A. Using less gas in the tube
- ○ B. Using more gas in the tube
- ○ C. Using a heavier fluid in the gauge
- ○ D. Using a lighter fluid in the gauge

Question 681

A group of pulmonologists attempting to describe expiratory $CO_2(g)$ noted several positive deviations from ideality. Which statement best accounts for this finding?

- ○ A. Real gases exhibit non-negligible intermolecular attractive and repulsive forces.
- ○ B. Compared to ideal gases, real gases have less kinetic energy due to imperfectly elastic collision.
- ○ C. Gases deviate from ideality in high pressure, low temperature environments.
- ○ D. $CO_2(g)$ molecules possess a non-zero volume.

Refer to the graph below to answer questions 682-684.

The graph below shows PV/RT versus pressure for 1 mole of nitrogen gas at three different temperatures T_1, T_2, and T_3.

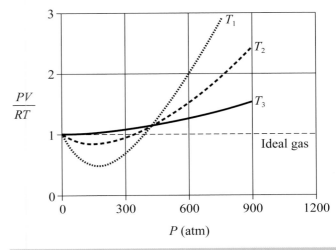

Question 682

Which of the following gives the temperatures in increasing order?

- ○ A. $T_1 < T_2 < T_3$
- ○ B. $T_3 < T_2 < T_1$
- ○ C. $T_2 < T_1 < T_3$
- ○ D. $T_1 < T_3 < T_2$

Question 683

At which temperature does the behavior of nitrogen most resemble that of an ideal gas?

- ○ A. T_1
- ○ B. T_2
- ○ C. T_3
- ○ D. The behavior of nitrogen resembles an ideal gas at all three temperatures.

Question 684

If 2 moles of nitrogen had been used instead of 1 mole, what would be the approximate value of PV/RT at T_1 and 600 atm?

- ○ **A.** 1
- ○ **B.** 2
- ○ **C.** 3
- ○ **D.** 4

Refer to the graph below to answer questions 685-687.

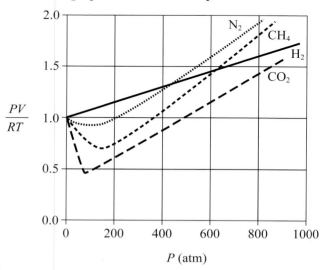

P (atm)

Question 685

According to the graph, at what pressure(s) of CO_2 is the ideal gas law most applicable and the proportionality constant R equal to 0.08206 L atm K^{-1} mol^{-1}?

- ○ **A.** 0 atm and 500 atm
- ○ **B.** 75 atm
- ○ **C.** 500 atm
- ○ **D.** 830 atm

Question 686

Which of the following would be true if the ideal gas law, $PV = nRT$, were used to calculate the volume of a sample of CH_4 gas from measured variables at 200 atm and 300 K, and again at 600 atm and 300 K?

- ○ **A.** The calculated volume would be less than the real volume for both calculations.
- ○ **B.** The calculated volume would be greater than the real volume for both calculations.
- ○ **C.** The calculated volume would be less than the real volume for the 200 atm sample and greater than the real volume for the 600 atm sample.
- ○ **D.** The calculated volume would be greater than the real volume for the 200 atm sample and less than the real volume for the 600 atm sample.

Question 687

Which of the following is indicated by the graph?

- ○ **A.** If temperature is sufficiently low, deviations due to molecular attractions dominate.
- ○ **B.** If temperature is sufficiently low, deviations due to molecular volume dominate.
- ○ **C.** If pressure is sufficiently high, deviations due to molecular attractions dominate.
- ○ **D.** If pressure is sufficiently high, deviations due to molecular volume dominate.

Use the van der Waals equation given below to answer questions 688–689.

The Van der Waals equation is used to predict the behavior of real gases. a and b are constants specific for a particular gas. Their values can be obtained by experiment or from a reference book.

$$\left[P + \left(\frac{n^2 a}{V^2}\right)\right](V - nb) = nRT$$

Van der Waals Equation

Question 688

The Van der Waals constants, *a* and *b*, tend to increase when which of the following changes are made to the gas molecules?

○ **A.** Increasing both molecular mass and structural complexity

○ **B.** Decreasing both molecular mass and structural complexity

○ **C.** Increasing molecular mass but decreasing structural complexity

○ **D.** Decreasing molecular mass but increasing structural complexity

Question 689

Which of the following would be expected to have the greatest value for *a* and *b*?

○ **A.** He

○ **B.** Ne

○ **C.** Ar

○ **D.** Kr

The Liquid and Solid Phases

Question 690

The primary interaction between molecules of acetone in the liquid phase is:

○ **A.** London dispersion forces.

○ **B.** hydrogen bonding.

○ **C.** covalent bonding.

○ **D.** dipole-dipole.

Question 691

Researchers exploring fluid dynamics noted that at STP, water is a liquid, while carbon dioxide is a gas. Which of the following statements best explains this phenomenon?

○ **A.** Water molecules have a greater dipole moment.

○ **B.** Water molecules exhibit a bent molecular geometry.

○ **C.** Carbon dioxide has a greater molar mass.

○ **D.** Carbon dioxide exhibits greater electron repulsion due to its large number of *p* orbitals.

Question 692

The primary interaction between molecules of cyclohexane in the liquid phase is(are):

○ **A.** London dispersion forces.

○ **B.** hydrogen bonding.

○ **C.** covalent bonding.

○ **D.** dipole-dipole.

Question 693

Many long-chain unsaturated hydrocarbons are liquids at room temperature, but when the molecules are hydrogenated, they become solids. Which of the following is the most likely explanation for this?

○ **A.** The hydrogenation enhances the amount of hydrogen bonding present.

○ **B.** The sigma bonds in the hydrogenated compound rotate more easily than the pi bonds in the unsaturated compound, allowing the molecules to pack together more easily.

○ **C.** The hydrogen atoms form dimers, doubling the size of the molecules.

○ **D.** The heat of hydrogenation provides the energy for the phase change.

Question 694

The fluidity of a lipid is reduced when degrees of unsaturation are added. Unsaturated lipid chains are shorter than the saturated lipid chain. What bonds determine the fluidity of the lipids?

○ **A.** Dipole-dipole

○ **B.** London dispersion

○ **C.** Hydrogen bonding

○ **D.** Pi interactions

Question 695

Which of the following most accurately describes the movement of molecules in a solid?

○ **A.** Held perfectly motionless by strong bonds with other molecules or atoms

○ **B.** Vibrating in place close to other molecules or atoms

○ **C.** Moving closely past each other in random directions vibrating, rotating, and forming and breaking bonds with other molecules or atoms

○ **D.** Moving past each other at a distance in random directions vibrating and rotating, without bonding

Question 696

When water melts, what kind(s) of bonds are breaking?

    I. Covalent

    II. Ionic

    III. Hydrogen

  ○ **A.** I only

  ○ **B.** III only

  ○ **C.** I and II only

  ○ **D.** I and III only

Calorimetry

Question 697

It takes 35 calories to increase the temperature of 5 grams of a material by 10°C. How much heat is required to raise the 5 grams of material by 10 K?

  ○ **A.** 0.0037 cal

  ○ **B.** 35 cal

  ○ **C.** 308 cal

  ○ **D.** 9600 cal

Question 698

Which of the following requires the most energy?

  ○ **A.** Bringing a small pot of water to a boil slowly

  ○ **B.** Bringing a small pot of water to a boil quickly

  ○ **C.** Bringing a large pot of water to a boil slowly

  ○ **D.** Bringing a large pot of water to a boil quickly

Question 699

Which of the following is the amount of energy that 1 g of a substance must absorb in order to change its temperature by 1 K?

  ○ **A.** Heat capacity

  ○ **B.** Specific heat

  ○ **C.** Molar heat capacity

  ○ **D.** Volume heat capacity

Question 700

Equal amounts of heat are added to 10 gram blocks of metal X and metal Y. The temperature of metal X is found to increase by twice as much as that of metal Y. Which of the following is the most likely explanation for this observation?

  ○ **A.** The specific heat of metal X is twice as great as that of metal Y.

  ○ **B.** The specific heat of metal X is half as great as that of metal Y.

  ○ **C.** The density of metal X is twice as great as that of metal Y.

  ○ **D.** The density of metal X is half as great as that of metal Y.

Question 701

The human body is 60% water. The specific heat of water allows the body to:

    I. stay warm longer in cold environments.

    II. cool off more quickly in hot environments.

    III. warm slowly in hot environments.

  ○ **A.** I only

  ○ **B.** I and II only

  ○ **C.** I and III only

  ○ **D.** I, II, and III

Question 702

The heat transfer in a coffee cup calorimeter corresponds to:

  ○ **A.** the enthalpy change.

  ○ **B.** the entropy change.

  ○ **C.** the Gibbs free energy change.

  ○ **D.** the energy change.

Question 703

A coffee cup calorimeter often consists of two nested Styrofoam cups with a lid. The primary purpose of using two coffee cups is to:

  ○ **A.** reduce convection through the Styrofoam by providing a thicker barrier.

  ○ **B.** reduce conduction through the Styrofoam by providing a thicker barrier.

  ○ **C.** increase the heat capacity of the calorimeter by increasing its mass.

  ○ **D.** reduce the likelihood of the cups tipping over by increasing their mass.

Question 704

An experimenter uses a coffee cup calorimeter to measure the ΔH of a reaction. During the experiment, she leaves the lid off of the cup, allowing a significant amount of convection. What effect does this have on the determination of the calculated magnitude of ΔH in an exothermic reaction?

○ **A.** It is too low.

○ **B.** It is too high.

○ **C.** It is correct.

○ **D.** It may be too high or too low, depending on the specific reaction.

Question 705

Which of the following values can be measured with a coffee cup calorimeter?

    I. Internal energy

    II. Enthalpy

    III. Change in enthalpy

○ **A.** I only

○ **B.** II only

○ **C.** III only

○ **D.** I, II, and III

Question 706

In careful calculations with calorimeters, the heat capacity of such items as the thermometer and the stirring rod must be considered. Suppose a coffee cup calorimeter is used to calculate the heat of solution for sodium hydroxide, but the experimenter does not include the heat capacity of the thermometer and stirrer. How would this affect the results?

○ **A.** The calculated value of the heat of solution would be too low.

○ **B.** The calculated value of the heat of solution would be too high.

○ **C.** The calculated value of the heat of solution would be unaffected.

○ **D.** The effect on the results depends on whether the reaction is endothermic or exothermic.

Phase Changes

Question 707

When an iron bar is heated, it gradually changes from the solid to liquid phase, eventually turning into a liquid completely. Which of the following is a true statement?

○ **A.** Melting iron is an exothermic process.

○ **B.** The temperature of iron remains constant as it is transformed from solid to liquid.

○ **C.** When iron is heated, the additional kinetic energy restrains molecules, preventing them from moving freely.

○ **D.** For iron, solid and liquid cannot be considered distinct phases.

Question 708

A glass of ice water sits in a room. The room, the water in the glass, and the ice are at 0°C. How many phases of water are there in the room?

○ **A.** One

○ **B.** Two

○ **C.** Three

○ **D.** The situation as described is physically impossible.

Question 709

Which of the following physical processes, when occurring in a pure substance, is accompanied by an increase in temperature?

    I. Melting

    II. Vaporization

    III. Sublimation

○ **A.** I only

○ **B.** I and II only

○ **C.** I, II, and III

○ **D.** None are accompanied by a temperature increase.

Question 710

Which of the following gives an approximate value for the heat of sublimation of a substance?

- **A.** Add the heat of vaporization and the heat of fusion.
- **B.** Subtract the heat of fusion from the heat of vaporization.
- **C.** Multiply the heat of formation by the heat of vaporization.
- **D.** Divide the heat of reaction by the heat of formation.

Question 711

Water has a heat of fusion of 80 cal/g and a heat of vaporization of 540 cal/g. How much heat is required to convert 100 grams of ice at 0°C to steam at 100°C?

- **A.** (80 + 540) cal
- **B.** (100)(80 + 540) cal
- **C.** (100)(1)(1000) cal
- **D.** (100)(80 + 100 + 540) cal

Question 712

Water has a heat of fusion of 80 cal/g and a heat of vaporization of 540 cal/g. If it takes 10 minutes to heat a pot of water from 20°C to 100°C, and the heat is delivered at a constant rate, how much longer does it take for all the water to be converted to steam?

- **A.** Less than 1 minute
- **B.** Between 1 minute and ten minutes
- **C.** Between ten minutes and one hour
- **D.** More than one hour

Use the phase diagram below to answer questions 713–714.

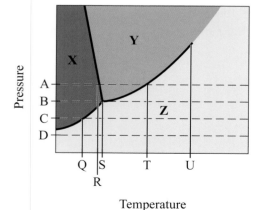

Question 713

From the diagram, which of the following represents solid, liquid, and gas respectively?

- **A.** X, Y, Z
- **B.** Y, X, Z
- **C.** Z, X, Y
- **D.** X, Z, Y

Question 714

If the phase diagram is for water, which line could represent 100°C?

- **A.** R
- **B.** S
- **C.** T
- **D.** U

Question 715

A heating curve for 10 grams of an unknown substance is shown below:

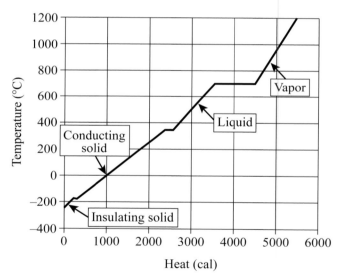

If the pressure exerted on the liquid is increased, the melting point:

- **A.** will increase.
- **B.** will decrease.
- **C.** will remain the same.
- **D.** cannot be determined from the information given.

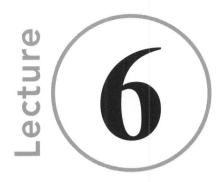

Lecture

6

Questions 716–858

Solutions and Electrochemistry

Solution Chemistry
Vapor Pressure
Solubility
Chemical Potential and Redox Reactions
Electrochemical Cells

Solution Chemistry

Question 716

Which of the following measures of concentration is/are NOT affected by changes in temperature?

   I. Molarity

   II. Molality

   III. Mole Fraction

- ○ **A.** I only
- ○ **B.** III only
- ○ **C.** II and III only
- ○ **D.** I, II, and III

Question 717

Which of the following is/are proper procedure(s) to follow when making a 2.000 M solution of sodium chloride?

   I. Measure out 116.88 grams of sodium chloride onto a tared weighing paper, transfer all of the sodium chloride into a 1.0000 L volumetric flask, and then add water up to the mark.

   II. Measure out 29.22 grams of sodium chloride onto a tared weighing paper, transfer all of the sodium chloride into a 250.0 mL volumetric flask, and then add water up to the mark.

   III. Fill a 500.0 mL volumetric flask to the mark, weigh 58.44 grams of sodium chloride onto a tared weighing paper, and then transfer the sodium chloride into the flask.

- ○ **A.** I only
- ○ **B.** III only
- ○ **C.** I and II only
- ○ **D.** I, II, and III

Question 718

18.0 grams of sucrose (molecular weight 180 amu) are dissolved in 1.8 kg of water at room temperature. What is the molarity of the sucrose solution? (Assume the sucrose does not significantly change the volume of the solution.)

- ○ **A.** 0.056 M
- ○ **B.** 0.091 M
- ○ **C.** 0.100 M
- ○ **D.** 0.180 M

Question 719

30 grams of NaOH are dissolved in 100 grams of water. What is the molality of NaOH in the resulting solution?

- ○ **A.** 0.0075 m
- ○ **B.** 0.30 m
- ○ **C.** 7.5 m
- ○ **D.** 300 m

Question 720

0.1 moles of NaCl are placed in a fish tank containing 60 liters of water. What is the ppm of NaCl in the water in the fish tank?

- ○ **A.** 0.00097 ppm
- ○ **B.** 0.097 ppm
- ○ **C.** 97 ppm
- ○ **D.** 970 ppm

Question 721

A naturally-occurring pure sample of which of the following has the lowest density at room temperature?

- ○ **A.** Aluminum
- ○ **B.** Magnesium
- ○ **C.** Sodium
- ○ **D.** Chlorine

Question 722

A naturally-occurring sample of which of the following has the lowest density at room temperature?

- ○ **A.** Carbon (diamond)
- ○ **B.** Fluorine gas
- ○ **C.** Nitrogen gas
- ○ **D.** Oxygen gas

Question 723

A naturally-occurring sample of which of the following has the lowest density at room temperature?

- ○ **A.** Argon
- ○ **B.** Chlorine
- ○ **C.** Phosphorus
- ○ **D.** Sulfur

Question 724

A 2.0 kilogram block has dimensions 3 cm × 5 cm × 8 cm. What is its density?

- A. 1.67×10^{-3} kg/m^3
- B. 1.67 kg/m^3
- C. 167 kg/m^3
- D. 1.67×10^4 kg/m^3

Question 725

Argon is the most common noble gas in the atmosphere at the surface of the Earth, despite the fact that helium is much more common in the universe. Why?

- A. Argon is a byproduct of the decay of radioactive xenon in the Earth's crust.
- B. Argon is the most stable of the noble gases.
- C. The production of argon is catalyzed by greenhouse gases.
- D. Argon has a similar density to nitrogen, the major component of the atmosphere.

Question 726

Which of the following will increase the maximum concentration of NaCl that can be dissolved in water?

- A. Increasing the temperature
- B. Decreasing the temperature
- C. Adding more NaCl to solution
- D. Adding more water to solution

Question 727

Which of the following is NOT true concerning the solubility product, K_{sp}?

- A. Its value depends upon temperature.
- B. Its value depends upon the solvent.
- C. Its value is independent of the concentration of the reactants.
- D. Its value is zero for insoluble compounds.

Use the solubility table below to answer questions 728-730.

Solid	K_{sp}	Solid	K_{sp}
NiCO$_3$	1.4×10^{-7}	Ba(OH)$_2$	5.0×10^{-3}
CaCO$_3$	8.7×10^{-9}	Ca(OH)$_2$	1.3×10^{-6}
BaCO$_3$	1.6×10^{-9}	Fe(OH)$_2$	1.8×10^{-15}
CuCO$_3$	2.5×10^{-10}	Ni(OH)$_2$	1.6×10^{-16}
MnCO$_3$	8.8×10^{-11}	BaCrO$_4$	8.5×10^{-11}
FeCO$_3$	2.1×10^{-11}	FeS	3.7×10^{-19}
Ag$_2$CO$_3$	8.1×10^{-12}	NiS	3.0×10^{-21}

Question 728

A textbook defines insoluble compounds as those compounds with a solubility less than 0.01 mol/L. Which of the following would be considered soluble by this definition?

    I. NiCO$_3$

    II. Ba(OH)$_2$

    III. FeS

- A. I only
- B. II only
- C. II and III only
- D. I, II, and III

Question 729

If compounds with a solubility of less than 0.01 mol/L are insoluble, Ca(OH)$_2$ should be insoluble. However, Ca(OH)$_2$ is, in fact, soluble. How can this discrepancy be reconciled?

- A. Ca^{2+} ions and OH$^-$ ions form ion pairs in solution.
- B. The reaction is exothermic, raising the temperature of the solution and increasing K_{sp}.
- C. Calcium hydroxide dissociates into three particles, not two.
- D. Calcium hydroxide creates a basic solution, shifting the equilibrium expression to the right.

Question 730

Comparing the K_{sp} of different solids, which of the following is the most soluble in 0.1 M silver nitrate solution?

- A. MnCO$_3$
- B. FeCO$_3$
- C. Ag$_2$CO$_3$
- D. BaCrO$_4$

Question 731

Which of the following statements is true of an unsaturated solution?

- **A.** If left for long enough, the solution will reach equilibrium.
- **B.** If a catalyst is added, a precipitate will form.
- **C.** If a very small amount of solid is added to the solution, the rate at which that solid dissolves will equal the rate at which new solid is formed.
- **D.** The solution may become saturated if the temperature is changed.

Question 732

100 mL of 0.1 M NaCl is mixed with 900 mL of 0.01 M $Pb(NO_3)_2$ solution. If the K_{sp} of $PbCl_2$ is 1.6×10^{-5}, what is the most likely result?

- **A.** An unsaturated solution
- **B.** A sodium nitrate precipitate
- **C.** A lead(II) chloride precipitate
- **D.** Both sodium nitrate and lead(II) chloride precipitate

Question 733

Which expression could be used to find the number of grams of solid NaCl that would have to be added to 20.0 mL of 6.0 M $AgNO_3$ to form a saturated solution of silver chloride? Silver chloride has a K_{sp} of 1.8×10^{-10}.

- **A.** $\dfrac{(1.8 \times 10^{-10})(6.0)(20.0)(58.4)}{(1000)}$
- **B.** $\dfrac{(1.8 \times 10^{-10})(6.0)(58.4)}{(20)(1000)}$
- **C.** $\dfrac{(1.8 \times 10^{-10})(58.4)}{(20)(6.0)(1000)}$
- **D.** $\dfrac{(1.8 \times 10^{-10})(20.0)(58.4)}{(6.0)(1000)}$

Question 734

Water has a higher heat capacity than many other molecules because:

- **A.** water molecules are light and thus able to move faster to absorb more heat energy.
- **B.** the atoms of water molecules are able to absorb a greater proportion of heat energy via vibration.
- **C.** the hydrogen bonds of water break to absorb heat energy.
- **D.** the hydrogen bonds of water form to absorb heat energy.

Question 735

Water and butanol are partially miscible. At room temperature, when equal amounts of water and butanol are poured into the same container, two phases are formed, one containing mostly water with a small amount of butanol, and one containing mostly butanol with a small amount of water. At some critical solution temperature water and butanol are completely miscible and only one phase exists for any mixture. The miscibility graph below shows temperature vs. mole fraction for a hypothetical organic Fluid X with water at a constant pressure of 1 atm. The shaded region represents the two phase system and the light region represents the one phase system.

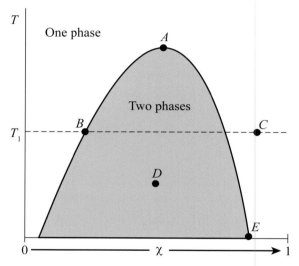

Fluid X is probably:

- **A.** nonpolar.
- **B.** polar, but less polar than water.
- **C.** exactly as polar as water.
- **D.** more polar than water.

Question 736

A container is partially filled with a mixture of ether and water. The space above the mixture is vacuumed and the container is sealed. The container is shaken and then allowed to sit. Which of the following is true after several hours have passed?

- **A.** Both the liquid portion and the gas portion of the container contain two phases.
- **B.** Both the liquid portion and the gas portion of the container contain one phase.
- **C.** The liquid portion has two phases and the gas portion has one phase.
- **D.** The liquid portion has two phases and there is no gas portion.

Question 737

Which of the following molecules, when poured into a beaker containing methanol, is LEAST likely to result in the formation of two solvent layers?

○ **A.**

○ **B.**

○ **C.**

○ **D.**

Question 738

Water is poured into a beaker containing diethyl ether at 25°C. Which of the following best describes the subsequent interaction that takes place?

○ **A.** Hydrogen bonds are broken as the solute dissociates in the solvent.

○ **B.** The intermolecular bonds of the solute cannot be broken by the polar solvent.

○ **C.** The nonpolar solvent exhibits weaker intermolecular interactions than the polar solute.

○ **D.** The solute's permanent dipole moment prevents the solvent from dissociating the solute.

Question 739

Researchers measured the boiling points of four linear alkanes. The data are presented in the table below.

Alkane	Boiling point (°C)
CH_4	−162.0
C_2H_6	−89.1
C_3H_8	−42.5
C_4H_{10}	1.04

Which statement best explains the collected data?

○ **A.** Increased Van der Waals' forces result in greater boiling points.

○ **B.** Molecular weight increases the boiling point.

○ **C.** Increased intramolecular interactions generate greater boiling points.

○ **D.** London dispersion forces increase the boiling point as a function of hydrogen ion concentration.

Vapor Pressure

Question 740

When cold water is placed in a glass, small bubbles can eventually be seen to form on the inside of the glass. Which of the following is the most likely explanation for this observation?

○ **A.** As the water warms up, oxygen from the air is absorbed into the water.

○ **B.** As the water warms up, oxygen in the water is released.

○ **C.** As the glass cools down, oxygen in the water condenses on to the sides of the glass.

○ **D.** As the glass cools down, oxygen in the glass is released into the water.

Question 741

Fractional distillation is a technique that allows for separation of two liquids by differences in vapor pressure. Below is a depiction of the fractional distillation of ethanol from water. What is the boiling point of the highest purity ethanol that can be distilled by this method?

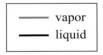

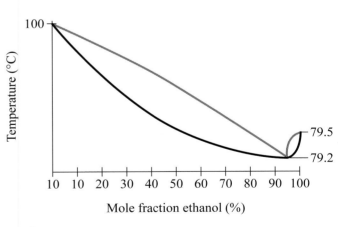

○ **A.** 79.2°C

○ **B.** 79.5°C

○ **C.** 84.3°C

○ **D.** 100°C

Question 742

A scientist inadvertently mixes two liquids. They are miscible but have different properties. Molecule A is highly volatile and molecule B is weakly volatile. Which of the following mole fractions and partial pressures would be expected of the gas directly above the mixture?

○ **A.**

Molecule	χ	P (atm)
A	0.5	0.5
B	0.5	0.5

○ **B.**

Molecule	χ	P (atm)
A	1.0	1.0
B	0.0	0.0

○ **C.**

Molecule	χ	P (atm)
A	0.1	0.1
B	0.9	0.9

○ **D.**

Molecule	χ	P (atm)
A	0.9	0.9
B	0.1	0.1

Question 743

If the phase diagram below is of water, and line A is one atm, can ice, liquid water, and water vapor exist in equilibrium at 0°C and 1 atm?

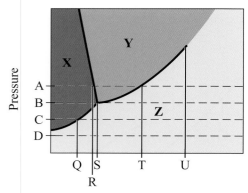

○ **A.** No, because the triple point is below 1 atm.
○ **B.** No, because the triple point is below 0°C.
○ **C.** Yes, because ice and water can have equilibrium with the vapor phase regardless of the pressure or temperature.
○ **D.** Yes, because 1 atm and 0°C is above the triple point.

Question 744

Why does the boiling point rise when a nonvolatile solute is added to a pure liquid?

○ **A.** Because the density of the solution becomes greater than the density of the pure liquid.
○ **B.** Because the kinetic energy of the molecules of the liquid in the solution is less than the kinetic energy of the molecules in the pure liquid.
○ **C.** Because adding a solute to a liquid cools the liquid.
○ **D.** Because solute molecules occupy surface area of the liquid and lower the vapor pressure.

Question 745

At 25°C, water has a vapor pressure of 23.8 torr and ethanol has a vapor pressure of 58.9 torr. If 50 grams of ethanol (M.W. 46 amu) are added to 200 grams of water, what is the approximate vapor pressure of the mixture?

○ **A.** 5.3 torr
○ **B.** 21.7 torr
○ **C.** 27.0 torr
○ **D.** 82.7 torr

Question 746

Which of the following is true concerning the hard boiling of an egg?

○ **A.** The egg will become hardboiled faster at low altitudes.
○ **B.** The water will boil sooner at low altitudes.
○ **C.** The water will get hotter at high altitudes.
○ **D.** The water will reach a higher vapor pressure at high altitudes.

Question 747

Which of the following is true?

○ **A.** A pure liquid will always have a greater vapor pressure than its solutions.
○ **B.** A pure liquid will always have a lower vapor pressure than its solutions.
○ **C.** If liquid X has a greater vapor pressure than liquid Y, then adding liquid X to liquid Y will always result in a vapor pressure greater than liquid Y.
○ **D.** If liquid X has a greater vapor pressure than liquid Y, adding liquid X to liquid Y may result in a vapor pressure greater or lower than liquid Y.

Question 748

A pure volatile liquid is placed in a sealed container. Which of the following accurately describes how an equilibrium is reached between the rate of evaporation and rate of condensation?

○ **A.** The rate of condensation rises and the rate of evaporation falls until the rates are equal.

○ **B.** The rate of condensation falls and the rate of evaporation rises until the rates are equal.

○ **C.** The rate of condensation rises and the rate of evaporation remains constant until the rates are equal.

○ **D.** The rate of condensation remains constant and the rate of evaporation falls until the rates are equal.

Question 749

Which of the following solutions has the greatest vapor pressure?

○ **A.** 20 mL of pure water at 30°C

○ **B.** 30 mL of pure water at 20°C

○ **C.** 40 mL of 3 M aqueous sodium chloride at 30°C

○ **D.** 50 mL of 3 M aqueous glucose at 20°C

Solubility

Question 750

20 grams of an unknown substance are dissolved in 70 grams of water. When the solution is transferred to another container, it is found to weigh 92 grams. Which of the following is a possible explanation?

○ **A.** The reaction was exothermic, resulting in an increase in the average molecular speed.

○ **B.** The solution reacted with the first container, causing some byproducts to be transferred with the solution.

○ **C.** The solution reacted with the second container, causing a precipitate to form.

○ **D.** Some of the solution was left in the first container.

Question 751

The chlorite ion is which of the following?

○ **A.** ClO^-

○ **B.** ClO_2^-

○ **C.** ClO_3^-

○ **D.** ClO_4^-

Question 752

The bicarbonate ion is which of the following?

○ **A.** CO_3^-

○ **B.** CO_3^{2-}

○ **C.** HCO_3^-

○ **D.** HCO_3^{2-}

Question 753

Which of the following types of compounds are insoluble in water?

○ **A.** Compounds containing the nitrate ion

○ **B.** Sulfate compounds other than those containing Ca^{2+}, Sr^{2+}, Ba^{2+}, Hg_2^{2+}, and Pb^{2+}

○ **C.** Compounds containing the carbonate ions excluding ammonium salts

○ **D.** Compounds containing the ammonium ion

Question 754

Which of the following metal ions forms a soluble compound with Cl^-, Br^-, and I^-?

○ **A.** Al^{3+}

○ **B.** Ag^{2+}

○ **C.** Hg_2^{2+}

○ **D.** Pb^{2+}

Question 755

Which of the following metal ions forms an insoluble compound with OH^-?

○ **A.** Ca^{2+}

○ **B.** Al^{3+}

○ **C.** Sr^{2+}

○ **D.** Ba^{2+}

Question 756

Which of the following metal ions forms an insoluble compound with S^{2-}?

○ **A.** NH_4^+

○ **B.** Al^{3+}

○ **C.** Sr^{2+}

○ **D.** Ba^{2+}

Question 757

Hydration involves:

○ **A.** the breaking of water-water bonds.

○ **B.** the breaking of solute-solute bonds.

○ **C.** the formation of solute-water bonds.

○ **D.** both the breaking of water-water bonds and the formation of solute-water bonds.

Question 758

Experimenters dissolve hydrochloric acid into water. The following reaction is expected to take place.

$$HCl(aq) + H_2O(l) \rightarrow H_3O^+(aq) + Cl^-(aq)$$

In this reaction, the hydronium ion acts as which of the following?

○ **A.** Acid

○ **B.** Base

○ **C.** Conjugate acid

○ **D.** Conjugate base

Question 759

Prolonged, intense exercise can lead to severe electrolyte depletion through sweat. Electrolyte replenishment is typically done via consumption of aqueous salts composed of the following ions with varying hydration numbers: Ca^{2+}, Na^+, Cl^-, SO_4^{2-}, and HCO_3^-. Which of the following best orders the hydration numbers from smallest to largest?

○ **A.** Na^+, SO_4^{2-}, Ca^{2+}

○ **B.** HCO_3^-, Na^+, SO_4^{2-}

○ **C.** Cl^-, Ca^{2+}, SO_4^{2-}

○ **D.** Na^+, HCO_3^+, SO_4^{2-}

Question 760

The hydration number of an ion is:

○ **A.** the number of ions that can dissolve in one liter of water.

○ **B.** the number of ions that bond to a water molecule when in aqueous solution.

○ **C.** the number of water molecules required to dissolve one liter of ions.

○ **D.** the number of water molecules that bond to an ion in an aqueous solution.

Question 761

The heat of hydration for any solute is:

○ **A.** always positive.

○ **B.** always negative.

○ **C.** always zero.

○ **D.** may be either positive or negative depending upon the solute.

Question 762

The solubility of $Ca(OH)_2$ in water:

○ **A.** is greatest in acidic solutions.

○ **B.** is greatest in neutral solutions.

○ **C.** is greatest in basic solutions.

○ **D.** does not change with pH.

Question 763

In which solution will sodium chloride be least soluble?

○ **A.** 3.0 M hydrochloric acid

○ **B.** 5.0 M sulfuric acid

○ **C.** 3.0 M lithium hydroxide

○ **D.** Sodium chloride will be equally soluble in all of these solutions.

▼

Use the information below to answer questions 764–765.

The solubility of CaF_2 is increased by adding acid to the solution. The process can be understood in terms of the following summation of reactions:

$$CaF_2(s) \rightleftharpoons Ca^{2+}(aq) + 2F^-(aq)$$
$$2\left\{2F^-(aq) + H^+(aq) \rightleftharpoons HF(aq)\right\}$$
$$\overline{CaF_2(s) + 2H^+(aq) \rightleftharpoons Ca^{2+}(aq) + 2HF(aq)}$$

Question 764

A saturated solution of CaF_2 is created by adding excess CaF_2 to water. The excess CaF_2 precipitate is filtered out of solution. 0.1 M HCl is added to the solution. Does a precipitate form?

○ **A.** Yes, because chloride ions from the dissociation of HCl act as a common ion causing precipitation.

○ **B.** Yes, because HCl is a strong acid.

○ **C.** No, because acid increases the solubility of CaF_2.

○ **D.** No, because protons push the equilibrium of the overall reaction to the right balancing out the leftward shift caused by HCl.

Question 765

A saturated solution of CaF_2 is created by adding excess CaF_2 to water. The excess CaF_2 precipitate is filtered out of solution. HCl is added to the solution. Next, a very small amount of a soluble calcium salt is added to solution. Is a precipitate likely to form?

- O **A.** Yes, because the solution was saturated before the addition of the calcium salt.
- O **B.** Yes, due to the common ion effect.
- O **C.** No, because the solution was not saturated when the calcium salt was added.
- O **D.** No, because the solution will become supersaturated.

Question 766

Parietal cells of the stomach can overproduce HCl and cause heartburn in many individuals. An inexpensive yet effective treatment for heartburn is consuming a liquid suspension of magnesium hydroxide. Compared to a pH 7 solution, magnesium hydroxide dissolved in the stomach:

- O **A.** reaches equilibrium at a faster rate due to increased solubility.
- O **B.** generates more Mg^{2+} per mole of magnesium hydroxide.
- O **C.** has reduced solubility due to the greater presence of H^+ ions.
- O **D.** generates $H_2(g)$.

Question 767

Iodine, which is only slightly soluble in pure water, dissolves readily in a 1 M sodium iodide solution. Which of the following is a possible explanation for this observation?

- O **A.** The presence of iodide ions in solution enhances the solubility of iodine.
- O **B.** Iodide is a powerful oxidizing agent: it reduces the iodine, bringing it into solution.
- O **C.** The iodine reacts with the iodide ions, thus keeping the concentration of iodine in the solution low.
- O **D.** The sodium ions balance the charge of the newly formed iodide ions.

Question 768

Scientists interested in determining the concentration of a hydrated iron complex, $[Fe(H_2O)_6]^{2+}$, would most likely:

- O **A.** mix iron and water and observe the reaction until it reaches completion.
- O **B.** mix iron and water and observe the reaction until the concentrations of the reactants remains constant.
- O **C.** mix iron, water, and the hydroxide ion and observe the reaction until it reaches completion.
- O **D.** mix iron, water, and the hydroxide ion and observe the reaction until the concentrations of the reactants remains constant.

Question 769

A chemist has a mystery aqueous solution. Which of the following compounds could the chemist add to obtain the most useful information about the ion in this solution?

- O **A.** AgCl
- O **B.** NaCl
- O **C.** Lysine
- O **D.** $AgClO_3$

Question 770

AgCl dissolves in water to form Ag^+ and Cl^- ($K_{sp} = 1.8 \times 10^{-10}$ at 25°C). Which of the following will increase the solubility of silver chloride in water?

- O **A.** Adding $AgNO_3$
- O **B.** Adding NH_3
- O **C.** Decreasing the temperature
- O **D.** Increasing the amount of AgCl added

Refer to the following information for questions 771-773.

Argyria is a serious health condition wherein individuals develop bluish-grey skin discoloration. This can be due to excessive consumption of solid silver iodide (AgI), which dissolves upon entry to the blood. Once dissolved, silver ion can react with cyanide in the following reaction:

$$Ag^+(aq) + 2CN^-(aq) \leftrightarrow Ag(CN)_2^-(aq)$$

Question 771

Controlling for quantity of solid silver iodide consumed, which of the following is most likely true of individuals with elevated blood levels of HCN? These individuals:

- ○ **A.** have less circulating $AgI(s)$.
- ○ **B.** also have elevated blood concentrations of $Ag^+(aq)$.
- ○ **C.** have a greater blood pH due to increased CN^- concentration.
- ○ **D.** have a greater degree of skin discoloration than individuals with normal blood levels of HCN.

Question 772

Subsequent to consuming a fixed quantity of $AgI(s)$, an individual immediately consumes large quantities of heavily iodized salt ($NaI(s)$). Compared to only consuming $AgI(s)$, how would the salt consumption most likely affect the individual's circulating blood chemistry?

- ○ **A.** The quantity of solid silver iodide will decrease.
- ○ **B.** The concentration of $Ag^+(aq)$ will increase.
- ○ **C.** The concentration of $Ag(CN)_2^-(aq)$ will decrease.
- ○ **D.** The addition of iodized salt will have a negligible effect on blood chemistry.

Question 773

What is the formation constant K_f of the complex ion formed following the solvation of solid silver chloride?

- ○ **A.** $[Ag(CN)_2^-]/[CN^-]^2[Ag^+]$
- ○ **B.** $[CN^-]^2[Ag^+]/[Ag(CN)_2^-]$
- ○ **C.** $[Ag^+][I^-]$
- ○ **D.** $[Ag^+][I^-]/[AgI(s)]$

▲

Question 774

A scientist is developing a new drug containing a metal ion, but when the drug is ingested, it is poorly soluble in the stomach of an average patient and does not get readily absorbed. Which of the following could be a solution?

- ○ **A.** Administer the drug with Vitamin C.
- ○ **B.** Administer the drug with a large ligand with a lone electron pair.
- ○ **C.** Administer the drug with sodium bicarbonate.
- ○ **D.** Administer the drug with a lipid.

Question 775

What is the expected outcome when attempting to dissolve silver chloride in an aqueous ammonia solution?

- ○ **A.** The lone electrons in the d orbital accept electrons from ammonia.
- ○ **B.** Ammonia is a non-polar solvent and will not dissolve silver chloride.
- ○ **C.** The empty orbitals in the s, p, and d levels accept electrons from ammonia.
- ○ **D.** Ammonia is a cation and will bind the chlorine ions.

Question 776

How does adding sodium chloride to pure water alter the solubility and K_{sp} of silver chloride in that solution?

- ○ **A.** Both the solubility and K_{sp} are lowered.
- ○ **B.** The solubility is lowered, but the K_{sp} remains the same.
- ○ **C.** The solubility remains the same, but the K_{sp} is lowered.
- ○ **D.** Neither are affected.

Question 777

The following equilibrium exists in the human body as a physiological acid/base buffer system.

$$CO_2(g) + H_2O(l) \leftrightarrow H_2CO_3(aq) \leftrightarrow HCO_3^-(aq) + H^+(aq)$$

Giving a patient sodium bicarbonate ($NaHCO_3$) would:

- ○ **A.** shift the equilibrium to the left, decreasing blood pH.
- ○ **B.** shift the equilibrium to the right, decreasing blood pH.
- ○ **C.** shift the equilibrium to the left, increasing blood pH.
- ○ **D.** not alter equilibrium or blood pH.

Question 778

How does increasing the partial pressure of a gas affect its solubility in water?

- ○ **A.** The solubility of the gas decreases.
- ○ **B.** The solubility of the gas increases.
- ○ **C.** The solubility of the gas remains the same.
- ○ **D.** The effect on the solubility of the gas depends on the gas.

Chemical Potential and Redox Reactions

Question 779

Consider the following redox reaction:

$$Cl_2 + Fe \rightarrow Fe^{2+} + 2Cl^-$$

Which of the following is the reducing agent in this reaction?

- ○ **A.** Cl_2
- ○ **B.** Fe
- ○ **C.** Fe^{2+}
- ○ **D.** Cl^-

Question 780

Consider the following reaction:

$$2NaClO_3 + SO_2 + H_2SO_4 \rightarrow 2NaHSO_4 + 2ClO_2$$

Which of the following is/are the reducing agent(s) in this reaction?

- I. $NaClO_3$
- II. SO_2
- III. H_2SO_4

- ○ **A.** I only
- ○ **B.** II only
- ○ **C.** III only
- ○ **D.** II and III only

Question 781

Consider the following reaction:

$$NaH + H_2O \rightarrow NaOH + H_2$$

What is the role of water in this redox reaction?

- ○ **A.** It is an oxidizing agent only.
- ○ **B.** It is a reducing agent only.
- ○ **C.** It is both an oxidizing and a reducing agent.
- ○ **D.** It is neither an oxidizing nor a reducing agent.

Question 782

What is the role of NO_2 in this redox reaction?

$$3NO_2 + H_2O \rightarrow 2HNO_3 + NO$$

- ○ **A.** It is an oxidizing agent only.
- ○ **B.** It is a reducing agent only.
- ○ **C.** It is both an oxidizing and a reducing agent.
- ○ **D.** It is neither an oxidizing nor a reducing agent.

Question 783

Which of the following is necessary to transform nitrogen gas into ammonia gas?

- ○ **A.** An acid
- ○ **B.** A base
- ○ **C.** An oxidizing agent
- ○ **D.** A reducing agent

Question 784

Magnesium disks are often attached to the (iron) hulls of ships to prevent them from rusting. Why does this work?

- ○ **A.** Magnesium is a better oxidizing agent than iron, thus the magnesium is oxidized preferentially.
- ○ **B.** Magnesium is a better oxidizing agent than iron, thus the magnesium is reduced preferentially.
- ○ **C.** Magnesium is a better reducing agent than iron, thus the magnesium is oxidized preferentially.
- ○ **D.** Magnesium is a better reducing agent than iron, thus the magnesium is reduced preferentially.

Question 785

When an atom is oxidized:

- ○ **A.** there is an actual transfer of electrons from the reductant to the atom.
- ○ **B.** there is an actual transfer of electrons from the atom to the reductant.
- ○ **C.** the oxidation state of the atom becomes more negative.
- ○ **D.** the oxidation state of the atom becomes more positive.

Question 786

What is the oxidation state of iron in Fe_2S_3?

- ○ **A.** 0
- ○ **B.** +1
- ○ **C.** +2
- ○ **D.** +3

Question 787

What is the oxidation number of xenon in potassium perxenate, K_4XeO_6?

- ○ **A.** +2
- ○ **B.** +8
- ○ **C.** +12
- ○ **D.** This compound cannot exist; it is impossible for xenon to be oxidized to this degree.

Question 788

In the compound $KHSO_4$, which element has the highest oxidation number?

- A. K
- B. H
- C. S
- D. O

Question 789

If a metal forms more than one oxide, the basicity decreases as the oxidation state of the metal increases. Which of the following is the strongest base?

- A. CrO
- B. CrO_2
- C. CrO_3
- D. Cr_2O_3

Question 790

Which of the following is true concerning oxidation and reduction half-reactions?

- A. A reduction half-reaction can occur by itself if the reduction half-reaction potential is applied across the reaction.
- B. A reduction half-reaction can occur by itself if the negative of the reduction half-reaction potential is applied across the reaction.
- C. Oxidation and reduction must take place simultaneously.
- D. Reduction can only occur by itself in the presence of a strong reducing agent.

Question 791

Which of the following statements is/are true for a galvanic cell at equilibrium at 298 K?

  I. $Q = K$
  II. $E = E°$
  III. $\Delta G° = \Delta G$

- A. I only
- B. III only
- C. II and III only
- D. I, II, and III

Question 792

Which of the following represents ΔG of a galvanic cell when all concentrations in the half cell solutions are 1.4 M? (Note: n = number of electrons transferred in a balanced redox reaction; F = 96,500 C/mol; E = the emf of the cell.)

- A. nFE
- B. $-nFE$
- C. $nFE°$
- D. $-nFE°$

Question 793

Consider a cell making use of the following half reactions:

Anode:

$$Mg \rightarrow Mg^{2+} + 2e^-$$

Cathode:

$$MnO_2 + 4H^+ + 2e^- \rightarrow MN^{2+} + 2H_2O$$

Under standard conditions, this cell yields a potential of 3.6 V. If the pH were then increased to 7 and the concentrations of the other ions maintained at 1 M, the cell potential would most likely:

- A. decrease.
- B. increase.
- C. stay the same.
- D. asymptotically approach 1 V.

Question 794

The standard potential of a galvanic cell is +2.03 V. Which of the following must be true of the cell?

  I. $K > 1$
  II. $\Delta S° > 0$
  III. $\Delta G° < 0$

- A. II only
- B. II and III only
- C. I and III only
- D. I, II, and III

Question 795

A galvanic cell with a standard cell potential of -0.02 V is designed so as to operate spontaneously when first used. Which of the following statements is/are true for this cell when first used?

    I. $K > 1$

    II. $Q < K$

    III. $\Delta G^\circ < 0$

- **A.** II only
- **B.** III only
- **C.** I and III only
- **D.** I, II, and III

Question 796

The standard potential of a reaction is $+0.38$ V. Which of the following can be concluded about this reaction?

- **A.** Under standard conditions, the free energy of the reaction is positive.
- **B.** At equilibrium, the free energy of the reaction is positive.
- **C.** Under standard conditions, the free energy of the reaction is negative.
- **D.** At equilibrium, the free energy of the reaction is negative.

Question 797

Which of the following will always increase the emf of a galvanic cell?

- **A.** Increasing the concentration of the oxidant at the anode
- **B.** Increasing the concentration of the oxidant at the cathode
- **C.** Decreasing the internal resistance of the cell
- **D.** Raising the temperature of the cell

Questions 798–800 depend on the following table:

Half-reaction	E°, V
$Ag^+ + e^- \rightarrow Ag$	$+0.80$
$Cd^{2+} + 2e^- \rightarrow Cd$	-0.40
$2F^- \rightarrow F_2 + 2e^-$	-2.87
$2I^- \rightarrow I_2 + 2e^-$	-0.54
$Na^+ + e^- \rightarrow Na$	-2.71
$Se^{2-} \rightarrow Se + 2e^-$	$+0.67$

Question 798

Based only on the half-reactions in the table, which of the following is the strongest oxidizing agent?

- **A.** Cd^{2+}
- **B.** F^-
- **C.** I^-
- **D.** Na^+

Question 799

Based only on the half-reactions in the table, which of the following is the strongest reducing agent?

- **A.** Cd^{2+}
- **B.** F^-
- **C.** I^-
- **D.** Na^+

Question 800

What would be the standard cell potential of a galvanic cell in which sodium and iodine electrodes are placed in a 1 M sodium iodide solution?

- **A.** 1.00 V
- **B.** 2.17 V
- **C.** 3.25 V
- **D.** 5.96 V

Use the table below to answer questions 801–804.

The table below is an activity series of metals in an aqueous solution. The half reactions are listed highest potential to lowest potential from top to bottom.

Metal	Oxidation reaction
Lithium	$Li \rightarrow Li^+ + e^-$
Potassium	$K \rightarrow K^+ + e^-$
Magnesium	$Mg \rightarrow Mg^{2+} + 2e^-$
Aluminum	$Al \rightarrow Al^{3+} + 3e^-$
Zinc	$Zn \rightarrow Zn^{2+} + 2e^-$
Hydrogen	$H_2 \rightarrow 2H^+ + 2e^-$
Copper	$Cu \rightarrow Cu^{2+} + 2e^-$
Silver	$Ag \rightarrow Ag^+ + e^-$

Question 801

Which of the following metals will not form hydrogen gas when placed in an acid solution?

- ○ **A.** Li
- ○ **B.** Al
- ○ **C.** Zn
- ○ **D.** Cu

Question 802

Which of the following is the strongest oxidizing agent?

- ○ **A.** Li
- ○ **B.** Li^+
- ○ **C.** Ag
- ○ **D.** Ag^+

Question 803

Which of the following is the strongest reducing agent?

- ○ **A.** Li
- ○ **B.** Li^+
- ○ **C.** Ag
- ○ **D.** Ag^+

Question 804

What is the balanced reduction half reaction as it would take place in an acidic solution?

- ○ **A.** $e^- + 2H^+(aq) + MnO_4^-(aq) \rightarrow MnO_2(s) + H_2O(l)$
- ○ **B.** $3e^- + 4H^+(aq) + MnO_4^-(aq) \rightarrow MnO_2(s) + 2H_2O(l)$
- ○ **C.** $e^- + H_2O(l) + MnO_4^-(aq) \rightarrow 2H^+(aq) + MnO_2(s)$
- ○ **D.** $5e^- + 6H^+(aq) + MnO_4^-(aq) \rightarrow MnO_2(s) + 3H_2O(l)$

Question 805

What is the balanced oxidation half reaction as it would take place in an acidic solution?

- ○ **A.** $e^- + 2H^+(aq) + CN^-(aq) \rightarrow CNO^-(aq) + H_2O(l)$
- ○ **B.** $CN^-(aq) + 2H_2O(l) \rightarrow CNO^-(aq) + 4H^+(aq) + 3e^-$
- ○ **C.** $CN^-(aq) + H_2O(l) \rightarrow CNO^-(aq) + H^+(aq) + e^-$
- ○ **D.** $CN^-(aq) + H_2O(l) \rightarrow CNO^-(aq) + 2H^+(aq) + 2e^-$

Question 806

Which of the following is the most probable application of iodometry?

- ○ **A.** To find the molarity of the reducing agent.
- ○ **B.** To find the molarity of the oxidizing agent.
- ○ **C.** To create an electrolytic cell.
- ○ **D.** To synthesize tetrathionate.

Question 807

Which of the following is NOT true regarding a redox titration?

- ○ **A.** At the equivalence point, the voltage of the solution is 0.
- ○ **B.** The equivalence point is where all the moles of the reducing agent have been completely oxidized.
- ○ **C.** The solution of unknown concentration is known as the analyte, and the standard solution is known as the titrant.
- ○ **D.** Either a voltmeter or an indicator can be used to monitor the equivalence point.

Question 808

50.0 mL of 0.200 M Fe^{2+} is titrated with 0.400 M Ce^{2+} in the following reaction:

$$Fe^{2+}(aq) + Ce^{4+}(aq) \rightleftharpoons Ce^{3+}(aq) + Fe^{3+}(aq)$$

At what volume of Ce^{2+} added will the equivalence point be reached?

- ○ **A.** 25 mL
- ○ **B.** 35 mL
- ○ **C.** 50 mL
- ○ **D.** 100 mL

Electrochemical Cells

Question 809

Suppose a galvanic cell operates using the following half-reactions:

Anode:

$$Zn(s) + 4NH_3(g) \rightarrow [Zn(NH_3)_4]^{2+}(aq) + 2e^-$$

Cathode:

$$MnO_2(s) + NH_4^+(aq) + e^- \rightarrow MnO(OH)(s) + NH_3(g)$$

If 3 moles of Zn are oxidized, how many moles of manganese(IV) oxide are reduced?

- ○ **A.** 1.5
- ○ **B.** 3
- ○ **C.** 4.5
- ○ **D.** 6

Question 810

The purpose of a galvanic cell is to:

○ **A.** metal plate.

○ **B.** purify solids.

○ **C.** transduce chemical energy to electrical energy.

○ **D.** allow for oxidation without reduction.

Question 811

Which of the following electrode pairs would cause electrons to flow from right to left if a galvanic cell is depicted?

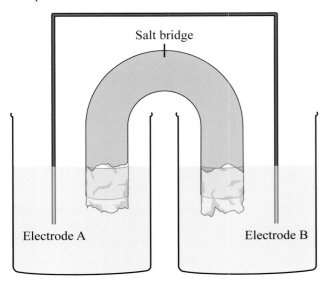

Salt bridge

Electrode A   Electrode B

Standard reduction potential table
(at 25°C, 101 kPa, 1 M)

Half-reaction	Volts
$Li^+ + e^- \rightarrow Li$	−3.04
$Zn^{2+} + 2e^- \rightarrow Zn$	−0.76
$Fe^{2+} + 2e^- \rightarrow Fe$	−0.44
$Ni^{2+} + 2e^- \rightarrow Ni$	−0.26
$Pb^{2+} + 2e^- \rightarrow Pb$	−0.13
$2H^+ + 2e^- \rightarrow H_2$	0.00
$Cu^{2+} + 2e^- \rightarrow Cu$	0.34
$Cu^+ + e^- \rightarrow Cu$	0.52
$Br_2 + 2e^- \rightarrow 2Br^-$	1.07

○ **A.** Electrode A is copper and electrode B is zinc.

○ **B.** Electrode A is zinc and electrode B is silver.

○ **C.** Electrode A is copper and electrode B is silver.

○ **D.** Electrode A is copper and electrode B is gold.

Question 812

Which of the following is the maximum amount of non pressure volume work available from a galvanic cell?

○ **A.** $-\Delta G$

○ **B.** $-\Delta G°$

○ **C.** E

○ **D.** $E°$

Question 813

Which of the following is a possible application of an electrochemical cell?

   I. A voltage source

   II. A pH meter

   III. A device for dissolving a gold bar and electro-plating the ions onto a nickel bar

○ **A.** II only

○ **B.** III only

○ **C.** I and II only

○ **D.** I and III only

Question 814

In an electrolytic cell, the cathode is:

○ **A.** negative and reduction takes place.

○ **B.** negative and oxidation takes place.

○ **C.** positive and reduction takes place.

○ **D.** positive and oxidation takes place.

Question 815

Which of the following statements does NOT accurately describe a Galvanic cell?

○ **A.** Electrodes tend to be strips of conductive material.

○ **B.** The oxidation half reaction takes place at the cathode; the reduction half reaction takes place at the anode.

○ **C.** Each component is present in more than one phase.

○ **D.** A strip of metal together with its electrolyte solution is often times called a half cell.

Question 816

Gel electrophoresis is a common laboratory technique used to separate negatively-charged nucleic acids, such as DNA or RNA, by size. In this technique, an electric field is sent through an agarose gel, with the cathode and anode on opposite sides of the gel. If this technique uses an electrolytic cell, which electrode should the nucleic acid travel towards?

○ **A.** Positively charged cathode

○ **B.** Positively charged anode

○ **C.** Negatively charged cathode

○ **D.** Negatively charged anode

Question 817

While running a polyacrylamide gel of her PCR products, a student observes that the dye band migrates upwards instead of down the gel. Which of the following best explains this result?

○ **A.** The student neglected to incubate the DNA with SDS prior to loading the gel.

○ **B.** The student used too low a concentration of polyacrylamide when making the gel.

○ **C.** The student reversed the anode and cathode of the apparatus used to run the gel.

○ **D.** The student applied a magnetic field opposite the necessary magnetic field when running the gel.

▼

Questions 818–821 use the following table of half-reaction potentials:

An electrolytic cell is constructed with a silver and a zinc electrode immersed in the same aqueous solution. The solution is 1 M in zinc and silver ions. The electrolytic cell is arranged so that the silver electrode is the anode.

Half-reaction	E°, V
$Ag^+ + e^- \rightarrow Ag$	+0.80
$Cd^{2+} + 2e^- \rightarrow Cd$	−0.40
$2F^- \rightarrow F_2 + 2e^-$	−2.87
$2I^- \rightarrow I_2 + 2e^-$	−0.54
$Na^+ + e^- \rightarrow Na$	−2.71
$Se^{2-} \rightarrow Se + 2e^-$	+0.67
$2H_2O \rightarrow O_2 + 4H^+ + 4e^-$	−1.23
$2H_2O + 2e^- \rightarrow H_2 + 2OH^-$	−0.83
$Zn^{2+} + 2e^- \rightarrow Zn$	−0.76

Question 818

What is oxidized in this cell?

○ **A.** The silver electrode

○ **B.** The zinc electrode

○ **C.** The water

○ **D.** The zinc ions

Question 819

What is reduced in this cell?

○ **A.** The zinc electrode

○ **B.** The water

○ **C.** The silver ions

○ **D.** The zinc ions

Question 820

If the silver electrode were replaced by a sodium electrode, and the silver ions in solution replaced by sodium ions, what would happen?

○ **A.** The sodium would be oxidized at the anode and reduced at the cathode, resulting in a layer of sodium metal on the cathode.

○ **B.** The sodium would be oxidized at the anode, but zinc ions would be reduced at the cathode. The result would be the replacement of zinc ions by sodium ions in solution.

○ **C.** Water would be oxidized at the anode, but sodium would be reduced at the cathode. The result would be the replacement of sodium ions in solution by hydrogen ions, accompanied by the release of oxygen gas.

○ **D.** Water would be oxidized at the anode and reduced at the cathode. The result would be the production of oxygen and hydrogen gas.

Question 821

Suppose both electrodes are removed from the original cell and replaced by platinum wires, which can neither be oxidized nor reduced. Likewise, the solution is replaced by pure water. If sufficient voltage is applied , what will the net reaction be?

○ **A.** $H^+ + OH^- \rightarrow H_2O$

○ **B.** $H_2O \rightarrow H^+ + OH^-$

○ **C.** $2H_2O \rightarrow 2H_2 + O_2$

○ **D.** No reaction will take place.

▲

Question 822

Corrosion is the oxidation of a metal. Iron may be coated with tin, zinc, or another metal to protect it against corrosion. If the surface coat on the iron breaks and the metals are exposed to water, corrosion occurs. The standard reduction potentials for tin, zinc, and iron ions are given below.

$$Sn^{2+}(aq) + 2e^- \rightarrow Sn(s) \qquad E° = -0.14 \text{ V}$$
$$Zn^{2+}(aq) + 2e^- \rightarrow Zn(s) \qquad E° = -0.76 \text{ V}$$
$$Fe^{2+}(aq) + 2e^- \rightarrow Fe(s) \qquad E° = -0.44 \text{ V}$$

Which metal, tin or zinc, will prevent the corrosion of iron even after the surface coat is broken?

- ○ **A.** Tin, because tin will oxidize more easily than iron.
- ○ **B.** Tin, because tin will reduce more easily than iron.
- ○ **C.** Zinc, because zinc will oxidize more easily than iron.
- ○ **D.** Zinc, because zinc will reduce more easily than iron.

Question 823

Which of the following is/are strong electrolytes?

    I. Salts
   II. Strong bases
  III. Weak acids

- ○ **A.** I only
- ○ **B.** I and II only
- ○ **C.** I and III only
- ○ **D.** I, II, and III

Question 824

Which of the following is a non-electrolyte?

- ○ **A.** Sucrose
- ○ **B.** Ammonia
- ○ **C.** Sodium chloride
- ○ **D.** Potassium hydroxide

Question 825

Hydrochloric acid contains:

- ○ **A.** covalent bonds and is a nonelectrolyte.
- ○ **B.** covalent bonds and is a strong electrolyte.
- ○ **C.** ionic bonds and is a weak electrolyte.
- ○ **D.** ionic bonds and is a strong electrolyte.

Question 826

Which of the following statements is true?

- ○ **A.** Strong electrolytes are highly soluble in water.
- ○ **B.** Weak electrolytes are insoluble in water.
- ○ **C.** The extent to which an electrolyte dissolves in solution does not indicate whether it is strong or weak.
- ○ **D.** Most electrolytes are insoluble in water.

Question 827

Potassium oxide contains:

- ○ **A.** covalent bonds and is a nonelectrolyte.
- ○ **B.** covalent bonds and is a strong electrolyte.
- ○ **C.** ionic bonds and is a weak electrolyte.
- ○ **D.** ionic bonds and is a strong electrolyte.

Question 828

In a galvanic cell, anions and cations move through the salt bridge, while electrons move through the load. In a galvanic cell:

- ○ **A.** anions and electrons move toward the anode.
- ○ **B.** anions and electrons move toward the cathode.
- ○ **C.** anions move toward the cathode, and electrons move toward the anode.
- ○ **D.** anions move toward the anode, and electrons move toward the cathode.

Question 829

An electron has a higher potential energy when it is at which electrode in a galvanic cell?

- ○ **A.** The anode because electrons flow toward the anode.
- ○ **B.** The anode because electrons flow away from the anode.
- ○ **C.** The cathode because electrons flow toward the cathode.
- ○ **D.** The cathode because electrons flow away from the cathode.

Question 830

If the image depicts an electrolytic cell where electrode A is gold and electrode B is silver, which of the following is true?

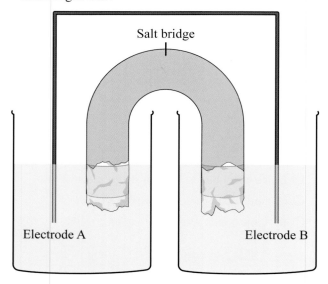

Salt bridge

Electrode A   Electrode B

Standard reduction potential table
(at 25°C, 101 kPa, 1 M)

Half-reaction	Volts
$Li^+ + e^- \rightarrow Li$	−3.04
$Zn^{2+} + 2e^- \rightarrow Zn$	−0.76
$Fe^{2+} + 2e^- \rightarrow Fe$	−0.44
$Ni^{2+} + 2e^- \rightarrow Ni$	−0.26
$Pb^{2+} + 2e^- \rightarrow Pb$	−0.13
$2H^+ + 2e^- \rightarrow H_2$	0.00
$Cu^{2+} + 2e^- \rightarrow Cu$	0.34
$Cu^+ + e^- \rightarrow Cu$	0.52
$Br_2 + 2e^- \rightarrow 2Br^-$	1.07

- **A.** The silver gets plated in gold.
- **B.** The gold gets plated with silver.
- **C.** The reduction potential is insufficient to move electrons.
- **D.** It would depend on the voltage of the battery.

Question 831

In an experiment, a solid zinc strip is placed in a copper sulfate solution. The strip dissolves and solid copper forms in its place. In a second experiment, a beaker of one molar copper sulfate solution is connected to a beaker of one molar zinc sulfate solution by a salt bridge. A zinc strip is placed in the zinc sulfate solution and a copper strip is placed in the copper sulfate solution. What happens when the strips are connected by a copper wire?

- **A.** Electrons flow from the cathode in the zinc sulfate solution to the anode in the copper sulfate solution.
- **B.** Electrons flow from the anode in the zinc sulfate solution to the cathode in the copper sulfate solution.
- **C.** Electrons flow from the cathode in the copper sulfate solution to the anode in the zinc sulfate solution.
- **D.** Electrons flow from the anode in the copper sulfate solution to the cathode in the zinc sulfate solution.

Question 832

A galvanic cell is created using silver and zinc electrodes, a 1.0 M aqueous silver solution, and a 0.1 M aqueous zinc solution. The reduction half reactions for silver and zinc are:

$$Ag^+(aq) + e^- \rightarrow Ag \qquad E° = 0.80 \text{ V}$$
$$Zn^{2+}(aq) + 2e^- \rightarrow Zn(s) \qquad E° = -0.76 \text{ V}$$

What is the EMF for this cell?

- **A.** 1.50 V
- **B.** 1.53 V
- **C.** 1.56 V
- **D.** 1.59 V

Question 833

Consider an electrochemical cell that utilizes lithium and zinc:

$$Li^+ + e^- \rightarrow Li \qquad E° = -3.05 \text{ V}$$
$$Zn^{2+} + 2e^- \rightarrow Zn \qquad E° = -0.76 \text{ V}$$

What is the standard voltage for this cell?

- **A.** 1.90 V
- **B.** 2.29 V
- **C.** 3.81 V
- **D.** 5.34 V

Question 834

A spontaneous redox reaction is indicated by:

- ○ **A.** a positive emf.
- ○ **B.** a negative emf.
- ○ **C.** a positive enthalpy.
- ○ **D.** a negative enthalpy.

Question 835

A particular voltaic cell is made with aqueous solutions in both half cells. The emf of the cell depends upon all of the following EXCEPT:

- ○ **A.** the temperature.
- ○ **B.** the concentrations of half cell reactants and products.
- ○ **C.** the specific reactions occurring in the half cells.
- ○ **D.** the volume of solutions used in each half cell.

Question 836

The emf of a galvanic cell depends upon all the following EXCEPT:

- ○ **A.** the temperature of the solutions in the half cells.
- ○ **B.** the concentrations of the solutions in the half cells.
- ○ **C.** the reactions in the solutions in the half cells.
- ○ **D.** the length of the wire connecting the half cells.

▼

Use the Nernst equation in the form given below to help answer questions 837–840.

$$E = E^\circ - \frac{0.06}{n} \log Q$$

Question 837

A concentration cell is created using silver electrodes and an aqueous silver solution. The reduction half reaction for silver is:

$$Ag^+(aq) + e^- \rightarrow Ag(s) \qquad E^\circ = 0.80$$

What value should be plugged in for E° to derive the E for the concentration cell?

- ○ **A.** 0
- ○ **B.** +0.80
- ○ **C.** −0.76
- ○ **D.** +1.60

Question 838

A concentration cell is created using silver electrodes and an aqueous silver solution. The reduction half reaction for silver is:

$$Ag^+(aq) + e^- \rightarrow Ag(s) \qquad E^\circ = 0.80$$

If the silver ion concentration at the cathode is 1 M, which of the following could be the silver ion concentration at the anode in a galvanic cell?

- ○ **A.** 0.1 M
- ○ **B.** 1 M
- ○ **C.** 10 M
- ○ **D.** A positive emf cannot be achieved because the oxidation and reduction potentials will cancel.

Question 839

A concentration cell is created using zinc electrodes and an aqueous zinc solution. The reduction half reaction for zinc is:

$$Zn^{2+}(aq) + 2e^- \rightarrow Zn(s) \qquad E^\circ = -0.76$$

If the zinc ion concentration at the cathode is 1 M, which of the following could be the zinc ion concentration at the anode in a galvanic cell?

- ○ **A.** 0.1 M
- ○ **B.** 1 M
- ○ **C.** 10 M
- ○ **D.** A positive emf cannot be achieved because the oxidation and reduction potentials will cancel.

Question 840

Which of the following describes Q in the Nernst equation for a concentration cell made with silver electrodes and an aqueous silver solution?

$$Ag^+ + e^- \rightarrow Ag \qquad E^\circ = 0.80$$

- ○ **A.** $[Ag^+]_{cathode}/[Ag^+]_{anode}$
- ○ **B.** $[Ag^+]_{anode}/[Ag^+]_{cathode}$
- ○ **C.** $[Ag]_{anode}[Ag^+]_{cathode}/[Ag]_{cathode}[Ag^+]_{anode}$
- ○ **D.** $[Ag]_{cathode}[Ag^+]_{anode}/[Ag]_{anode}[Ag^+]_{cathode}$

Question 841

A pH meter can be thought of as a hydronium concentration cell. The reference half-cell is kept at a pH of 2.0. The other half-cell consists of a platinum probe placed into the sample being tested. If electrons flow from the reference half-cell into the sample, which of the following is true? (The applicable half-reaction is: $2H^+ + 2e^- \rightarrow H_2$)

○ **A.** The probe is the anode, and the sample solution has a pH less than 2.0.

○ **B.** The probe is the anode, and the sample solution has a pH greater than 2.0.

○ **C.** The probe is the cathode, and the sample solution has a pH less than 2.0.

○ **D.** The probe is the cathode, and the sample solution has a pH greater than 2.0.

Question 842

Attempts to obtain solid sodium by the electrolysis of aqueous sodium chloride inevitably fail, producing hydrogen gas at the cathode rather than sodium. Which of the following is a possible explanation?

○ **A.** Chlorine ions are oxidized more easily than sodium.

○ **B.** Chlorine is reduced more easily than sodium ions.

○ **C.** Water is oxidized more easily than sodium.

○ **D.** Water is reduced more easily than sodium ions.

Question 843

Suppose an electrolytic cell utilizes the following half-reactions:

Anode: $Mg \rightarrow Mg^{2+} + 2e^-$

Cathode: $Cu^+ + e^- \rightarrow Cu$

How many moles of magnesium need to be oxidized in order to reduce three moles of copper ions?

○ **A.** ⅔

○ **B.** 3/2

○ **C.** 3

○ **D.** 6

Question 844

Electrolytic cells are involved in all of the following situations EXCEPT:

○ **A.** causing metal to plate onto an electrode.

○ **B.** recharging an electrochemical cell.

○ **C.** powering an electrical device.

○ **D.** decomposing a salt into its constituent elements.

Question 845

Many electrolytic cells involve reactions with positive free energies of reaction. How is this possible?

○ **A.** Chemical thermodynamics does not apply to electrical systems.

○ **B.** The entropy of free electrons is not accounted for in reaction free energies.

○ **C.** The nonspontaneous reactions are driven by spontaneous reactions.

○ **D.** Since electrons are negatively charged, the flow of free energy is reversed.

Question 846

Which of the following is/are a possible application of an electrolytic cell?

   I. A voltage source

   II. A pH meter

   III. A device for dissolving a gold bar and electroplating the ions onto a nickel bar

○ **A.** II only

○ **B.** III only

○ **C.** I and II only

○ **D.** I and III only

Questions 847–850 use the following table of half-reaction potentials:

Half-reaction	$E°$, V
$Ag^+ + e^- \rightarrow Ag$	+0.80
$Cd^{2+} + 2e^- \rightarrow Cd$	−0.40
$2F^- \rightarrow F_2 + 2e^-$	−2.87
$2I^- \rightarrow I_2 + 2e^-$	−0.54
$Na^+ + e^- \rightarrow Na$	−2.71
$Se^{2-} \rightarrow Se + 2e^-$	+0.67
$2H_2O \rightarrow O_2 + 4H^+ + 4e^-$	−1.23
$2H_2O + 2e^- \rightarrow H_2 + 2OH^-$	−0.83
$Zn^{2+} + 2e^- \rightarrow Zn$	−0.76

An electrolytic cell is constructed with a silver and a zinc electrode immersed in the same aqueous solution. The solution is 1 M in zinc and silver ions. The electrolytic cell is arranged so that the silver electrode is the anode.

Question 847

What is the net reaction for this cell?

- **A.** $2Ag^+ + Zn \rightarrow 2Ag + Zn^{2+}$
- **B.** $2Ag + Zn^{2+} \rightarrow 2Ag^+ + Zn$
- **C.** $4Ag^+ + 2H_2O \rightarrow 4Ag + O_2 + 4H^+$
- **D.** No net chemical reaction takes place.

Question 848

What is the minimum theoretical voltage necessary to run this electrolytic cell (neglect the overvoltage)?

- **A.** −1.56 V
- **B.** 0 V
- **C.** 0.43 V
- **D.** 1.56 V

Question 849

Suppose a cell was constructed out of two half-cells, one made of a zinc electrode in 1 M aqueous zinc nitrate, and the other a silver electrode in 1 M aqueous silver nitrate. The two electrodes are connected by a salt bridge. An external power supply is attached in such a way as to make the silver electrode the anode. Assume the nitrate is neither oxidized nor reduced. Which of the following would most likely occur?

- **A.** Zinc would be oxidized at the anode, and silver ions would be reduced at the cathode.
- **B.** Silver would be oxidized at the anode, and zinc ions would be reduced at the cathode.
- **C.** Silver would be oxidized at the anode, and water would be reduced at the cathode, accompanied by the production of hydrogen gas.
- **D.** No reaction would occur, since the resulting cell voltage would be negative.

Question 850

The cell described in the previous question is:

- **A.** a galvanic cell.
- **B.** an electrolytic cell.
- **C.** a concentration cell.
- **D.** a fuel cell.

Question 851

If a current of 3 amperes is used to reduce Cu^{2+} to Cu, how many seconds will it take for 5 grams of copper to be reduced? (The charge on one mole of electrons is equal to 96,485 C.)

- **A.** $\dfrac{(5)(3)(96,485)}{(63.5)}$
- **B.** $\dfrac{(5)(96,485)}{(3)(63.5)}$
- **C.** $\dfrac{(5)(2)(96,485)}{(3)(63.5)}$
- **D.** $\dfrac{(5)(96,485)}{(2)(3)(63.5)}$

Question 852

A solution of $ZnSO_4(aq)$ is subjected to a 10 A current flow. How long does the current need to be sustained in order to generate 130.0 g of solid zinc? ($F = 96,485$ C/mole e^-)

- **A.** 8,300 seconds
- **B.** 19,200 seconds
- **C.** 39,000 seconds
- **D.** 48,200 seconds

Question 853

Suppose an electrolytic cell utilizes the following cathode reaction to silver-plate a piece of jewelry:

$$Ag^+ + e^- \rightarrow Ag \qquad E° = +0.80 \text{ V}$$

If 0.108 grams of silver is to be plated using a 2.0 A current, for how long should the cell be run? (One Faraday = 96,485 C/mol e^-.)

- **A.** 48 seconds
- **B.** 108 seconds
- **C.** 3 minutes
- **D.** 17 minutes

Question 854

A cup is plated with gold in an electrolytic process. The reduction half reaction for gold is:

$$Au^{3+}(aq) + 3e^- \rightarrow Au(s) \qquad E° = 1.50$$

If the current is 2 amps and the plating lasts for 30 seconds, what mass of gold is deposited onto the cup? (Faraday's constant is 96,500 C/mole e⁻.)

- ○ **A.** $\dfrac{(197)(2)(30)}{(96,500)(3)}$

- ○ **B.** $\dfrac{(197)(2)(30)(3)}{(96,500)}$

- ○ **C.** $\dfrac{(197)(3)(30)}{(96,500)(2)}$

- ○ **D.** $\dfrac{(197)(3)(96,500)}{(30)(2)}$

Question 855

One spoon is plated with gold and another with copper. If a current generator is used to plate both spoons at a constant current, which spoon will acquire 1 gram of plating the fastest? The reduction half reactions are:

$$Au^{3+}(aq) + 3e^- \rightarrow Au(s) \qquad E° = 1.50$$
$$Cu^{2+}(aq) + 2e^- \rightarrow Cu(s) \qquad E° = 0.34$$

- ○ **A.** The copper spoon because copper has a lower emf.
- ○ **B.** The copper spoon because copper reduces with fewer electrons.
- ○ **C.** The gold spoon because gold is heavier.
- ○ **D.** The gold spoon because gold reduces with more electrons.

Question 856

Car batteries act as:

- ○ **A.** galvanic cells.
- ○ **B.** electrolytic cells.
- ○ **C.** electrolytic cells when discharging, but galvanic cells when charging.
- ○ **D.** galvanic cells while discharging, but electrolytic cells when charging.

Question 857

In an ordinary lead automobile battery, lead anodes and lead(IV) oxide cathodes are placed directly in a solution of sulfuric acid. The half-reactions are:

$$Pb(s) + SO_4^{2-} \rightarrow PbSO_4(s) + 2e^-$$
$$PbO_2(s) + H_2SO_4(aq) + 2H^+ + 2e^- \rightarrow PbSO_4(s) + 2H_2O(l)$$

Why is a salt bridge unnecessary?

- ○ **A.** Lead sulfate is insoluble in water, so it does not contribute additional ions to solution.
- ○ **B.** The acidic conditions would dissolve a salt bridge.
- ○ **C.** Lead and lead(IV) oxide are insoluble in water, so they do not have to be kept in separate half-cells to prevent them from reacting.
- ○ **D.** The electrons generated by the battery are consumed by the electrical equipment of the car.

Question 858

Which of the following options describe(s) a property of nickel-cadmium batteries?

   I. Rechargeable

   II. Acts as a galvanic cell

   III. Acts as a electrolytic cell

- ○ **A.** I only
- ○ **B.** I and II only
- ○ **C.** I and III only
- ○ **D.** I, II, and III

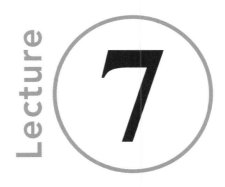

Lecture

7

Questions 859–1001

Acids and Bases

Acids and Bases
Water and Acid-Base Chemistry
Titration
Salts and Buffers

Acids and Bases

Question 859

Which of the following is NOT a definition of an Arrhenius acid?

- ○ **A.** An Arrhenius acid is a substance that increases the H^+ concentration in aqueous solution.
- ○ **B.** An Arrhenius acid is a substance that increases the pH of an aqueous solution.
- ○ **C.** An Arrhenius acid is a substance that increases the pOH of an aqueous solution.
- ○ **D.** An Arrhenius acid is a substance that decreases the OH^- concentration in an aqueous solution.

Question 860

Which of the following is/are Arrhenius acids?

- I. HCl
- II. CH_3CH_2OH
- III. BF_3

- ○ **A.** I only
- ○ **B.** III only
- ○ **C.** I and II only
- ○ **D.** I, II, and III

Question 861

A warning sign in an industrial laboratory says "Do not store acids with bases! Acids go in cabinet A, bases in cabinet B." The definition of acid and base that this sign is using is most likely:

- ○ **A.** the Arrhenius definition, since unlike the Brønsted-Lowry and Lewis definitions, it is not possible for a substance to be sometimes an acid and sometimes a base.
- ○ **B.** the Brønsted-Lowry definition, since it is the definition most commonly used.
- ○ **C.** the Lewis definition, since it involves reactions between substances.
- ○ **D.** the Lewis definition, since it can be applied to almost all substances.

Question 862

Which of the following can act as Brønsted-Lowry acids in some circumstances?

- I. HCl
- II. CH_3CH_2OH
- III. BF_3

- ○ **A.** I only
- ○ **B.** III only
- ○ **C.** I and II only
- ○ **D.** I, II, and III

Question 863

In the following reaction, which substance is acting as a Brønsted-Lowry acid?

$$NH_3 + H^- \rightarrow NH_2^- + H_2$$

- ○ **A.** NH_3
- ○ **B.** H^-
- ○ **C.** NH_4^+
- ○ **D.** NH_2^-

Question 864

Which of the following is NOT possible?

- ○ **A.** A Lewis acid that is not a Brønsted-Lowry acid.
- ○ **B.** A Brønsted-Lowry acid that is not a Lewis acid.
- ○ **C.** A substance that is sometimes a Lewis acid and sometimes a Lewis base.
- ○ **D.** A substance that is sometimes a Brønsted-Lowry acid and sometimes a Brønsted-Lowry base.

Question 865

Which of the following molecules is a Lewis base?

- ○ **A.** CH_4
- ○ **B.** NH_3
- ○ **C.** $AlCl_3$
- ○ **D.** BH_3

Question 866

Which of the following molecules could NOT be a Lewis base?

- ○ **A.** $NH(CH_3)_2$
- ○ **B.** NH_4^+
- ○ **C.** H_2O
- ○ **D.** OH^-

Question 867

Consider the following reaction:

$$CaH_2 + 2BH_3 \rightarrow 2BH_4^- + Ca^{2+}$$

What type of reaction is this?

- **A.** Lewis acid/Lewis base
- **B.** Brønsted-Lowry acid/base
- **C.** Oxidation/reduction
- **D.** Combustion

Question 868

Which of the following can act as Lewis acids in some circumstances?

   I. HCl

   II. CH_3CH_2OH

   III. BF_3

- **A.** I only
- **B.** III only
- **C.** I and II only
- **D.** I, II, and III

Question 869

Consider the following reaction:

$$Fe^{3+} + 6H_2O \rightarrow [Fe(H_2O)_6]^{3+}$$

In this reaction, water acts as a/an:

- **A.** Lewis acid.
- **B.** Lewis base.
- **C.** oxidizing agent.
- **D.** reducing agent.

Question 870

Which of the following is necessary to transform the nitrite ion (NO_2^-) into nitrous acid (HNO_2)?

- **A.** An acid
- **B.** A base
- **C.** An oxidizing agent
- **D.** A reducing agent

Question 871

If HA is a stronger acid than H_3O^+:

- **A.** HA will transfer its proton to H_2O more effectively than H_3O^+ will transfer its proton to A^-.
- **B.** H_3O^+ will transfer its proton to H_2O more effectively than HA will transfer its proton to A^-.
- **C.** HA will transfer its proton to A^- more effectively than H_3O^+ will transfer its proton to H_2O.
- **D.** HA will transfer its proton to H_3O^+ more effectively than H_2O will transfer its proton to A^-.

Question 872

Which of the following is the strongest acid?

- **A.** HF
- **B.** HCl
- **C.** HBr
- **D.** HI

Question 873

What is a hydride?

- **A.** A metal atom without a hydration shell.
- **B.** Compounds that have been formed by the removal of water.
- **C.** Compounds containing only two elements where one of the elements is hydrogen.
- **D.** Compounds containing hydrogen.

Question 874

Which of the following oxyacids is the strongest acid in aqueous solution?

- **A.** HClO
- **B.** $HClO_2$
- **C.** $HClO_3$
- **D.** $HClO_4$

Question 875

Rank the following oxyacids from strongest acid to weakest acid in aqueous solution?

   I. HClO

   II. HBrO

   III. HIO

- **A.** I, II, III
- **B.** II, III, I
- **C.** III, II, I
- **D.** III, I, II

Question 876

Why are oxyacids with more oxygens around the central atom stronger acids?

- ○ **A.** Because each oxygen can take on a proton
- ○ **B.** Because oxygens are electron withdrawing and can neutralize hydroxide ions
- ○ **C.** Because oxygens around the central atom strengthen the bond between the oxygen and the acidic hydrogen
- ○ **D.** Because oxygens around the central atom withdraw electrons, increasing the polarity of the bond between the oxygen and the acidic hydrogen

Question 877

Which of the following is generally true concerning hydrides (other than NH_3)?

- ○ **A.** All hydrides are acidic or neutral.
- ○ **B.** All hydrides are basic or neutral.
- ○ **C.** Metal hydrides are acidic or neutral, while nonmetal hydrides are basic or neutral.
- ○ **D.** Metal hydrides are basic or neutral, while nonmetal hydrides are acidic or neutral.

Question 878

Which of the following is NOT a strong base in aqueous solution?

- ○ **A.** LiH
- ○ **B.** CaH_2
- ○ **C.** H_2
- ○ **D.** KH

Question 879

Which of the following statements is/are true?

   I. NaH is a stronger base than NaOH.
   II. CaH_2 is a stronger base than $Ca(OH)_2$.
   III. HCl is a stronger acid than HClO.

- ○ **A.** I only
- ○ **B.** I and II only
- ○ **C.** I and III only
- ○ **D.** I, II, and III

Question 880

Which of the following is the weakest acid?

- ○ **A.** Hydrochloric acid
- ○ **B.** Sulfuric acid
- ○ **C.** Nitric acid
- ○ **D.** Formic acid

Question 881

Which of the following is NOT true?

- ○ **A.** Strong acids have weak conjugate bases.
- ○ **B.** Weak acids have strong conjugate bases.
- ○ **C.** The stronger the acid, the weaker its conjugate base.
- ○ **D.** The weaker the acid, the stronger the conjugate base.

Question 882

Which of the following is the weakest acid?

- ○ **A.** $HClO_4$
- ○ **B.** H_3O^+
- ○ **C.** HBr
- ○ **D.** HNO_3

Question 883

Which of the following is the weakest base?

- ○ **A.** H^-
- ○ **B.** Na_2O
- ○ **C.** N_3^-
- ○ **D.** OH^-

Question 884

Which of the following is the weakest base in aqueous solution?

- ○ **A.** KOH
- ○ **B.** $Ca(OH)_2$
- ○ **C.** $Mg(OH)_2$
- ○ **D.** OH^-

Question 885

Place the following in order from strongest to weakest base?

   I. ClO^-
   II. H_2O
   III. Cl^-

- ○ **A.** I, II, III
- ○ **B.** I, III, II
- ○ **C.** II, I, III
- ○ **D.** III, I, II

Question 886

Which of the following oxides forms a base when dissolved in water?

- ○ **A.** K_2O
- ○ **B.** CO_2
- ○ **C.** SO_2
- ○ **D.** NO_2

Question 887

Hydrofluoric acid is a weak acid ($pK_a = 3.1$). In terms of its ionization in water, fluoride is:

- ○ **A.** a weak acid.
- ○ **B.** a weak base.
- ○ **C.** a strong acid.
- ○ **D.** a strong base.

Question 888

Benzoic acid is a weak acid with a pK_a of 4.19. Its conjugate, the benzoate ion, is:

- ○ **A.** a strong acid.
- ○ **B.** a strong base.
- ○ **C.** a weak acid.
- ○ **D.** a weak base.

Question 889

What is the conjugate base of ammonia?

- ○ **A.** NH_2^-
- ○ **B.** NH_3
- ○ **C.** NH_4^+
- ○ **D.** OH^-

Question 890

What is the conjugate base of HCO_3^-?

- ○ **A.** H_2CO_3
- ○ **B.** CO_3^{2-}
- ○ **C.** H_2O
- ○ **D.** OH^-

Question 891

What is the conjugate base of H_3O^+?

- ○ **A.** H_2O
- ○ **B.** H_3O^+
- ○ **C.** OH^-
- ○ **D.** H_2O_2

Question 892

What is the conjugate acid of phosphoric acid?

- ○ **A.** $H_2PO_4^-$
- ○ **B.** H_3PO_4
- ○ **C.** $H_4PO_4^+$
- ○ **D.** H_3O^+

Question 893

Which of the following is NOT true concerning conjugate bases?

- ○ **A.** Every acid has a conjugate base.
- ○ **B.** The conjugate base of a Brønsted-Lowry acid is that acid minus its acidic proton.
- ○ **C.** Some conjugate bases are acidic.
- ○ **D.** OH^- is the conjugate base of H_3O^+.

Question 894

Which of the compounds has the largest base strength?

- ○ **A.** IO_3^-
- ○ **B.** NO_2^-
- ○ **C.** $C_6H_5COO^-$
- ○ **D.** CH_3COOH

Question 895

Researchers interested in identifying an unknown compound are able to determine that the K_b of the compound's conjugate base at 25°C is 2.5×10^{-11}. What is the identity of the unknown compound?

- ○ **A.** Iodic acid ($K_a = 1.6 \times 10^{-1}$)
- ○ **B.** Nitrous acid ($K_a = 4.0 \times 10^{-4}$)
- ○ **C.** Acetic acid ($K_a = 1.76 \times 10^{-5}$)
- ○ **D.** Cannot be determined

Question 896

H^+ represents the acidic proton on conjugate base X^-. Which of the following tends to decrease the acidity of HX?

- ○ **A.** A polar H–X bond.
- ○ **B.** A strong H–X bond.
- ○ **C.** A stable conjugate base X^-.
- ○ **D.** A high temperature.

Question 897

The definition of pH is:

- A. $\log[H^+]$.
- B. $-\log[H^+]$.
- C. 7.
- D. the number of hydrogen ions in solution.

Question 898

Which of the following defines a neutral solution?

- A. $pH = 7$
- B. $[H^+] = [OH^-]$
- C. $[H^+] = 0$
- D. A solution where acids do not donate protons and bases do not accept protons

Question 899

What is the pH of a solution with a hydrogen ion concentration of 3.0×10^{-4} M?

- A. 3.0
- B. 3.5
- C. 4.0
- D. 4.5

Question 900

Compared to a solution with a pH of 5, how many H^+ ions are in a solution with a pH of 3?

- A. 4 times as many
- B. 10 times as many
- C. 20 times as many
- D. 100 times as many

Question 901

What is the pH of a 0.01 M solution of KOH?

- A. 0.01
- B. 1.0
- C. 2.0
- D. 12.0

Question 902

What is the pOH of a 0.01 M solution of KOH?

- A. 0.01
- B. 1.0
- C. 2.0
- D. 12.0

Question 903

What is the hydrogen ion concentration in a solution with a pH of 11.26?

- A. 5.5×10^{-12}
- B. 5.5×10^{-11}
- C. 5.5×10^{-10}
- D. 1.12×10^{-6}

Question 904

1 mL of a strong acid solution has a pH of 2.3. It is diluted with water to make a 100 mL solution. What is the new pH?

- A. 0.023
- B. 2.3
- C. 4.3
- D. 230

Question 905

What is the pH of a 0.1 M solution of acetic acid? ($pK_a = 4.74$)

- A. 1.0
- B. 2.9
- C. 11.1
- D. 13.0

Question 906

Substance X is amphiprotic with a $pK_a = 5.7$. Which of the following is true about the pH of a 3.0 M solution of substance X?

- A. The pH is less than 7.
- B. The pH is 7.
- C. The pH is more than 7.
- D. It is impossible to determine anything about the pH without more information.

Question 907

Given the pK_a table below, which of the following choices is the strongest base?

Acid	pK_a
HSCN	−1.8
HBF$_4$	0.5
HIO	10.5

- A. SCN^-
- B. BF_4^-
- C. IO^-
- D. Cannot determine from the information provided

Question 908

Which of the following pK_as would be indicative of a weak acid?

    I. −3.0

    II. 4.5

    III. 11.2

○ **A.** I only

○ **B.** II only

○ **C.** I and II only

○ **D.** II and III only

Question 909

Acetic acid has a pK_a of 4.74. What is the pK_b of the acetate ion?

○ **A.** 2.26

○ **B.** 4.74

○ **C.** 9.26

○ **D.** Cannot be determined from the information given

Question 910

Hydrocyanic acid has a pK_a of 9.31. What is the pK_b of the cyanide ion?

○ **A.** 2.31

○ **B.** 4.69

○ **C.** 9.31

○ **D.** Cannot be determined from the information given

Question 911

The pK_a of the amphoteric hydrogen carbonate ion is 10.25. What is the pK_b of this ion?

○ **A.** 3.25

○ **B.** 3.75

○ **C.** 10.25

○ **D.** Cannot be determined from the information given

Question 912

Which of the following factors determine the percent ionization of an acid?

    I. Temperature of solution

    II. Identity of acid

    III. Concentration of another acid

○ **A.** II only

○ **B.** I and II only

○ **C.** II and III only

○ **D.** I, II, and III

Question 913

Which of the following is true concerning the percent dissociation of an acid?

○ **A.** Percent dissociation increases with concentration.

○ **B.** Percent dissociation is 100% for strong acids regardless of concentration.

○ **C.** Percent dissociation typically decreases as temperature increases.

○ **D.** Percent dissociation is greater for stronger acids.

Question 914

Which of the following techniques could be used to find the pK_a of a weak acid?

    I. Measure the amount of base needed to neutralize the acid.

    II. Measure the pH of a given concentration of the acid.

    III. Find the pK_b of its conjugate base.

○ **A.** I only

○ **B.** I and II only

○ **C.** II and III only

○ **D.** I, II, and III

Question 915

Hydroiodic acid has a much higher K_a than hydrochloric acid. In aqueous solution, however, equal concentrations of each produce essentially the same pH. Which of the following is the most reasonable explanation for this observation?

○ **A.** Hydroiodic acid is less soluble in water than hydrochloric acid.

○ **B.** Both acids are much weaker than water, so essentially no dissociation takes place.

○ **C.** Both acids are much stronger than water, so dissociation is essentially 100% in both cases.

○ **D.** Both acids are much stronger than hydronium, so dissociation is essentially 100% in both cases.

Question 916

Hydroiodic acid has a much higher K_a than hydrochloric acid. In aqueous solution equal concentrations of each produce essentially the same pH. However, in acetic acid, hydroiodic acid produces a lower pH. Which of the following is the most reasonable explanation for this observation?

- ○ **A.** Hydroiodic acid is a stronger acid than acetic acid.
- ○ **B.** The conjugate base of hydrochloric acid is a stronger base than water.
- ○ **C.** Acetic acid is a weaker base than water.
- ○ **D.** Acetic acid is a stronger base than water.

Question 917

Which of the following is NOT true of diprotic acids?

- ○ **A.** It is always easier to remove the first proton than the second.
- ○ **B.** On a titration curve for a polyprotic acid, there is one equivalence point for each acidic proton.
- ○ **C.** In concentrated solutions, the second proton does not affect the pH.
- ○ **D.** The K_a values increase for successive acidic protons on a single polyprotic acid.

Question 918

The K_a for HSO_4^- is 1.2×10^{-2}. At a pH of about 2, the HSO_4^- concentration is about equal to the concentration of:

- ○ **A.** H_2SO_4.
- ○ **B.** SO_4.
- ○ **C.** H^+.
- ○ **D.** it depends upon the concentration of HSO_4 because the percent dissociation changes with concentration.

Question 919

Propanol has a much higher K_a than ethane. In an aqueous solution, however, equal concentrations of each produce essentially the same pH. Which of the following is a reasonable explanation for this observation?

- ○ **A.** Propanol is less soluble than ethane in water.
- ○ **B.** Both acids are much weaker than water, so essentially no dissociation takes place.
- ○ **C.** Both acids are much stronger than water, so dissociation is essentially 100% in both cases.
- ○ **D.** Both acids are much stronger than hydronium, so dissociation is essentially 100% in both cases.

Water and Acid-Base Chemistry

Question 920

Water is capable of autoionization due to the molecule's:

- ○ **A.** ability to act as an amphoteric substance.
- ○ **B.** large heat capacity.
- ○ **C.** two lone pairs of electrons.
- ○ **D.** ability to hydrogen bond with itself.

Question 921

The autoionization of water (shown below) is an endothermic reaction.

$$2H_2O \rightarrow H_3O^+ + OH^-$$

As the temperature of pure water increases, the pH:

- ○ **A.** decreases because $[H^+]$ increases.
- ○ **B.** increases because $[OH^-]$ increases.
- ○ **C.** increases because $[H^+]$ increases.
- ○ **D.** remains at 7 because $[H^+]$ equals $[OH^-]$ even after an equilibrium shift.

Question 922

Which of the following reactions would occur in an aqueous solution upon the addition of a weak acid, HA?

　I. $HA + H_2O \rightleftharpoons A^+ + H_3O^+$
　II. $A^+ + H_2O \rightleftharpoons HA + OH^-$
　III. $H_2O + H_2O \rightleftharpoons H_3O^+ + OH^-$

- ○ **A.** I only
- ○ **B.** I and II only
- ○ **C.** I and III only
- ○ **D.** I, II, and III

Question 923

Which of the following is true of the equilibrium for the autoionization of water (shown below)?

$$2H_2O \leftrightarrow H_3O^+ + OH^-$$

- ○ **A.** The equilibrium lies slightly to the left.
- ○ **B.** The equilibrium lies far to the left.
- ○ **C.** The equilibrium lies far to the right.
- ○ **D.** The equilibrium is balanced evenly between the left and the right.

LECTURE 7

Researchers heated pure water in a vessel and recorded the pH at varying temperatures. Data are shown in the table below.

Temperature (°C)	pH
10	7.27
20	7.08
25	7.00
30	6.92
40	6.77

Question 924

Water at 30°C is:

○ **A.** neutral.

○ **B.** more acidic than water at 10°C.

○ **C.** has a smaller pOH than water at 20°C.

○ **D.** contains less hydronium ions than water at 25°C.

Question 925

The researchers later sought to record the pOH at every temperature level. Which results are most likely?

○ **A.** pOH will increase as temperature increases.

○ **B.** pOH will remain the same.

○ **C.** pOH will decrease as temperature increases.

○ **D.** This cannot be determined without more information.

Question 926

The autoionization of water (see below) is an endothermic reaction. As the temperature of pure water increases, its K_w is expected to:

$$H_2O + H_2O \rightleftharpoons H_3O^+ + OH^-$$

○ **A.** increase.

○ **B.** remain the same.

○ **C.** decrease.

○ **D.** be unable to be determined.

Question 927

0.001 M HCl is added to a beaker of pure water at 25°C. What is the pOH of the resulting solution?

○ **A.** 3

○ **B.** 7

○ **C.** 11

○ **D.** 14

Question 928

Acetic acid is a weak acid with a K_a of 1.76×10^{-5} at 25°C. What is the K_b of the acetate ion at 25°C?

○ **A.** 1.76×10^{-5}

○ **B.** 1.34×10^{-9}

○ **C.** 5.68×10^{-10}

○ **D.** Cannot be determined

Question 929

What is the acid dissociation constant (K_a) of water?

○ **A.** 1.0×10^{-14}

○ **B.** 1.8×10^{-16}

○ **C.** 1

○ **D.** 10

Question 930

A glass of pure water sits at room temperature. Which of the following is true?

○ **A.** There is about one hydrated H^+ for every one million water molecules in the glass.

○ **B.** There are roughly equal numbers of hydrated H^+ ions and water molecules in the glass.

○ **C.** There are roughly equal numbers of hydrated OH^- ions and water molecules in the glass.

○ **D.** The total number of hydrated H^+ ions and OH^- ions exceeds the total number of water molecules.

Question 931

The K_w of pure water at 40°C is 2.916×10^{-14}. What is the pH of pure water at this temperature?

○ **A.** 6.04

○ **B.** 6.77

○ **C.** 7.00

○ **D.** 7.96

Question 932

The K_b of benzoate ($C_6H_5COO^-$) at 25°C is 1.55×10^{-10}. What is the pK_a of benzoic acid (C_6H_5COOH) at 25°C?

○ **A.** −3.82

○ **B.** 4.19

○ **C.** 7.02

○ **D.** 9.81

LECTURE 7

Question 933

Researchers heated a basin of water and calculated the K_w at varying temperatures. The results are shown in the table below.

Temperature (°C)	K_w
10	0.293×10^{-14}
20	0.681×10^{-14}
25	1.01×10^{-14}
30	1.47×10^{-14}
40	2.92×10^{-14}

Which of the following conclusions is best supported by the researchers' results?

- **A.** Water remains neutral as temperature increases.
- **B.** Water autoionizes more readily with decreasing temperature.
- **C.** Temperature has no effect on the autoionization of water.
- **D.** The hydronium and hydroxide ion concentrations increase with temperature.

Titration

Question 934

What is the most accurate classification of the reaction occurring during titration?

- **A.** Double replacement
- **B.** Single replacement
- **C.** Neutralization
- **D.** Redox

Question 935

What is the most common reason for performing a titration?

- **A.** To dilute an acid or base
- **B.** To adjust the pH of an acid or base
- **C.** To discover the concentration of an unknown solution
- **D.** To discover the endpoint of an indicator

Question 936

30.0 mL of sodium cyanide is titrated with 21.0 mL of 7.0 M HCl. What was the concentration of the original sodium cyanide solution?

- **A.** 4.9 M
- **B.** 5.1 M
- **C.** 7.0 M
- **D.** 10.0 M

Question 937

50 mL of a weak acid is titrated with 5.0 M NaOH. If 25 mL of NaOH is needed to reach the equivalence point, what is the molarity of the acid?

- **A.** 2.5 M
- **B.** 5.0 M
- **C.** 10 M
- **D.** The pK_a of the weak acid is required to answer this question.

Question 938

In a titration, 30 mL of 7 M NaOH is needed to reach the equivalence point with 100 mL of HF solution. What is the molarity of the HF solution?

- **A.** 2.1 M
- **B.** 3.1 M
- **C.** 10 M
- **D.** 23.3 M

Question 939

If 30 mL of 3 M acetic acid ($pK_a = 4.7$) were added to 50 mL of 2 M sodium hydroxide, the resulting solution would have a pH:

- **A.** less than two.
- **B.** between two and seven.
- **C.** equal to seven.
- **D.** greater than seven.

Question 940

If 30 mL of 3 M acetic acid ($pK_a = 4.7$) were added to 45 mL of 2 M sodium hydroxide, the resulting solution would have a pH:

- **A.** less than two.
- **B.** between two and seven.
- **C.** equal to seven.
- **D.** greater than seven.

Question 941

If 30 mL of 3 M acetic acid (pK_a = 4.7) is added to 40 mL of 2 M sodium hydroxide, the resulting solution has a pH:

○ **A.** less than two.

○ **B.** between two and seven.

○ **C.** equal to seven.

○ **D.** greater than seven.

Question 942

If an experimenter mixed an equal number of moles of hydrochloric acid (a strong acid) with ammonia (a weak base), which of the following would be expected?

○ **A.** Since hydrochloric acid is a strong acid, the reaction goes nearly to completion, resulting in a solution with pH 7.

○ **B.** Since hydrochloric acid is a strong acid, the reaction goes nearly to completion, resulting in a solution with pH less than 7.

○ **C.** Since ammonia is a weak base, the reaction should be represented as an equilibrium. The unreacted hydrochloric acid then gives a solution with pH less than 7.

○ **D.** Since ammonia is a weak base, the reaction should be represented as an equilibrium. The hydrochloric acid, however, dissociates completely. The unreacted ammonia then gives a solution with pH greater than 7.

Question 943

A known volume of an unknown weak acid is titrated with sodium hydroxide. Which of the following can be determined from a titration curve?

   I. The initial concentration of the acid

   II. The pK_a of the acid

   III. The molecular weight of the acid

○ **A.** I only

○ **B.** I and II only

○ **C.** II and III only

○ **D.** I, II, and III

Use the graph below to answer questions 944–953.

The graph below shows titration curves of 50 mL of the six acids, Q, R, S, T, U, and V. In each case, the titrant used was 0.1 M NaOH.

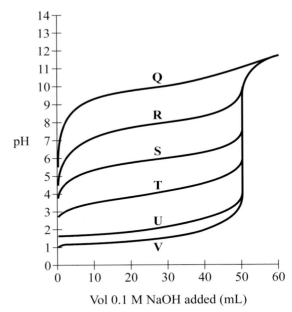

Vol 0.1 M NaOH added (mL)

Question 944

What was the concentration of acid S before the titration?

○ **A.** 0.05 M

○ **B.** 0.1 M

○ **C.** 0.2 M

○ **D.** 1 M

Question 945

What is the approximate K_a of acid T?

○ **A.** 1×10^{-10}

○ **B.** 1×10^{-6}

○ **C.** 1×10^{-4}

○ **D.** 1×10^{-3}

Question 946

What is the hydrogen ion concentration of acid U after 45 mL of 0.1 M NaOH has been added during the titration?

○ **A.** 0.0001 M

○ **B.** 0.001 M

○ **C.** 0.003 M

○ **D.** 3 M

Question 947

A 0.05 M solution of the conjugate base of acid S would have a pH of approximately:

- ○ **A.** 4.
- ○ **B.** 6.
- ○ **C.** 9.
- ○ **D.** 12.

Question 948

The choices below give an indicator followed by the pH where a color change occurs. Which of these would be the best indicator to use for the titration of acid R?

- ○ **A.** Bromocresol green, 3.6–5.5
- ○ **B.** Thymol blue, 7.8–9.6
- ○ **C.** Alizarin yellow, 8.7–11.4
- ○ **D.** Sodium indigo sulfonate, 11.8–13.9

Question 949

What is the approximate percent dissociation of acid S at the beginning of the titration?

- ○ **A.** 0.1%
- ○ **B.** 2.5%
- ○ **C.** 10%
- ○ **D.** 25%

Question 950

What is the pH of the equivalence point of the titration of acid V?

- ○ **A.** 6
- ○ **B.** 7
- ○ **C.** 8
- ○ **D.** 9

Question 951

If the conjugate base of acid S were titrated with acid V, which of the following represents the titration curve that would result?

○ **A.**   ○ **B.**

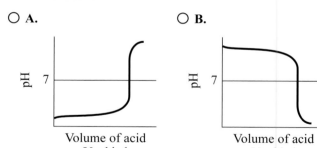

○ **C.**   ○ **D.**

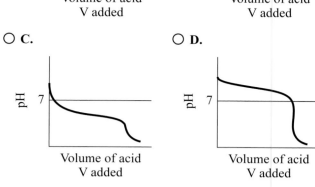

Question 952

Acid Q is probably:

- ○ **A.** water.
- ○ **B.** a weak acid.
- ○ **C.** a weak base.
- ○ **D.** a strong base.

Question 953

Which acid would be the most appropriate for producing a buffer solution at a pH of 4?

- ○ **A.** Q
- ○ **B.** S
- ○ **C.** T
- ○ **D.** V

Question 954

Which of the following describes the spacing of the equivalence points when a triprotic acid is titrated with a strong base?

- **A.** As each proton is removed, the acid becomes weaker, thus each successive equivalence point will require a smaller volume of base to be added.
- **B.** As each proton is removed, the acid becomes weaker, thus each successive equivalence point will require a larger volume of base to be added.
- **C.** The ratio of base added to proton removed in a titration is one-to-one; therefore, each successive equivalence point will require the same volume of base to be added as the previous one.
- **D.** The ratio of base added to proton removed in a titration is one-to-one; therefore, each successive equivalence point will experience the same change in pH as the previous one.

Question 955

A diprotic acid is titrated with a strong base. At the first equivalence point, the pH will be:

- **A.** below 7.
- **B.** 7.
- **C.** above 7.
- **D.** unable to be determined without more information.

Question 956

A diprotic acid is titrated with a strong base. At the second equivalence point, the pH will be:

- **A.** below 7.
- **B.** 7.
- **C.** above 7.
- **D.** unable to be determined without more information.

Question 957

The K_{a1} for H_2CO_3 is 4.3×10^{-7}. The K_{a2} for the H_2CO_3 is 5.6×10^{-11}. Which of the following depends upon the concentration of acid and conjugate base?

- **A.** The pH of the first equivalence point
- **B.** The pH of the first half equivalence point
- **C.** The pH of the second half equivalence point
- **D.** The pK_{a1}

Question 958

A monoprotic weak acid is titrated with a strong base. In the middle of the first buffer region, the pH will be:

- **A.** less than 7.
- **B.** 7.
- **C.** more than 7.
- **D.** unable to be determined without more information.

Question 959

Which of the following titration curves could NOT involve a reaction which emits CO_2?

A.

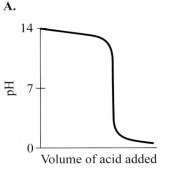

B.

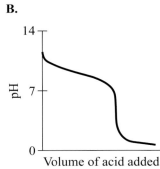

C.

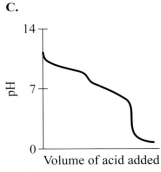

D.

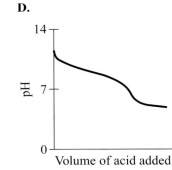

- **A.** Curve A
- **B.** Curve B
- **C.** Curve C
- **D.** Curve D

Question 960

Which of the following titration curves cannot involve HCl?

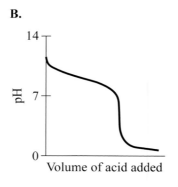

A.

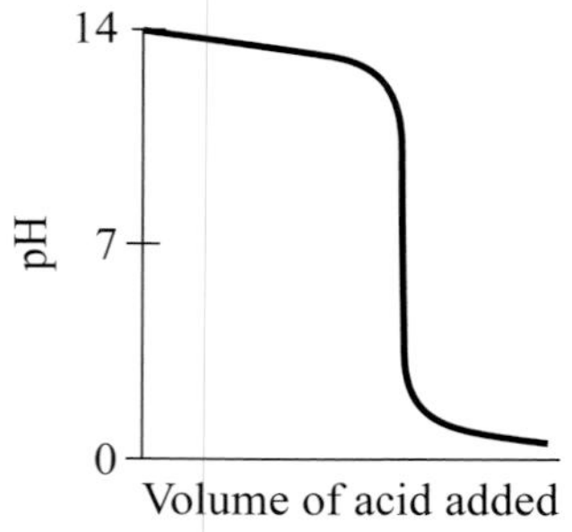

B.

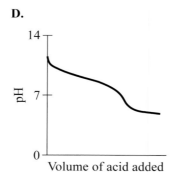

C.

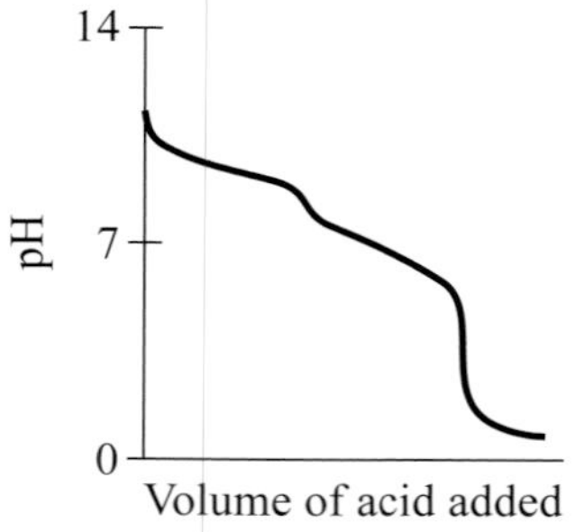

D.

- ○ **A.** Curve A
- ○ **B.** Curve B
- ○ **C.** Curve C
- ○ **D.** Curve D

Question 961

What is the pH of the second equivalence point when H_2SO_4 is titrated with NaOH?

- ○ **A.** 1.69
- ○ **B.** 2.98
- ○ **C.** 7.14
- ○ **D.** 9.85

Question 962

The pK_a of an indicator used in a weak acid-strong base titration should ideally be closest to:

- ○ **A.** 1.57.
- ○ **B.** 4.90.
- ○ **C.** 7.13.
- ○ **D.** 8.97.

Question 963

The pK_a of an indicator used in the titration of HCl with NaOH should ideally be closest to:

- ○ **A.** 1.57.
- ○ **B.** 4.90.
- ○ **C.** 7.13.
- ○ **D.** 8.97.

Question 964

The pK_a of an indicator used in a strong acid-weak base titration should ideally be closest to:

- ○ **A.** 1.57.
- ○ **B.** 4.90.
- ○ **C.** 7.13.
- ○ **D.** 8.97.

Question 965

In a standard titration, where is the indicator, such as phenolphthalein, always added?

    I. The titrant

    II. The analyte

    III. The reference solution

- ○ **A.** I only
- ○ **B.** II only
- ○ **C.** I and II only
- ○ **D.** II and III only

Question 966

In titration, the indicator changes color after a certain amount of titrant is added to the analyte. What is the point at which this occurs?

- ○ **A.** The endpoint
- ○ **B.** The half-equivalence point
- ○ **C.** The equivalence point
- ○ **D.** The buffer point

Question 967

Indicators are weak acids that change color over a fairly narrow pH range. In order to be used in a titration, an indicator should change color at a pH:

- ○ **A.** roughly equal to the pK_a of the acid being titrated.
- ○ **B.** roughly equal to the pH at the equivalence point.
- ○ **C.** of 7.
- ○ **D.** The pH at which the indicator changes color is irrelevant.

Question 968

Which of the following is measured directly in a titration?

- ○ **A.** The degree of dissociation of the titrant
- ○ **B.** The pK_a of the indicator
- ○ **C.** The equivalence point for the titration
- ○ **D.** The endpoint of the titration

Question 969

The equivalence point of a titration is at a pH of 7. Which of the following is the most appropriate indicator?

- ○ **A.** Alazarin yellow, $K_a = 1.6 \times 10^{-11}$
- ○ **B.** Phenolphthalein, $K_a = 1.0 \times 10^{-8}$
- ○ **C.** Bromthymol blue, $K_a = 7.9 \times 10^{-8}$
- ○ **D.** Methyl orange, $K_a = 3.2 \times 10^{-4}$

Salts and Buffers

Question 970

Which of the following acids is LEAST likely to dissociate completely in water?

- ○ **A.** Perchloric acid
- ○ **B.** Chloric acid
- ○ **C.** Acetic acid
- ○ **D.** Nitric acid

▼

Refer to the information below for questions 971-973.

Without proper electrolyte rehydration, marathon runners often experience cramps, dizziness, and increased muscle fatigue as a result of an internal fluid imbalance. Researchers interested in electrolyte replenishment methods noted that many electrolytes are in fact derived from biological acids, and the researchers analyzed the extent to which varying acids dissociate in water at 25°C. Results are displayed in the table below.

Acid	K_a
NH_4^+	5.6×10^{-10}
H_2CO_3	4.4×10^{-7}
HF	7.2×10^{-4}
CH_3COOH	1.8×10^{-5}

Question 971

Based on the researchers' results, which of the following compounds is most likely to be the strongest base at 25°C?

- ○ **A.** $NH_4^+(aq)$
- ○ **B.** $F^-(aq)$
- ○ **C.** $HCO_3^-(aq)$
- ○ **D.** $CH_3COO^-(aq)$

Question 972

How will the addition of NH_4Cl salt and KF salt affect the equilibrium concentrations of the acids analyzed?

- ○ **A.** The concentration of all acids will increase.
- ○ **B.** The concentration of NH_4^+ will decrease.
- ○ **C.** The concentration of HF will increase.
- ○ **D.** Equilibrium concentrations will not be affected because K_a is a constant.

Question 973

In a subsequent experiment, the researchers added sodium acetate salt (CH_3COONa) to the reaction vessel. Will the researchers be able to use the conclusions drawn from their previous experiment to analyze the effects of the salt addition?

- ○ **A.** No, the K_a values are dependent on initial concentrations of reactants.
- ○ **B.** No, the addition of CH_3COONa will force the dissociation of CH_3COOH in the reverse direction.
- ○ **C.** Yes, the addition of the salt will not affect equilibrium concentrations.
- ○ **D.** Yes, the K_a values function independently of reactant/product concentrations.

▲

Question 974

In a 1 M solution of acetic acid ($pK_a = 4.7$), the vast majority of the acetic acid is undissociated. Aspartic acid resides in proteins, and has an acetic acid group on its side chain. Why is aspartic acid found in proteins almost completely dissociated when acetic acid is not?

- ○ **A.** In aspartic acid, nearby hydrophobic residues activate the acid.
- ○ **B.** Proteins are generally found in extremely acidic environments, increasing the dissociation of residues such as aspartic acid.
- ○ **C.** Proteins contain basic residues stronger than water, which deprotonate the aspartic acid.
- ○ **D.** The many acidic residues found in a typical protein increase the effective concentration to above 1 M.

Question 975

Which of the following cations is a weak acid in an aqueous solution?

- ○ A. Sr^{2+}
- ○ B. Ca^{2+}
- ○ C. Ba^{2+}
- ○ D. Mg^{2+}

Question 976

Which of the following cations is a weak acid in an aqueous solution?

- ○ A. Na^+
- ○ B. Al^{3+}
- ○ C. Cs^+
- ○ D. Ca^{2+}

Question 977

Which of the following salts is(are) basic?

   I. $NaNO_3$
   II. $NaCN$
   III. Na_2CO_3

- ○ A. I only
- ○ B. II only
- ○ C. II and III only
- ○ D. I, II, and III

Question 978

Which of the following salts will be less soluble in acidic solutions than in basic solutions?

- ○ A. NaOH
- ○ B. NaCl
- ○ C. KCl
- ○ D. NH_4Cl

Question 979

Hydrochloric acid is a strong acid. A solution of sodium chloride should have a pH of:

- ○ A. less than seven.
- ○ B. seven.
- ○ C. more than seven but less than fourteen.
- ○ D. more than fourteen.

Question 980

What is the pH of a 0.02 M solution of benzoic acid ($K_a = 6 \times 10^{-5}$) in water?

- ○ A. 1.2
- ○ B. 2.9
- ○ C. 6.0
- ○ D. 7.8

Question 981

What is the pH of a 0.5 M solution of ammonium in water? (The K_a of ammonium is 5.8×10^{-10})

- ○ A. 8.3
- ○ B. 4.8
- ○ C. 1.7
- ○ D. 9.5

Question 982

A strong acid and a weak base are mixed to produce salt and water. The salt is dried and added to pure water. The pH of the salt solution:

- ○ A. is less than seven.
- ○ B. is seven.
- ○ C. is greater than seven.
- ○ D. depends upon the concentration of the salt.

Question 983

Consider the polyprotic acid H_2CO_3 ($pK_{a1} = 6.37$, $pK_{a2} = 10.25$). An aqueous solution of $NaHCO_3$ would have a pH:

- ○ A. of less than seven.
- ○ B. of seven.
- ○ C. of greater than seven.
- ○ D. that depends on the concentration of the salt.

Question 984

The digestive tract requires an acidic environment for optimal food degradation and enzyme function. Which salt(s), once dissolved in water, could artificially mimic the pH requirements of the digestive tract?

   I. NH_4Cl
   II. $NaCH_3COO$
   III. $KHSO_4$

- ○ A. I only
- ○ B. II only
- ○ C. I and III only
- ○ D. I, II, and III

Question 985

The K_a of NH_4^+ is 5.6×10^{-10}. The K_b of CN^- is 2×10^{-5}. The pH of an aqueous solution of the salt NH_4CN is:

- **A.** below 7 because NH_4^+ is more acidic than CN^- is basic.
- **B.** below 7 because NH_4^+ is more basic than CN^- is acidic.
- **C.** above 7 because CN^- is more basic than NH_4^+ is acidic.
- **D.** above 7 because CN^- is more acidic than NH_4^+ is basic.

Question 986

What is the pH of a solution containing 1 M sodium bicarbonate ($NaHCO_3$)? (The K_a of carbonic acid is 4.4×10^{-7})

- **A.** 10.3
- **B.** 3.8
- **C.** 1.5
- **D.** 9.5

Question 987

$NaClO$ salt is dissolved in a beaker of water at 25°C forming a 0.20 M solution. What is the pH of this newly formed solution? (K_a of $HClO = 3.0 \times 10^{-8}$)

- **A.** 3.59
- **B.** 7.00
- **C.** 10.41
- **D.** 13.28

Question 988

What is the ideal pK_a of the acid found in the buffer system of blood? (The pH of blood is about 7.4)

- **A.** 0.87
- **B.** 6.37
- **C.** 10.3
- **D.** 4.0

Question 989

Which of the following is NOT needed to determine the capacity of a buffer solution?

- **A.** An acid or base of known concentration
- **B.** The concentration of the buffer
- **C.** The volume of acid added
- **D.** The pH of the solution after acid is added

Question 990

In the blood, bicarbonate serves as a(n):

- **A.** acid.
- **B.** base.
- **C.** buffer.
- **D.** catalyst.

Question 991

Which of the following acids mixed with the appropriate conjugate base makes the best buffer solution?

- **A.** Oxalic acid in a solution of pH 4
- **B.** Hydrochloric acid in a solution of pH 7
- **C.** Histidine in solution of pH 12
- **D.** Hydrofluoric acid in solution of pH 8

Question 992

Which of the following statements best describes the properties of a buffer?

- **A.** It functions to buffer pH at the half equivalence point.
- **B.** It functions to buffer pH at the equivalence point.
- **C.** It functions to indicate the endpoint of a reaction at the half equivalence point.
- **D.** It functions to indicate the endpoint of a reaction at the equivalence point.

Question 993

Which of the four acids would be most ideal in a solution designed to buffer acids at pH 5.1?

	K_a
Acid 1	1.3×10^6
Acid 2	1.0×10^3
Acid 3	4.8×10^{-11}
Acid 4	1.75×10^{-5}

- **A.** Acid 1
- **B.** Acid 2
- **C.** Acid 3
- **D.** Acid 4

Question 994

Which of the following expressions gives the pH of a buffered solution?

○ **A.** $\log[H^+]$

○ **B.** $-\log[H^+]$

○ **C.** $pK_a - \log([A^-]/[HA])$

○ **D.** $pK_b + \log([A^-]/[HA])$

Question 995

Which of the following pairs would not make a good buffer if placed in the same aqueous solution?

○ **A.** HCl and KCl

○ **B.** H_2S and NaHS

○ **C.** NH_4Cl and NH_3

○ **D.** $KHCO_3$ and K_2CO_3

Question 996

A buffer is made by combining 30 mL of a 2.0 M acidic solution with 42.0 grams of its salt. The resulting solution has a pH of 7.5. If the solution is then diluted to a total volume of 300 mL, what will be the new value of the pH?

○ **A.** 6.5

○ **B.** 7.5

○ **C.** 8.5

○ **D.** Cannot be determined from the information given

Question 997

An aqueous solution is created from equal amounts of 1 M HCl (a strong acid) and 0.01 M sodium chloride. What is the approximate pH of the solution?

○ **A.** 0

○ **B.** 1

○ **C.** 2

○ **D.** The pH of the solution cannot be estimated without the volumes of solution.

Question 998

A solution is composed of equal concentrations of aqueous ammonia ($pK_b = 4.74$) and ammonium chloride ($pK_a = 9.26$). What would be the pH of the resulting solution?

○ **A.** 4.74

○ **B.** 7.00

○ **C.** 9.26

○ **D.** The pH of the solution cannot be determined from the information given.

Question 999

An aqueous solution is composed of 2 M ammonia ($pK_b = 4.74$) and 0.2 M ammonium chloride ($pK_a = 9.26$). What is the pH of the solution?

○ **A.** 4.74

○ **B.** 8.26

○ **C.** 9.26

○ **D.** 10.26

Question 1000

Which of the following would be an equation that could be used to find the pH of a buffer if the pK_b of the base and the concentrations of base and acid are known?

○ **A.** $pH = pK_b + \log([base]/[acid])$

○ **B.** $pH = pK_b + \log([acid]/[base])$

○ **C.** $pH = pK_b - \log([base]/[acid])$

○ **D.** $pH = 14 - pK_b + \log([base]/[acid])$

Question 1001

Solution A contains a buffer formed of 2.0 M acetic acid and 0.8 M potassium acetate. Solution B contains a buffer formed of 0.2 M acetic acid and 0.08 M potassium acetate. How do the solutions compare?

○ **A.** The pH and buffer capacity of both solutions are the same.

○ **B.** The pH of solution A is lower than that of solution B, but the buffer capacity is the same.

○ **C.** The pH of solution A is the same as that of solution B, but solution A has a greater buffer capacity.

○ **D.** The pH of solution A is lower than that of solution B, and solution A has a greater buffer capacity than solution B.

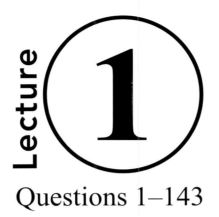

Lecture 1

Questions 1–143

Introduction to General Chemistry

ANSWERS & EXPLANATIONS

ANSWER KEY										
1. C	14. C	27. B	40. A	53. B	66. C	79. A	92. D	105. C	118. A	131. C
2. C	15. A	28. D	41. A	54. D	67. C	80. B	93. B	106. D	119. A	132. B
3. B	16. A	29. B	42. B	55. D	68. A	81. B	94. C	107. B	120. D	133. B
4. D	17. B	30. C	43. B	56. B	69. A	82. D	95. C	108. D	121. C	134. A
5. C	18. C	31. B	44. A	57. A	70. C	83. C	96. B	109. C	122. D	135. B
6. C	19. D	32. C	45. C	58. C	71. D	84. D	97. C	110. D	123. B	136. D
7. B	20. A	33. D	46. A	59. C	72. A	85. C	98. A	111. C	124. B	137. B
8. B	21. C	34. B	47. D	60. D	73. D	86. A	99. C	112. D	125. A	138. B
9. B	22. C	35. C	48. A	61. A	74. A	87. A	100. A	113. C	126. D	139. A
10. D	23. D	36. C	49. D	62. A	75. C	88. C	101. B	114. C	127. B	140. B
11. B	24. C	37. D	50. D	63. A	76. C	89. A	102. D	115. D	128. C	141. A
12. A	25. D	38. D	51. A	64. A	77. B	90. B	103. B	116. C	129. D	142. B
13. A	26. C	39. C	52. D	65. B	78. A	91. C	104. D	117. D	130. D	143. A

Atoms

1. **C is the best answer.** The number of protons and the number of neutrons is represented by Z on the elemental symbol and is called the atomic number. Choices A and B can be eliminated. The mass number is written to the upper left of the elemental symbol. The mass number is the number of protons plus neutrons. Choice C is a strong answer choice. The number of electrons in a neutral atom is the same as the number of protons because the -1 charge of an electron cancels out the $+1$ charge of a proton. This means the number of electrons would also be represented by Z if the element is neutral. Choice D can be eliminated.

2. **C is the best answer.** In a neutral element, the number of electrons is the same as the number of protons because the -1 charge of an electron would cancel out the $+1$ charge of a proton. The number of protons is represented by Z on the elemental symbol, which will also be the number of electrons in a neutral element. Choices A and B can be eliminated. The charge is written to the upper right of the elemental symbol. The charge is the number of protons minus electrons. Choice C is a strong answer. The number of neutrons plus the number of protons is the atomic mass, which is represented by A on the elemental symbol. Choice D can be eliminated.

3. **B is the best answer.** The mass number, which is the number of protons plus the number of neutrons, is represented by A on the elemental symbol. Choice A can be eliminated. The atomic number is written to the lower left of the elemental symbol and is represented by Z on the elemental symbol. Choice B is a strong answer choice. The overall charge on the element, calculated as the number of protons minus the number of electrons, is represented as C on the elemental symbol. Choice C can be eliminated. Choice D, the mass number plus the atomic number, is not found on the elemental symbol. Choice D can be eliminated.

4. **D is the best answer.** Since Z is the number of protons and A is the number of protons plus neutrons, Z will be equal to or less than A. Choice A can be eliminated. All elements have atoms with neutrons except for hydrogen, which has only one proton and one electron. For hydrogen, A and Z are equal to one, which eliminates choice B. An isotope is an atom with the same number of protons but one or more additional neutrons. The additional neutrons would increase A but not increase Z, which represents the number of protons. Choice C can be eliminated. Because A is the number of protons plus the number of neutrons, and Z is the number of protons, A minus Z is the number of neutrons. Choice D is the best answer.

5. **C is the best answer.** An element is defined by the number of protons it has, which is represented by Z on the elemental symbol. A on the elemental symbol can vary depending on the number of neutrons an atom has, which is common for elements that have isotopes. Choice A can be eliminated. C on the elemental symbol represents the charge on the element. Electrons can be gained or lost from a particular element, meaning the value of C can change. Choice B can be eliminated. The atomic number represents the number of protons an element has and does not change. Choice C is a strong answer choice. Because the atomic weight can change with the addition of more neutrons, as seen in isotopes, there is more than one possible value for $A + Z$. Choice D can be eliminated.

6. **C is the best answer.** If the two atoms have different atomic masses but are both the same element, they must have differing numbers of neutrons. Remember that an atom is defined by the number of protons it has, meaning these two atoms are the same element. Choice A can be eliminated. An atom that does not have the same number of protons and electrons is called an ion. Electrons have negligible mass compared to protons and electrons and are not included in the calculation of A. Choice B can be eliminated. Atoms with the same atomic number but different mass numbers must have different numbers of neutrons. This makes these two atoms isotopes. Choice C is most likely the best answer. Isomers are two or more atomic nuclei that have the same atomic number and same mass number but different energy states. The question implies that the atoms have the same atomic number because they are the same element. Choice D can be eliminated.

7. **B is the best answer.** A bond stores energy between two atoms. When a bond is formed, the entropy of the system decreases and energy, usually in the form of heat, is released. Choice A can be eliminated. Energy must be put into the system in order to pull the two atoms apart, meaning energy is absorbed when a bond is broken. Remember that breaking a bond is endothermic, meaning it requires energy. Choice B is likely the best answer. Regardless of whether the bond is strong or weak, energy is required in order to break it apart. Choices C and D are weak answer choices and can be eliminated.

Elements and the Periodic Table

8. B is the best answer. Elements that fall in the same column on the periodic table belong to the same family (also called a group). Sodium and potassium belong in Group 1. The alkaline earth metals correspond to Group 2, eliminating choice A. The alkali metals correspond to Group 1, making choice B most likely to be the best answer. The transition metals are found in Groups 3-12 and do not contain sodium and potassium. Choice C can be eliminated. The halogens are found in Group 17 and contain elements like fluorine and chlorine. Choice D can be eliminated.

9. B is the best answer. Atoms that are part of the same column of the periodic table (also called a group or a family) have similar chemical reactivity. K is found in Group 1, so the best answer will likely be another element also in Group 1. Ca is found in Group 2, eliminating choice A. Cs is found in Group 1, making choice B most likely to be the best answer. Ar is found in Group 18, eliminating choice C. O is found in Group 16, eliminating choice D.

10. D is the best answer. Catching fire when exposed to water suggests extreme reactivity, probably due to the ease with which alkali metals lose their electrons. Elements in the same column on the periodic table (also called a group or a family) share similar chemical properties, which often makes them react in similar ways. The best answer will likely be an element found in Group 1 of the periodic table. Nitrogen is found in Group 15, eliminating choice A. Beryllium is found in Group 2, eliminating choice B. Titanium is found in Group 4, eliminating choice C. Potassium, along with sodium, is found in Group 1 of the periodic table and is the best answer.

11. B is the best answer. Ions typically form by taking on a noble gas electron configuration. The alkaline earth metals are found in Group 2 of the periodic table and would lose two electrons to gain a noble gas configuration. Alkali metals in Group 1 would lose one electron to get a charge of +1, while the alkaline earth metals would lose two electrons to get a charge of +2. Choice A can be eliminated, and choice B is most likely to be the best answer. The halogens, found in Group 17, often gain an electron to get a charge of −1. Choice C can be eliminated. Elements in Group 16, such as oxygen and sulfur, often gain two electrons to get a charge of −2. Choice D can be eliminated.

12. A is the best answer. Magnesium, Mg, is found in Group 2 on the periodic table. Group 2 corresponds to the alkaline earth metals, making choice A most likely to be the best answer. The alkali metals are found in Group 1, eliminating choice C. The transition metals are found in Groups 2-12, eliminating choice C. The noble gases are found in Group 18, eliminating choice D.

13. A is the best answer. Electron affinity increases up and to the right on the periodic table. Electronegativity follows the same trend. As chlorine is the element that is closest to the upper right corner of the table, choice A is the best answer. Barium, tin, and silver are not as close to the upper right corner as chlorine, eliminating choices B, C, and D.

14. C is the best answer. When atoms become ions, they typically adopt a noble gas configuration with eight electrons in the outer subshells. The alkali metals are found in Group 1 of the periodic table and tend to lose one electron, eliminating choice A. The alkaline earth metals are found in Group 2 and tend to lose two electrons. Choice B can be eliminated. Halogens are found in Group 17 and tend to gain one electron, making choice C a strong answer choice. Elements in Group 16 tend to gain two electrons, eliminating choice D.

15. A is the best answer. Group 1 of the periodic table contains the alkali metals. When the alkali metals form compounds, they tend to lose one electron to have a +1 charge. The halogens are found in column 17 and tend to gain one electron to have a charge of −1. This means a compound with an alkali metal and a halogen would form in a one-to-one manner, making choice A the best answer. Elements of Group 16 tend to gain two electrons when they enter a compound, eliminating choice B. Elements of Group 2, the alkaline earth metals, give up two electrons when they form compounds. Choice C can be eliminated. All alkali metals form +1 ions and all halogens form −1 ions, meaning the exact identity of X and Y do not impact the ratio of atoms that form the compound. Choice D can be eliminated.

16. A is the best answer. Halogens are often leaving groups in organic chemistry, especially those with higher molecular weight. Halogens can function as nucleophiles when negatively charged, not electrophiles, so choice B is not the best answer. The halogen group does not contain oxygen, so choice C is not the best answer. Halogens are often gases when diatomic but some are liquids, so choice D is not the best answer.

17. B is the best answer. The correct answer must be true of halogens and somehow relate to iodine functioning as an antiseptic. Halogens are electronegative but that would not help with being an antiseptic, so choice A is not the best answer. Halogens also have a strong electron affinity. This means they are likely to pick up electrons, or be reduced, meaning they are strong oxidizing agents. It is this property that makes iodine an antiseptic. Choice B is likely the best answer. Being a gas would not help, so choice C is not the best answer. Halogens are not enzyme inhibitors; they destroy proteins and lipids by oxidation, so choice D is not the best answer.

18. **C is the best answer.** Argon, Ar, is a noble gas that is found on row three and column eighteen of the periodic table. Noble gases are considered unreactive, as they contain a full octet in their outer orbitals, eliminating choice A. The $4p$ subshell corresponds to row four, not row three, eliminating choice B. Loss of one electron from K, potassium, would give it 18 electrons, which is the same number of electrons that Ar has. Remember that a neutral atom has the same number of protons and electrons, and that the number of protons defines the atomic number. Choice C is the best answer. Atomic radius increases as one moves down and to the left on the periodic table. Kr is below Ar on the periodic table, meaning choice D can be eliminated.

19. **D is the best answer.** It is reasonable to assume that the manufacturers of anesthetics would not want their products to react with other elements in the environment. The least reactive elements on the periodic table are the ideal gases, which are found in column 18. The best answer will likely be one of these elements. Oxygen and nitrogen are both components of the atmosphere, which could likely react with other molecules. Choices A and B can be eliminated. The halogens are often considered some of the most reactive elements, as they have one orbital that is half-filled. Choice C can be eliminated. Neon is a noble gas, likely making choice D the best answer.

20. **A is the best answer.** Radon, Rn, is found in row six column eighteen of the periodic table and is a noble gas. Remember that the orbitals are always listed with the primary orbital in an ascending manner, with the outermost s and p orbitals listed last. This means choices A and B are better answer choices than choices C and D. Rn has completely full orbitals, as it is a noble gas. The f orbitals can hold a maximum of 14 electrons and must be filled before the d, s, and p orbitals. This makes choice A a more likely answer than choice B. Additionally, the d orbital can only hold 10 electrons, not 12, further eliminating choice B.

21. **C is the best answer.** Iron, silver, and mercury are found in Groups 3-12 on the periodic table. The representative elements are Groups 1, 2, and 13-18, eliminating choice A. The halogens are found in Group 17, eliminating choice B. The transition elements are found in Groups 3-12, making choice C the best answer. The alkaline earth metals are found in Group 2, eliminating choice D.

22. **C is the best answer.** The alkali metals, like sodium, almost always adopt a +1 state by losing an electron. Choice A is a weak answer choice. He has a noble gas configuration and is unlikely to be found as an ion. Choice B can be eliminated. The transition metals are more likely to form more than one possible ion because they have d-orbitals that can hold or lose electrons. Choice C is a strong answer choice. Sr is an alkaline earth metal that almost always adopts a +2 charge by losing two electrons. Choice D can be eliminated.

23. **D is the best answer.** Solutions are likely to be colored when they are either unable to absorb some wavelengths of light and instead reflect them or absorb some wavelengths of light and emit a different wavelength. One property of transition metals is that they often absorb and reflect light due to their partially filled d orbitals. When an electron absorbs light, it jumps to a higher energy level. When this electron relaxes back to a lower energy level, it gives off light at a different wavelength. The best answer will be the compound that contains a transition metal. Transition metals are found in Group 3-12 on the periodic table. Choices A-C do not have any elements found in Groups 3-12, eliminating them as possible answer choices. Iron is a transition metal and is found in Group 8. Choice D is the best answer.

24. **C is the best answer.** A group, also known as a family, is defined as a column in the periodic table. Periods are rows in the periodic table. Representative elements are elements other than transition elements. So, the representative elements include Groups 1, 2, 13, 14, 15, 16, 17, 18, making choice C is the best answer. A mnemonic for this is the House of Representatives who are a group of people, not a period of people.

25. **D is the best answer.** Representative elements consist of the elements found within Groups 1, 2, and 13-18 of the periodic table. Groups 3-12 make up the transition metals. Choice A is an accurate statement and choice B is as well, the primary goal of forming a noble-gas configuration is to maintain stability of the ion. Choice C is also accurate as the representative elements are found outside of Groups 3-12. Choice D is the best answer as it is the antithesis of choice B.

26. **C is the best answer.** Choices A and B are both true but are physical, not chemical properties of metals. Choice C is the only accurate chemical property of metals. Metals are often reducing agents because they tend to be oxidized (lose electrons), so choice D can be eliminated.

27. **B is the best answer.** Table salt includes sodium which is a metal, so choice A can be eliminated. Glucose contains H, C, and O, which are all nonmetals, so choice B is the best answer. Hemoglobin contains proteins which are composed of amino acids which have H, C, N, O, and S. Those are all nonmetals. However hemoglobin also has a heme group that includes iron, a metal. Choice C can be eliminated. Tap water includes H and O for water but often has trace amounts of metals like Ca and Fe, so choice D is not the best answer. Hints that tap water is not pure are left by hard water stains and iron deposits in sinks and toilets. Heavy metals are also the reason people purify tap water with filtration systems.

28. **D is the best answer.** Nonmetals are found on the right side of the periodic table and are prone to gain electrons to make negative ions. Also, unlike metals, nonmetals often form covalent bonds with each other. So, choice D is the best answer.

29. **B is the best answer.** A family, also known as a group, is a column of the periodic table. The best answer will be the two elements that are found in the same column. Cr is found in Group 6, while Fe is found in Group 8. Choice A can be eliminated. Both O and Se are part of Group 16, making choice B the best answer. B is found in Group 13, while C is found in Group 14. Choice C can be eliminated. Ir is found in Group 9, while Pt is found in Group 10. Choice D can be eliminated.

30. **C is the best answer.** The chalcogen group is the name for the group (or column) that includes oxygen. Choice C is the best answer. The MCAT® has referred to the chalcogens in the past, so this is a fact worth memorizing.

31. **B is the best answer.** The attraction of the nucleus on the outer most electron is related to the ionization energy which increases to the right and up on the periodic table. The ionization energy increases moving from left to right across the periodic table, eliminating choice A. Because the ionization energy decreases when moving from right to left and top to bottom on the periodic table, choice B is the best answer. The ionization energy increases moving from bottom to top on the periodic table, eliminating choice C. The ionization energy increases moving from right to left and bottom to top on the periodic table, eliminating choice D.

32. **C is the best answer.** This question is equivalent to asking which element has the greatest first ionization energy. In order to remove an electron from an atom, the electron has to be pulled against the attractive force from the positively charged nucleus. First ionization energy increases from left to right and bottom to top across the periodic table, meaning an electron in an element that is found in the upper right corner of the periodic table experiences the greatest electrostatic force. Na is found on the upper left corner of the periodic table, eliminating choice A. Cs is found in the bottom left corner of the periodic table, eliminating choice B. F is the element found in the upper right portion of the periodic table, likely making choice C the best answer. Mg is also found in the upper left on the periodic table. Choice D can be eliminated.

33. **D is the best answer.** The process of removing an electron is called ionization energy. As each successive electron is removed, the force felt by the remaining electrons grows. This is because the number of protons has remained the same while the number of electrons they are attracted to decreases, increasing the effective nuclear charge. The best answer will be the one that has the most electrons removed. With each successive electron removal, the atom becomes more positive. Choice D is the most positive, meaning it has lost the most electrons. Choice A, B, and C can be eliminated, and choice D is the best answer.

34. **B is the best answer.** Atoms often adopt an electron configuration similar to a noble gas with a full octet in their outer subshells. The energy required to remove an electron is called the ionization energy. Removing one electron from Na would give a noble gas configuration, making choice A a weaker answer choice. Na^+ has lost an electron to adopt a noble gas configuration. Elements that have a noble gas configuration are highly stable, meaning it would take a significant amount of energy to remove an additional electron. Choice B is a strong answer choice. Mg often loses two electrons to achieve a noble gas configuration, so losing an electron from Mg or an additional electron from Mg^+ would require less energy than removing an electron from an atom like Na^+ that has a noble gas electron configuration. Choices C and D can be eliminated.

35. **C is the best answer.** The second ionization energy of lithium is significantly larger than the first ionization energy because after one electron is removed the resulting ion has a noble gas configuration. Noble gas configurations are highly stable, so removing an additional electron requires significant energy. Metals tend to have lower ionization energies than nonmetals, as their valence electrons are further from the nucleus than nonmetal valence electrons due to increased atomic radius. While element X does not have the same jump in second ionization energy, its first ionization energy is relatively similar to that of Li. This suggests that it is a metal and would not achieve a noble gas configuration upon removal of the first electron but might upon removal of the second electron. Oxygen is a nonmetal, which means it would likely have a higher first ionization energy. Choice A is a weak answer choice. Sodium, like lithium, would be expected to have a very high second ionization energy, as removal of an electron from sodium allows it to adopt a noble gas configuration. Choice B can be eliminated. Calcium is a metal and does not achieve a noble gas configuration upon the removal of one electron but does upon the removal of two. Choice C is most likely the best answer. Xenon is a noble gas, so removal of an electron would require a high amount of first ionization energy. Choice D can be eliminated.

36. **C is the best answer.** Fe^{2+} has lost two electrons, meaning it is smaller than the neutral atom. Choice A can be eliminated. Removing additional electrons from a positive ion requires more energy than removing the first electron, eliminating choice B. Choice C suggests that each outer electron is more tightly held in Fe^{2+} than in Fe, which is true and explains the increased ionization energy in Fe^{2+}. The greater effective nuclear charge is the result of the same number of protons pulling on fewer electrons after two electrons have been lost. Choice D indicates that Fe^{2+} is higher in energy than Fe, which is true but does not address the issue of how hard it is to remove an additional electron from Fe^{2+}.

37. **D is the best answer.** A row runs from left to right across the periodic table. Electronegativity increases left to right, so atom A would have a lower electronegativity. Option I is not part of the best answer. Ionization energy also increases from left to right across the periodic table. Option II is not part of the best answer. Atomic weight increases from left to right across the periodic table as additional protons and neutrons are added. Option III is not part of the best answer. Choice D is the best answer because it does not include any of the options.

38. **D is the best answer.** Ionization energy is the energy required to remove an electron from an atom. The trend increases when moving to the right across a row and up a column. In choices A and B, the element with the lowest ionization energy should be sodium. Neither choice A nor choice B has sodium with the lowest ionization energy, so choices A and B can be eliminated. In choices C and D, either sodium or calcium should have the lowest ionization energy (actually, it is sodium but that is hard to predict since calcium is diagonal to sodium). Choice C can be eliminated because it shows that nitrogen has the lowest ionization energy.

39. **C is the best answer.** Choice A is the electron configuration for helium, choice B is boron, choice C is rubidium and choice D is iodine. However, figuring that out is a waste of time. Ionization energy is the energy required to remove an electron from an atom. The lowest ionization energy will be removing an unpaired electron in a distant (high n) electron shell. Choice A has paired electrons in a near shell so this is not the best answer. Choice B has an unpaired electron, but it is in a shell close to the nucleus, so choice B is not a strong answer. Choice C has an unpaired electron in a distant shell, so choice C is the best answer. Removal of an electron would also give a full $4p$ orbital similar to that of a noble gas, further making it favorable to remove an electron. Choice D has unpaired electrons in distant shells, but when a shell is mostly full, it becomes more difficult to remove one electron as the energetically favorable option would be to add an electron. Choice D is not the best answer.

40. **A is the best answer.** Group 1 is the first column in the periodic table. Sometimes it includes hydrogen whereas other periodic tables do not include hydrogen in this group. There are 7 data points, so this plot must be including hydrogen. The ionization energy trend increases when moving up a row, so choices B and D can be eliminated. It is worth knowing that the ionization energy of the first group is all about the same except the ionization energy of hydrogen, which is about triple that of sodium. Choice A is the best answer.

41. **A is the best answer.** Electron affinity increases up and to the right on the periodic table. Electronegativity follows the same trend. As chlorine is the element that is closest to the upright corner of the table, choice A is the best answer.

42. **B is the best answer.** Electron affinity is the willingness of an element to accept a new electron into one of its orbitals. Electron affinity is measured as a negative value. Electron affinity becomes more negative up and to the right of the periodic table with the exception of the noble gases. Choice B is the best answer as fluorine would have the lowest electron affinity. Choice D can be eliminated as noble gases have complete octets, which makes their electron affinity essentially zero.

43. **B is the best answer.** Ionization to an anion occurs by picking up an electron. This question is really asking which atom has the greatest electron affinity. Electron affinity is a negative value and becomes more negative when moving to the right and up the periodic table. The halogens have particularly strong electron affinities because the electron configuration mirrors that of a noble gas when one electron is added, so iodine is the best answer. Oxygen would be the second best answer. Calcium and hydrogen have electron affinities near 0, meaning they rarely exist as anions, so choices C and D are not the best answers.

44. **A is the best answer.** Electron affinity is an atom's propensity to accept an electron and become an anion. By convention, release of energy is a negative value. So, electron affinity is a negative value and the most negative value is the greatest propensity to accept electrons. Of note, electron affinities for a second or third electron may be positive because energy is required. The halogens have the most negative electron affinity. Many students memorize that the trend for electron affinity is up and to the right but there are exceptions as stated in the question stem. Atoms with *d* orbitals can be found in the transition metals block, Groups 3-12. The atoms with nearly full *d* orbitals are in Group 11 because these have 9/10 electrons in the *d* orbital. Gold is in Group 11, so based on the question stem, gold must have an electron affinity that is unexpected. One would expect gold to have a weak electron affinity based on the periodic trend. But, since its *d* orbital is one electron away from being full, gold's electron affinity is probably much more negative than expected, although it is not likely greater than a halogen. The electron affinity for calcium should be near zero since calcium has no interest in obtaining an electron as this electron would be unpaired. The best answer should list calcium near zero, so choices B, C and D can all be eliminated. In choice A, notice how the electron affinity for gold is much more negative than would be expected from the trend.

45. **C is the best answer.** Electron affinity is a negative number, so the correct definition is based on energy released, and choices A and B can be eliminated. Electron affinity is defined in kJ/mol based on adding electrons to individual atoms. Choice D is not the best answer because it implies an electron can only be added to an uncharged entity, because the word "element" refers to the uncharged atom. Electrons can be added to ionized atoms, so choice D can be eliminated.

46. **A is the best answer.** Ionization energy is the amount of energy needed to detach an electron from an individual atom. Moving up and to the right of the periodic table, more energy is needed to detach electrons. Choice A is the best answer as lithium would possess the least amount of ionization energy since it's a member of Group 1 and row 1. Choice B would require the most energy input, followed by choice D, then choice C.

47. **D is the best answer.** Converting the electron configurations is not necessary but choices A, B, C, and D are rhodium, palladium, silver, and cadmium respectively. Electron affinity should increase across a row, so cadmium should have the greatest (most negative) electron affinity. However, cadmium has a full *d* and *s* orbital and the willingness to add one sole electron to the next *p* orbital is very small. So, the electron affinity for cadmium is essentially zero, which is less than expected based on the trend, making choice D is the best answer. Atoms with full orbitals have electron affinities near zero, where atoms with orbitals that lack one electron have electron affinities much higher than the periodic table trend would predict. Although memorizing trends is helpful for the MCAT®, it is also important to be able to use reasoning to answer questions like this. Choice B, palladium would also have a lower electron affinity than expected but adding one electron to the 5*s* orbital is easier than adding it to the 5*p* orbital because 5*p* is higher energy than 5*s*. So, choice D is the best answer.

48. **A is the best answer.** The question is asking which of the answer choices has the greatest electron affinity. Non-metals are more likely to accept an electron than metals. Remember that electron affinity generally increases moving up a group and across a period to the right. Additionally, recall that elements with a completed octet of valence electrons are particularly stable. Choice A is a strong answer, as adding another valence electron to chlorine would give it a complete octet. Choice B can be eliminated, as it is near the bottom of the group and an additional electron will be far from the nucleus and subject to the repulsive forces of the other negatively charged electrons. Choice C can be eliminated, as it is a noble gas. Adding another electron to choice D would move it further from a complete octet, making it an unlikely answer.

49. **D is the best answer.** Atomic radius is the only periodic trend that increases as one moves down and to the left of the periodic table. All the other periodic trends, such as electronegativity, electron affinity, and energy of ionization, increase as one goes up and to the right. Choice A and B can be eliminated, as the element from Group 1 would have a greater atomic radius than the element from Group 7. Choice C, while tempting, is not the best answer as the element from Group 1 would not possess more energy of ionization. Choice D is the best answer as it most accurately follows the periodic trends.

50. **D is the best answer.** Electronegativity increases as one moves towards the upper right hand corner of the periodic table. The element with the highest electronegativity is fluorine, which makes choice D the best answer.

51. **A is the best answer.** Electronegativity is the tendency of an atom to attract a bonding pair of electrons. Atoms with high electronegativity will pull electrons towards itself during a bond. Choice A is the best answer as it provides the definition of electron affinity instead of electronegativity. Electron affinity is the probability of an atom accepting an additional electron. Choices B, C, and D accurately describe electronegativity and can be eliminated.

52. **D is the best answer.** Electronegativity can be used to predict the type of bonds that will form between two atoms. Large differences in electronegativity usually lead to the formation of an ionic bond. Specifically, bonds between metals and nonmetals form ionic bonds as well. Choice A is the best answer as Element A and Element C possess the greatest difference in electronegativity. Note that Element C is likely a metal as well.

53. **B is the best answer.** Small differences in electronegativity between two atoms lead to covalent bonds. Elements that are very similar in their electronegativity values tend to form nonpolar covalent bonds. As Elements B and D have the closest electronegativity values, choice B is the best answer. While choice C is tempting, Elements A and E would form a polar covalent bond. A difference of 0.5 and under leads to a nonpolar covalent bond, while a difference between 0.5 and 1.5 leads to a polar covalent bond.

54. **D is the best answer.** Electronegativity measures the attraction of an element for electrons within a chemical bond. In order to measure electronegativity, the element needs to form bonds with other atoms. The small size of an element would not prevent it from bonding, so choice A is a weak answer choice. Helium does have inner-shell electrons, such as those that populate the $1s$ orbital. Choice B is a weak answer choice. Even though a helium atom is neutral, this would not prevent it from bonding with other elements. Choice C is a weak answer choice. Helium has a full electron shell, which prevents nearly any element from bonding with it. Because helium does not form bonds with other elements, its electronegativity cannot be measured. Choice D is the best answer.

55. **D is the best answer.** Electronegativity increases from left to right and bottom to top across the periodic table. The element that is in the upper right corner of the periodic table is F, which eliminates choices A-C and makes choice D the best answer.

56. **B is the best answer.** Electronegativity increases from left to right and bottom to top across the periodic table. This generally makes electronegativity higher for non-metals than for metals. While Be is near the top of the periodic table, it is an alkaline earth metal. Choice A is a possible answer, but it is probably not the best answer. Br is a halogen and is located on the right of the periodic table. Choice B is a strong answer choice. Cs is located in the bottom left of the periodic table, eliminating choice C. Noble gases tend not to form bonds due to their full outer electron shells. Even though they are on the right on the periodic table, they have low electronegativities. Choice D can be eliminated, and choice B is the best answer.

57. **A is the best answer.** The attraction of electrons to a particular atom in a bond is defined by the atoms electronegativity. Thus, this question is really asking for the highest electronegativity, which increases from left to right and bottom to top on the periodic table. Cl is the element on the top right of the periodic table from the choices listed, making choice A the best answer. Rb is located in the bottom left of the periodic table, eliminating choice B. He is generally considered to have no measurable electronegativity because it does not form bonds with other atoms due to its full outer electron shell. Choice C can be eliminated. I is also on the right side of the periodic table, but it is found further towards the bottom than Cl. Choice D can be eliminated.

58. **C is the best answer.** Electronegativity is the likelihood of an atom to attract electrons shared in a covalent bond. Generally, the closer an element is to fluorine on the periodic table, the more electronegative the element. Choice A is the furthest of all of the answer choices from fluorine and is the unlikely to be the best answer. Choice B is not the best answer; although it is adjacent to fluorine, the chlorine atom contains a filled $3s$ orbital and an almost filled $3p$ orbital. These additional electrons increase the distance from chlorine's nucleus to the covalently shared electrons, while also exerting repulsive forces on the negatively charged covalent electrons. Choice C is the strongest answer. Oxygen's small size and fewer electrons allow it to exert a stronger attractive force on covalently shared electrons, making it the most likely to have the highest electronegativity value. Choice D can also be eliminated since noble gases do not readily bond with other elements and do not have well defined electronegativity values.

59. **C is the best answer.** Atomic radius increases as more principle shells are added and grows larger moving from right to left and top to bottom across the periodic table. Of the choices listed, K is found furthest to the left and bottom on the table, eliminating choices A, B, and D and making choice C the best answer.

60. D is the best answer. The atomic radius increases moving from right to left and top to bottom across the periodic table. Since atoms get smaller moving to the right across the periodic table, but get larger moving down, the size is not likely to change as much moving down and to the right (or up and to the left). This "diagonal relationship" is not an unbreakable rule, but it is a good basis for estimates. Phosphorous is represented by P on the periodic table, and Se is located down and to the right, making choices A, B, and C less likely to be the best answer. Choice D is the best answer.

61. A is the best answer. Atomic radium increases down a column and decreases moving to the right across a row. Sodium and cesium are at opposite ends of a column and would have a large difference in atomic radius. Lithium and fluorine are at opposite ends of a row and would also have a large difference in atomic radius. It is worth knowing the difference in atomic radius is much more pronounced when moving down a column than across a row, so choice A is the best answer. Hydrogen and helium have atomic radii that are very similar with He being only slightly smaller due to increased nuclear charge pulling the electrons closer. Choice C can be eliminated. Aluminum and antimony also have similar atomic radii because, although antimony has more electrons and higher energy shells, it has a more positive nucleus that keeps the electrons close. Choice D can be eliminated.

62. A is the best answer. Atomic radius decreases when moving across a row because the nucleus becomes more positive and attracts the electrons closer. The images depict s orbitals which are round and p orbitals which are 3 sets of dumbbells. For atomic radius to decrease across the row, each orbital must shrink smaller and smaller, so choice A is the best answer. Choice B assumes that there is no trend for atomic radius and orbitals are always a set size. Choice C is the opposite of the best answer. Choice D shows p orbitals that are larger than the previous s orbital. If this was the case, the atomic radius of boron would be larger than that of beryllium which is not the case. Choice D can be eliminated.

63. A is the best answer. These atoms are all isoelectronic with one another, meaning they have the same number of electrons. Negative ions are much larger than their neutral counterparts due to the extra electron-electron repulsion, while positive ions are much smaller due to increased effective nuclear charge. The atom with the least number of protons will be the best answer. Cl^- has 17 protons, Ar has 18 protons, K^+ has 19 protons, and Ca^{2+} has 20 protons. Choice A will be the largest because it has the least number of protons and is the best answer.

64. A is the best answer. The largest atomic radius will belong to the atom with the least positive nucleus. Oxygen has the fewest number of protons in its nucleus, so choice A is the best answer.

65. B is the best answer. Positive ions are much smaller than their neutral counterparts, while negative ions are much larger. Since the size of neutral atoms decreases moving from left to right across the periodic table, neutral aluminum is bigger than neutral sulfur, eliminating choice A and making choice B a strong answer choice. Al^{3+} has lost three electrons, which would make it smaller than S, eliminating choices C and D.

66. C is the best answer. Mg^{2+} is isoelectronic with Na^+, meaning it has the same number of electrons, eliminating choice A. Mass is almost irrelevant to chemical behavior, which is why different isotopes of the same element still behave similarly in chemical reactions. Choice B can be eliminated. Mg^{2+} has more protons for the same number of electrons, meaning the effective nuclear charge is greater. This makes an atom smaller, and choice C is the best answer. It is much more difficult to continue removing electrons with each additional removal. Mg^{2+} has already had two electrons removed compared to Na^+, meaning its ionization energy would be greater not less. Choice D can be eliminated.

Quantum Mechanics

67. C is the best answer. An electron can move from a lower energy state to a higher energy state by absorbing a photon. Choice A can be eliminated. The spacing between energy levels changes as the principle quantum number, n, increases. Choice B can be eliminated. The energy of each level can be computed using a known formula, $E_n = -\dfrac{m_0 q^4}{8 e_0^2 h^2 n^2}$ where n is the principle quantum number. Choice C is likely the best answer. Hydrogen and helium have different numbers of protons, which would make the values of the energy levels different between the two atoms. Choice D can be eliminated.

68. A is the best answer. The Bohr atomic model depicted the atom as a nucleus surrounded by electrons in discrete electric shells. The energy level is characterized by the rotation of the electron about the nucleus. Choice A is a strong answer as it defines the model well. Choice B can be eliminated as electrons can increase or decrease in energy. Choices C and D are not the best answers because the nucleus of an atom is just the protons and neutrons. Adding electrons changes atomic radius but not nuclear radius.

69. **A is the best answer.** The Pauli exclusion principle describes that two electrons cannot occupy the same quantum state in one atom. The quantum state is expressed by the letters n, ℓ, m_ℓ and m_s. The best answer should be the situation where the two electrons have exact same quantum numbers. This is the case in choice A. The other answer choices do have issues but none are related to the Pauli exclusion principle. Choice B describes two electrons that do not exist. The azimuthal number (l) must be from 0 to $n - 1$. So if $n = 1$ then l must be 0. Again this is not related to the Pauli exclusion principle, so choice B is not the best answer. Choice C has a similar problem as choice B except that m_l must always be an integer between –l and l. Since l is 2, m_l bust be –2, –1, 0, 1 or 2. Again this is not related to the Pauli exclusion principle, so choice B is not the best answer. Choice D represents two possible electrons in an atom. They have opposite spins, so they do not violate the Pauli exclusion principle, meaning choice D is not the best answer.

70. **C is the best answer.** Choice A is an oversimplification. Two electrons in different orbitals can have different spins without violating the Pauli exclusion principle. The Pauli exclusion principle refers to electrons, not photons, so choice B can be eliminated. The Pauli exclusion principle states that two electrons (which are fermions because their spin states are not expressed as an integer) cannot occupy the same quantum state, so choice C is the best answer. Knowing the word fermion is not necessary because this question could be answered by process of elimination. Choice D describes a mixture of the Aufbau principle and Hund's rule. Neither the Aufbau principle nor Hund's rule are consistent with the Pauli exclusion principle.

71. **D is the best answer.** There are four quantum numbers, and each electron must have a unique combination of the quantum numbers. The principle quantum number is n and describes the size of the orbital. The azimuthal quantum number is l and describes the shape of the orbital. The magnetic quantum number is m_ℓ and describes the orientation of the orbital in space. The fourth quantum number is m_s and describes the spin of the electron. Choice D is the best answer.

72. **A is the best answer.** The principle quantum number is n and describes the size of the orbital and thus the shell level of an electron within it. Choice A is likely the best answer. The azimuthal quantum number is ℓ and describes the shape of the orbital, eliminating choice B. The magnetic quantum number is m_ℓ and describes the orientation of the orbital in space, eliminating choice C. The fourth quantum number is m_s and describes the spin of the electron, eliminating choice D. Choice A is the best answer.

73. **D is the best answer.** For $n = 3$, there are s, p, and d orbitals. Two electrons can fit in the s orbitals, six in the p orbitals, and ten in the d orbitals. Remember that there are three sub-orbitals in the p orbital that can each hold two electrons, and there are five sub-orbitals in the d orbitals that can each hold two electrons. The total is therefore 18. Choice D is the best answer.

74. **A is the best answer.** The energy of an electron primarily depends on which shell it is in. This means the electron that has the highest principle quantum number will also have the highest energy. Choice A described an electron with a principle quantum number, n, of 3. This is the highest principle quantum number of the choices listed, eliminating choice B-D and making choice A the best answer.

75. **C is the best answer.** There are a few rules to calculating quantum numbers. The azimuthal quantum number, ℓ, can take a value from 0 to $n - 1$, so it must be less than n. Choice A can be eliminated. m_ℓ can be any integer between –l and +l, so it must be less than or equal to l. Choices B and D can be eliminated. Choice C contains quantum numbers that are properly calculated, making it the best answer.

76. **C is the best answer.** An electron is much smaller than a nucleus, eliminating choice A. The fact that an electron can move between orbits does not help answer the question of why modeling an electron in a known position is not accurate. Choice B is a weak answer choice. As described by the Heisenberg Uncertainty Principle, it is impossible to know both the position and momentum of an electron simultaneously. This means the exact orbit cannot be determined. Choice C is a strong answer choice. While it is difficult to describe an orbit experimentally, the precise orbit of an electron cannot be determined at all, experimental or not, due to the Heisenberg Uncertainty Principle. Choice D is a weaker answer than choice C.

77. **B is the best answer.** The Heisenberg uncertainty principle relates position and momentum, not position and velocity. Thus, objects with large mass can have smaller uncertainties in their momenta than smaller mass objects with the same position uncertainty. This is why a nucleus can be localized much more accurately than an electron. The smaller uncertainty in a basketball's momentum makes it easier to describe its path, eliminating choice A and likely making choice B the best answer. The Heisenberg Uncertainty Principle applies to all objects, no matter how large or small. Choices C and D can be eliminated.

78. A is the best answer. Elements within the same group of the periodic table tend to have similar chemical properties due to equivalent amounts of valence electrons in their outermost shell. Choice A is the best answer as it most accurately describes valence electrons. Choice B is not the best answer as valence electrons are found in the outermost shell. Choices C and D can be eliminated as elements within the same group have the exact same number of valence electrons.

79. A is the best answer. Alkali metals comprise Group 1 of the periodic table. These are metals with only one valence electron and ionize to a positive 1 charge (K^+, Na^+). The first electron in the valence shell falls under the s orbital. This is represented by a configuration that ends in s^1. Choice B represents a generic member of the second group, alkaline earth metals. Choice C represents a possible metalloid or nonmetal in the p block, not an alkali metal. Choice D is the generic formula for a d block transition metal.

80. B is the best answer. The figure shows the trends of melting point across a period (horizontal section of the periodic table), and these trends extend to other periods as well. Groups, or the vertical columns of elements in the table, share similar properties due to a shared valence shell number. Since K belongs to the alkali metals group, and Ca belongs to the alkaline earth metals group, their relationship should be analogous to that of Cs to Ba. K has a significantly lower melting point than Ca, so expect that Cs has a significantly lower melting point (171.6 Kelvin) than Ba (1,000 Kelvin, in fact). Choice A reflects the opposite relationship. Choice C is a weaker answer because there is an observable difference, on a different level of magnitude even, in the melting points between Group 1 and Group 2 metals. Choice D can be eliminated because periodic trends do provide enough information to allow us to infer this relationship.

81. B is the best answer. The key here is to remember that valence electrons, or the bonding electrons, ultimately guide the chemical and electric characteristic of an atom. An element that forms the same cationic charge number is in the same group as element X. In a buffering solution, the substitute will bear the same charge and act similarly to element X. Choice A is not the best answer because elements close to each other in atomic number or mass on the periodic table do not necessarily behave similarly in bonding—take the very reactive chlorine (12) and the very stable argon (13). Choice C is not the best answer because elements in the same period do not behave similarly in bonding—as you go down the period the number of valence electrons is different. Choice D can be eliminated because isotopes are dictated by the number of neutrons in an atomic nucleus, not the electrons. Electrons dictate bonding and ion formation over any of these features.

82. D is the best answer. Electrons fill the lowest energy levels first before filling higher shells. The next smallest noble gas can stand in for the full electron configuration of previous shells in the abbreviated electron configuration. Argon is the next smallest for Fe. Fe is found in row 4, meaning it has $3d$ and $4s$ subshells. This eliminates choices A and C. Because Fe is found in row 4, its principle quantum number is $n = 4$. Choice B can be eliminated and choice D is the best answer. Remember that the coefficient in front of the d subshells is the principle quantum number minus one, or $n - 1$.

83. C is the best answer. Notice this question is asking about the iodide ion, I^-. Iodine likely gains an additional electron to have a noble gas configuration, which is especially stable. The d orbitals can only contain 10 electrons, two in each of the five sub-orbitals. Choices A and B can be eliminated. The electron configuration of iodine is $[Kr]4d^{10}5s^25p^5$ and becomes $[Kr]4d^{10}5s^25p^6$ when it picks up the additional electron. Choice C is a strong answer. Choice D fails to include the d orbitals, making it a weak answer.

84. D is the best answer. There is a special rule for positive ions—remove the electrons with the highest principal quantum number first. Since the ground state of the chromium atom is $[Ar]4s^23d^4$, then according to the rule, the first two electrons come from the $4s$-orbital and only then are the electrons in the $3d$ orbitals removed. Choice A is the electron configuration of Cr, eliminating it as the best answer. Choice B does not remove the electrons from the $4s$ orbital first, eliminating it as the best answer. Choice C is the configuration of the Cr^{3-} ion, which would have gained not lost three electrons. Choice C can be eliminated. Choice D removes the electrons from the $4s$ orbital before the $3d$ orbital, making it the best answer.

85. C is the best answer. Each electron must have a unique combination of quantum numbers. The addition of a third possible spin state means that three electrons could now go into an orbital instead of two. An atom with an atomic number of 16 would have 16 electrons, assuming it is neutral. Choice A fails to account for the additional spin state and the $1p$ orbital does not exist. Choice A can be eliminated. Choice B forgets to fill the $2p$ orbital before the $3s$ orbital and does not account for the third spin state. Choice B can be eliminated. Choice C accounts for the third spin state and includes the $2p$ orbital before the $3s$ orbital. Choice C is likely the best answer. Choice D forgets to fill the lowest energy levels first, including the $n = 1$ and $n = 2$ orbitals. Choice D can be eliminated.

86. A is the best answer. An atom with an excited electron would have an electron that moves from one energy state to the next, often due to the absorption of a photon. In the ground state of an atom, the $2s$ subshell should be followed by the $2p$ subshell. If an electron becomes excited, it could skip the $2p$ shell and move into the $3s$ shell, making choice A a possible answer. If this is the configuration of a neutral atom, it represents an excited state of boron. Choices B, C, and D all fill the electron configuration in a predictable manner, which would not represent an atom with an electron that moved to a higher energy orbital. Choices B, C, and D can be eliminated, and choice A is the best answer.

87. A is the best answer. An atom that has absorbed light most likely has one or more electrons that have moved into higher orbitals due to the absorption of a photon. In the ground state, the $3p$ orbitals fill before the $3d$ orbitals, so an atom that has electrons in the $3d$ orbitals instead of the $3p$ orbitals is likely excited. Choice A is a strong answer choice. Choice B is the ground state electron configuration for potassium, eliminating it as a possible answer. Choice C fills the $3p$ orbitals before the $3d$ orbitals, which would represent vanadium in its ground state. Choice C can be eliminated. Choice D fills the orbitals in their lowest energy levels first, following the normal Aufbau order for filling. Choice D can be eliminated, and choice A is the best answer.

88. C is the best answer. The ground state configuration of sulfur is $[Ne]3s^23p^4$. According to Hund's rule, the p-orbitals fill up separately first, then start to pair. This means that the first three p electrons go into different orbitals, and the fourth doubles up, leaving two still unpaired. Choice C is the best answer.

89. A is the best answer. Electrons are able to absorb and release photons, but only at discrete energy values. This is because the various energy levels are not continuous and can only take certain values. Emission of 4.1 eV would be the electron relaxing back to the ground state. The other alternative is the electron could relax to the intermediate state, which has an energy of 2.3 eV. The difference between 4.1 eV and 2.3 eV would be the energy of the emitted photon: 4.1 eV − 2.3 eV = 1.8 eV. Choice A is the best answer.

90. B is the best answer. Paramagnetic elements are elements with an incomplete shell and unpaired electrons. Since the spin of each unpaired electron is parallel to one another, the electrons will align with an external magnetic field. Choice A can be eliminated as a complete subshell would not have unpaired electrons. Choice B is a strong answer as it closely matches the definition of paramagnetic elements. Choice C is not the best answer as it describes diamagnetic elements, or elements that do not react to an external magnetic field. Choice D can be eliminated as an incomplete subshell would have unpaired electrons.

91. C is the best answer. As the orbital diagram shows an incomplete orbital, the element is paramagnetic. Choices A and B are both true statements as paramagnetic elements react to external magnetic fields, which would allow for attraction or repulsion to other paramagnetic elements. Choice C is the best answer as it describes diamagnetic compounds. Choice D is also a true statement for paramagnetic elements.

92. D is the best answer. Remember that to be absorbed, the photon must have exactly the right energy to boost the electron from one level to another, or enough energy to ionize the atom. It's also important to realize the question asks for the photons that could be absorbed by an electron in its ground state at the −14.9 eV (or lowest-energy) level. Choice A lists the energy levels of various electron states not the photon energies, eliminating it as a possible answer. Choice B lists photon energies that would be absorbed between intermediate states, not beginning with the ground state each time. Choice B can be eliminated. Choice C lists the energy levels of various electron states but also in positive eV. Choice C can be eliminated. From the ground state, it takes 6.7 eV to raise the electron to the next level, 9.6 eV for the level after that, and so on. Choice D is the best answer. The last two entries in choice D (15.0 eV and 16.1 eV) have enough energy to ionize the atom, and are thus allowed.

93. B is the best answer. Every atom has every energy level and every orbital available, eliminating choice A. The higher energy levels are rarely used, unless the lower ones are full or a lot of energy has been added to the atom to start promoting electrons into the higher levels. Ionizing an atom requires promoting an electron to the "$n =$ infinity" energy level. That may sound very high, but also remember that as the values of n get bigger the energy levels get closer and closer to each other. So once there is enough energy to reach $n = 6$, little additional energy is required to reach the $n =$ infinity ionized state. One the electron has left, it cannot relax back down to lower energy states, so no spectral lines would be seen. Choice B is a strong answer choice. It is unlikely that giving the electron a little energy (but not even enough to ionize it) is going to result in a nuclear reaction where the nuclei would decompose. Choice C is a weak answer choice. The question says the atom starts at STP, and the temperature is raised, meaning the atom is no longer at STP. While it is true that temperatures higher than STP would be needed to reach $n = 7$, this does not answer the question of why the spectral lines are not visible. Choice D can be eliminated.

94. **C is the best answer.** The photoelectric effect is the excitation of electrons by photons, so choice A is an implication and is not the best answer. The light frequency, not intensity, is proportional to the kinetic energy of emitted electrons, so choice B is not the best answer. Choice C is false—metals and nonmetals can undergo the photoelectric effect. One of the greatest implications of the photoelectric effect was that light is composed of particles, which are now called photons, so choice D can be eliminated.

95. **B is the best answer.** The kinetic energy of an electron excited by a photon is given by the equation $KE = hf - \Phi$ where KE is kinetic energy, h is Planck's constant, f is the frequency of the light and Φ is the work function of the element. The table refers to different color light where blue light has a slightly higher frequency than red light. Calculating the frequency is not required for this question. By the formula $KE = hf - \Phi$, the metal with the lowest work function should have the highest energy ejection. The highest energy ejection is from K, so choice B is the best answer.

Bonding

96. **B is the best answer.** Sodium is a metal and chlorine is a nonmetal. Covalent bonds form between two nonmetals, eliminating option I. Ionic bonds form between a metal and a nonmetal. Option II is part of the best answer. Dipole-dipole bonds are intermolecular bonds that form between molecules, not intramolecular bonds that form within a molecule. Option III can be eliminated. Choice B is the best answer because it contains only option II.

97. **C is the best answer.** Ionic compounds generally consist of a metal and a nonmetal. Sodium is a metal and both chlorine and hydrogen are nonmetals, eliminating choices A and B. Because both hydrogen and chlorine are nonmetals, choice C contains no ionic bonds. Choice C is the best answer. Choice D contains both metals and nonmetals, eliminating it as a possible answer.

98. **A is the best answer.** Electronegativity decreases when moving down a group (column). This means that sulfur is less electronegative than oxygen, which rules out choices C and D. Intramolecular forces determine bond energies whereas intermolecular forces determine physical properties like boiling point. Choice B can be eliminated, and choice A is the best answer.

99. **C is the best answer.** The data presented in the table show H_2O with the largest boiling point. H_2O exhibits hydrogen bonding, which occurs between a hydrogen that is covalently bound to a fluorine, oxygen, or nitrogen atom and a fluorine, oxygen, or nitrogen atom from another molecule. Hydrogen bonding the strongest type of dipole-dipole interaction. H_2O is the only molecule capable of hydrogen bonding. Choice A can be eliminated. Although molecular weight correlates with boiling point for H_8S, H_2Se, and H_2Te, this trend does not continue for H_2O. Choice B can be eliminated. H_2O is the only molecule with hydrogen bonding (a form of dipole-dipole interaction), and it has the largest boiling point. Choice C is a strong answer. Although greater quantities of electron orbitals seem to explain the boiling point trend for H_8S, H_2Se, and H_2Te, this is not the case for H_2O. Choice D can be eliminated. Choice C is the best answer.

100. **A is the best answer.** Note that dimethylformamide contains two electronegative atoms (oxygen and nitrogen) bound to a less electronegative atom (carbon). This will generate two dipole moments within the dimethylformamide molecule, placing partial negative charges on oxygen and nitrogen and a partial positive charge on carbon. These partial charges can interact with other partial charges of the opposite charge via dipole-dipole interactions. Choice A is a strong answer. Covalent bonding represents intramolecular interactions, not intermolecular interactions. Choice B can be eliminated. Hydrogen bonding occurs between a hydrogen that is covalently bound to a fluorine, oxygen, or nitrogen atom and a fluorine, oxygen, or nitrogen atom from another molecule. Dimethylformamide is not capable of hydrogen bonding. Choice C can be eliminated. Induced dipoles occur in all molecules, including nonpolar molecules, as a result of electrons moving freely between a bond. At a given moment, electron density may be greater on one side of the bond than the other, generating an instantaneous dipole that can further induce neighboring bonds to exhibit induced dipoles. Induced dipole interactions are amongst the weakest of intermolecular interactions, and because dimethylformamide is capable of dipole-dipole interactions, induced dipole interactions are not the primary source of intermolecular interactions. Choice D can be eliminated. Choice A is the best answer.

101. B is the best answer. Although iodine is an electronegative atom, I_2 is nonpolar and does not have a permanent dipole because both atoms involved in the covalent bond have equal electronegativities. Choice A can be eliminated. Instantaneous dipoles can arise spontaneously in nonpolar molecules because at any given moment, the electrons within a covalent bond are not evenly distributed. This uneven distribution generates a momentary dipole that can induce neighboring molecules to sequentially generate a short-lived dipole, called an induced dipole. Choice B is the best answer. Hydrogen bonding occurs between a hydrogen that is covalently bound to a fluorine, oxygen, or nitrogen atom and a fluorine, oxygen, or nitrogen atom from another molecule. Choice C can be eliminated. Covalent bonds are intramolecular interactions, not intermolecular interactions. Choice D can be eliminated. Choice B is the best answer.

102. D is the best answer. Van der Waal's forces are the weakest dipole-dipole force between two instantaneous dipoles. Instantaneous dipoles occur spontaneously because, as electrons move about, at any given moment they may not be evenly distributed between two bonding atoms. This uneven distribution generates a dipole which, when combined with another instantaneous dipole, generates a Van der Waals' interaction. Because this interaction occurs between two bonded atoms, Van der Waals' forces can exist in all molecules, even when they are capable of stronger intermolecular interactions. Choice D is the best answer.

Reactions and Stoichiometry

103. B is the best answer. Use the units to help guide the conversion: 18 g/mol × 1 mol/(6.02 × 10^{23} molecules) × 1 kg/1,000 g. Choice A does not divide by Avogadro's number, eliminating it as a possible answer. Choice B closely matches the calculation, making it the best answer. Choice C can be eliminated because it multiplies, not divides, by 1000. Choice D does not convert g to kg, eliminating it as the best answer.

104. D is the best answer. The mass of one nitrogen atom is 14 amu, so the mass of two nitrogen atoms is 28 amu. If nitrogen makes up 10% of the compound multiply 28 amu by 10 to get 280 amu for the molecular weight of the compound. Choice D is the best answer.

105. C is the best answer. The best approach to this question is through process of elimination, where the molecular weight of each compound is calculated based on the amu values listed in the periodic table. Choice A has a molecular weight of 61 amu, while choice B has a molecular weight of 49 amu. These are much lighter than 98.96 amu, eliminating them as possible answers. Choice C looks about right: (2 × 35.5 amu) + (2 × 12 amu) + (4 × 1 amu) = 99 amu, which is close to the molecular weight of the molecule. Choice C is likely the best answer. Adding another chlorine, carbon, and four additional hydrogen atoms makes choice D too heavy, eliminating it as the best answer.

106. D is the best answer. The best approach to this question is through process of elimination, where the molecular weight of each compound is calculated based on the amu values listed in the periodic table. Choice A has a molecular weight of 110 amu, while choice B has a molecular weight of 142 amu. These are much lighter than 283.88 amu, eliminating them as possible answers. Choice C has a molecular weight of 174 amu, which is also too light. Choice D has a molecular weight of 284 amu, which matches the question stem. Choice D is the best answer.

107. B is the best answer. The periodic table lists the masses of atoms in atomic mass units (amu), which is also 1 g/mol. Water contains two hydrogen atoms, each with a mass of 1 amu, and one oxygen atom, with a mass of 16 amu. The water molecule then has a mass of 1 + 1 + 16 amu = 18 amu. Choice B is the best answer. The other answer choices do not have the proper units from the periodic table.

108. D is the best answer. Carbon tetrachloride is CCl_4. The atomic mass is about 12 amu + (4 × 35.5 amu) = 154 amu. Of that, the chlorine is 4 × (35.5 amu) = 142 amu. The percent by mass is 142 amu/154 amu × 100 = 92%. Choice D is the best answer, as it matches the calculated value.

109. C is the best answer. The overall molecular weight of NO_2 is 46 amu, and N is 14 amu. To calculate the percent mass, divide the atomic weight of nitrogen by the overall molecular weight and multiply by 100: 14 amu/46 amu × 100 = 30.4%. Choice C matches the calculated answer and is the best answer.

110. D is the best answer. Methane is CH_4, which is not included in choices A or B, eliminating them as the best answer. Choice C is not balanced. Notice that there are five H in the reactants but only four H in the products. Choice C can be eliminated. In addition, a combustion reaction includes oxygen. Choice D is appropriately balanced and contains methane and molecular oxygen. Choice D is the best answer.

111. C is the best answer. The best approach to answering this question is process of elimination. The carbon is not balanced in choice A, the hydrogen is not balanced in choice B, and the hydrogen is not balanced in choice D. These can be eliminated as potential answers. Choice C is appropriately balanced, making it the best answer.

112. D is the best answer. All of the reactions are properly balanced—the problem is in the nomenclature and ions. The "(II)" in copper(II) chloride means copper has a charge of +2. Chloride, being a halogen, has a charge of −1. So copper(II) chloride is $CuCl_2$. This eliminates choices A and C. Likewise, carbonate has a charge of −2, so iron(II) carbonate is $FeCO_3$. Choice B can be eliminated, and choice D is the best answer.

113. C is the best answer. The first step in solving this problem is balancing the reaction.

$$C_{12}H_{22}O_{11}(l) + 12O_2(g) \rightarrow 12CO_2(g) + 11H_2O(g)$$

From there, use the coefficients in front of the molecules to determine how many moles of oxygen are required. 1 mole of gas requires 12 moles of oxygen. Choice C is the best answer.

114. C is the best answer. The first step in solving this problem is balancing the reaction.

$$C_6H_{12}O_6(s) + 6O_2(g) \rightarrow 6CO_2(g) + 6H_2O(g)$$

From there, use the coefficients in front of the molecules to determine how many moles of oxygen are required. 1 mole of the solid requires 6 moles of oxygen. Choice C is the best answer.

115. D is the best answer. The first step in solving this problem is balancing the reaction.

$$2C_6H_{14}(g) + 19O_2(g) \rightarrow 12CO_2(g) + 14H_2O(g)$$

From there, use the coefficients in front of the molecules to determine how many moles of oxygen are required. 2 moles of hexane require 19 moles of oxygen. Choice D is the best answer.

116. C is the best answer. This question tests knowledge of reaction writing conventions. "Word" reactions are acceptable typically, but not in this case since words are not consistently used. A reverse arrow is likewise not appropriate in this case since peroxidase cannot reverse this reaction without the addition of other reagents. Peroxidase is an enzyme, not a reactant, and because it does not have a stoichiometric role, should only be written above the arrow, not to the left of it. This reaction is not missing coefficients, since it is already balanced and peroxidase does not require a coefficient as an enzyme.

117. D is best answer. A conventional reaction scheme is written with the participating (stoichiometrically important) reactants to the left of the arrow, although all reactants may be written to the left of the arrow as well. In a single step reaction, the solvent and heat or temperature change are noted below the arrow, and reagents are noted above. In a multistep reaction the first reaction is noted as "1) reagent, solvent" above the arrow and the second is noted as "2) reagent, solvent" below the arrow. The only choice that follows these conventions is choice D.

118. A is the best answer. Phase changes are considered physical changes. Boiling of a liquid turns it into a gas, so choice A is a strong answer choice. Because the reactant is already a gas, combustion of gas also forms a gas. Choice B can be eliminated. Dehydration of a solid stays a solid, eliminating choice D. Elimination is the formation of a double bond from a single bond or a triple bond from a double bond. This would not change the phase, eliminating choice D.

119. A is the best answer. Intermolecular bonds can be broken during physical changes, but the molecules themselves should not change. Choice A is a strong answer. Peptide bonds, covalent bonds, and other types of intramolecular bonds are within the molecule and should not be broken during phase change reactions like physical reactions. Choices B, C, and D can be eliminated.

120. D is the best answer. The reaction shown above is a combustion reaction because it reacts a molecule with oxygen. Choice A can be eliminated. Any reaction of one molecule with another is a chemical reaction, eliminating choice C. Oxidation-reduction reactions occur whenever molecules gain or lose electrons. The carbon loses four hydrogens and gains two oxygens, meaning methane is oxidized and oxygen is reduced. Choice C can be eliminated. Physical reactions do not form new molecules but are phase change reactions. Because intramolecular bonds are broken and formed in this reaction, it is not a physical reaction. Choice D is the best answer.

121. C is the best answer. First, the unbalanced reactions—choice A—can be eliminated. Next, choice D does not have a naturally occurring form of an iron and chlorine compound without a charge. Of the two remaining, both ferric and ferrous chloride are reasonable and are balanced. However, in choice B the charge of the iron chloride ion and tetraethylammonium chloride do not match up, leaving choice C as the best answer.

122. D is the best answer. Hydrogen peroxide is decomposed into water and oxygen, which is a redox reaction in which both reduction and oxidation of the same substrate occurs. In this case, this reaction is decomposition, but is more specifically disproportional. Likewise, while this is a catalyst mediated reaction, "catalytic" is not a standard reaction type. Due to the lack of ion transfer, this is not a single replacement. This makes choice D the most specific and best answer.

123. B is the best answer. This is an example of a disproportionation reaction, where one molecule is both oxidized and reduced. In the reactants, the chlorine gas has an oxidation state of 0. In the products, it has an oxidation state of −1 and +1 for HCl and HClO respectively. Choice B is the best answer.

124. B is the best answer. First, balance the reaction:

$$2Fe(s) + 1.5O_2(g) \rightarrow Fe_2O_3(s)$$

Note that although balanced equations are "supposed" to have integer coefficients, it is not necessary for doing stoichiometry. According to the reaction, 2 moles of iron should reaction with 1.5 moles of oxygen. If two moles of oxygen were available and 1.5 moles were used, 0.5 moles of oxygen will be left over. Choice B is the only answer choice that contains 0.5 moles of oxygen, making it the best answer.

125. A is the best answer. The limiting reagent is the one that runs out the earliest in a chemical reaction, meaning it must be a reactant. This eliminates choices C and D, meaning the best answer is either choice A or choice B. To determine which reactant is limiting, balance the reaction: $Au_2S_3(s) + 3H_2(g) \rightarrow 2Au(s) + 3H_2S(g)$. According to the balanced reaction, one mole of $Au_2S_3(s)$ reacts with three moles of hydrogen gas. If there are five moles of hydrogen gas, then there is more than enough hydrogen, and the $Au_2S_3(s)$ will run out first. Choice B can be eliminated, and choice A is the best answer.

126. D is the best answer. The equation is balanced, so multiplying the equation by 3 gives 36 moles of water and gives 12 moles of $N_2H_3(CH_3)(l)$. Choice A would be true if only 12 moles of water were produced, while choice B would be true if 24 moles of water were produced. Choice C would be true if 30 moles of water were produced. Multiplying the equation by 3 gives 36 moles of water and 12 moles of $N_2H_3(CH_3)(l)$, making choice D the best answer.

127. B is the best answer. The reaction that is presented is balanced. In order to see how many moles of water should have been produced, the entire reaction can be multiplied by two to get 10 moles of $N_2O_4(l)$. Multiplying 12 moles of water by two means the reaction should have produced 24 moles of water, but did not. This means that the other reactant must have run out first. Choice A can be eliminated, and choice B is most likely the best answer. Water is a product, not a reactant, eliminating choice C. Because 23 moles of water were produced instead of 24 moles, there is a limiting reagent. Choice D can be eliminated.

128. C is the best answer. The first step in solving this problem is identifying the limiting reagent. Because 4.5 moles of nitrogen gas were reacted, multiply the reaction by 4.5 to get:

$$4.5N_2(g) + 13.5H_2(g) \rightarrow 9NH_3(g).$$

Hydrogen is the limiting reagent because 13.5 moles are required for 4.5 moles of nitrogen gas to react, but only 11 moles of hydrogen were used in the reaction. For every 3 moles of hydrogen gas that reacts, two moles of ammonia are formed. Eleven moles of hydrogen should produce 11 moles × (2 moles ammonia/3 moles hydrogen gas) = 7.3 moles of ammonia. If it actually produces 6 moles, the yield is 6 moles/7.3 moles, which is around 82%. Choice C best matches this calculation, making it the best answer choice.

129. D is the best answer. HCl has a molar mass of 36.5 g/mol, so 328 grams is 9 moles. The question says that the reaction has a yield of 75%, so four every 4 moles of reactant that were used, only three of them produced a product. If 9 moles of HCl were produced in a 75% efficient reaction, this means that there should have been enough PCl_3 to produce 12 moles of HCl if the reaction was 100% efficient. Multiply the balanced reaction by 4 to get 12 moles of HCl in the products and 4 moles of PCl_3 in the reactants. Choice D is the best answer.

130. D is the best answer. The atomic mass listed on the periodic table has units of amu, which is also g/mol. The atomic mass of sodium is 23 amu meaning that the mass of one mole of sodium is 23 grams. Thus, 3 moles have a mass of 69 grams. Choice D is the best answer.

131. C is the best answer. The periodic table shows the atomic masses listed in amu, which is also g/mol. From the periodic table, magnesium has a molar mass of 24.3 g/mol, which means that 48 grams of magnesium would contain approximately 2 moles. Each mole has a number of atoms defined by Avogadro's number, 6.02×10^{23}. Because 48 g of Mg contains 2 moles, the number of atoms can be calculated as $2 \times 6.02 \times 10^{23}$. Choice C is the best answer.

132. B is the best answer. The charge on one electron is *e*, so one mole is Avogadro's number multiplied by *e*. Choice B is the best answer. Choice A is the charge on one electron, eliminating it as the best answer. A coulomb, C, is equal to about 6.2×10^{18} electrons, so choices C and D can be eliminated.

133. B is the best answer. The first step is figuring out how many moles of helium are in 2 g. Since helium has a molar mass of 4.0 g/mol, 2 grams is half a mole. Each mole of helium has 2 electrons since helium has an atomic number of 2 and the number of electrons and protons are equal in a neutral atom. Half of a mole of helium multiplied by 2 electrons per mole gives one mole of electrons. According to the question stem, there are 96,500 C/mol of electrons, so choice B is the best answer.

134. A is the best answer. A half-life is defined as the time required for half the amount of a substance to decay. This closely matches choice A, making it the best answer. A half-life is not half the time required for half of the substance to decay, eliminating choice B. Similarly, a half-life is defined as the time required for half the amount of a substance to decay, not all of the substance. Choices C and D can be eliminated.

135. B is the best answer. The best approach is to divide 384 grams by 2 until around 12 g of the substance remain. 384/2 = 192; 192/2 = 96; 96/2 = 48; 48/2 = 24; 24/2 = 12. This represents 5 half-lives. 5 half-lives × 10 hrs/half-life = 50 hrs. Choice B is the best answer.

Radioactive Decay

136. D is the best answer. A neutrino is an electrically neutral particle, eliminating choice A. A gamma particle is the product of radioactive atoms, eliminating choice B. A photon is a packet of light, eliminating choice C. A beta particle is a high-energy electron emitted during radioactive decay. Choice D is the best answer.

137. B is the best answer. Radioactive decay occurs when energy is released from an unstable atom, converting the atom to a more stable form. Beta decay, alpha decay, and positron emission are all forms of radioactive decay. Radioactive decay is a property of an atom, not a molecule, eliminating choice A and making choice B a strong answer. Radioactive decay is not a property of individual protons, neutrons, or electrons, eliminating choices C and D.

138. B is the best answer. Notice the mass number has decreased by four. A gamma particle has no mass, eliminating choice A. An alpha particle is a helium nucleus and has a mass number of four. Choice B is a strong answer. Both a beta particle, which is an electron, and a positron are considered to have no mass. Because the mass number changes, choices C and D can be eliminated.

139. A is the best answer. Beta decay occurs when an element releases an electron during radioactive decay. Release of an electron does not change the mass number, eliminating choices B and D. Beta decay increases the atomic number by one, changing U to Np. Choice D can be eliminated, and choice A is the best answer.

140. B is the best answer. A positron is a subatomic particle with the same mass as an electron but is positively charged. Because a positron is considered to have negligible mass, positron emission does not change the mass number. Choices A and C can be eliminated. Positron emission results in a decrease of 1 in the atomic number, changing C to B. Choice B is the best answer.

141. A is the best answer. Alpha decay releases a helium nucleus, removing 4 from the mass number and 2 from the atomic number. Each beta decay adds 1 to the atomic number. The net result is a decrease of 4 in the mass number and no change in the atomic number. This means the identity of the element stays the same, making choice A the best answer.

142. B is the best answer. Electron capture results in a decrease of 1 in atomic number and no change in mass number, as electrons are generally considered massless. Choices A and D can be eliminated because the mass number changed. A decrease of 1 in atomic number changes Hg to Au, making choice B the best answer.

143. A is the best answer. An alpha decay occurs by loss of a helium atom. The alpha decays remove 4 from the mass number and 2 from the atomic number with each decay. 7 times 4 is 28 and 7 times 2 is 14. Each beta decay adds 1 to the atomic number. The net result is a decrease of 28 in the mass number and a decrease of 8 in the atomic number. Count backwards 8 elements from U to find the identity of the new element, which is Po. Choice A is the best answer.

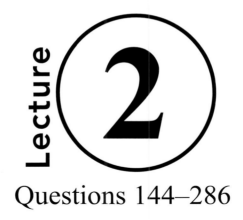

Lecture

②

Questions 144–286

Introduction to Organic Chemistry

ANSWERS & EXPLANATIONS

ANSWER KEY

144. B	157. A	170. C	183. B	196. C	209. C	222. B	235. B	248. D	261. C	274. B
145. C	158. D	171. B	184. A	197. B	210. A	223. C	236. C	249. A	262. B	275. C
146. A	159. B	172. C	185. C	198. A	211. D	224. D	237. C	250. B	263. D	276. C
147. D	160. B	173. A	186. D	199. A	212. B	225. A	238. A	251. B	264. A	277. C
148. A	161. B	174. C	187. D	200. B	213. C	226. D	239. C	252. D	265. D	278. C
149. A	162. B	175. D	188. A	201. B	214. B	227. B	240. C	253. B	266. A	279. A
150. A	163. C	176. D	189. C	202. C	215. C	228. C	241. C	254. B	267. B	280. D
151. C	164. C	177. B	190. B	203. D	216. D	229. C	242. D	255. B	268. B	281. C
152. C	165. C	178. A	191. C	204. A	217. C	230. D	243. A	256. C	269. A	282. C
153. B	166. C	179. D	192. D	205. B	218. B	231. D	244. C	257. D	270. A	283. B
154. D	167. D	180. D	193. A	206. A	219. D	232. C	245. B	258. A	271. D	284. C
155. A	168. C	181. D	194. A	207. D	220. A	233. B	246. C	259. B	272. A	285. C
156. A	169. C	182. D	195. B	208. C	221. D	234. C	247. C	260. B	273. D	286. C

Representations of Organic Molecules

144. B is the best answer. Double bonds contain one sigma bond and one pi bond. Each of these bonds has two electrons. The Lewis dot structure includes two double bonds; thus, it contains two pi bonds with a total of four electrons. Choice B is the best answer.

145. C is the best answer. There is one sigma bond, also known as a single bond, between the carbon and the nitrogen. Because the atoms share electrons, each atom contributes one electron to the bond for a total of 2 electrons. Choice C is the best answer.

146. A is the best answer. A carbon makes four bonds to complete its octet. Each pair of electrons represents one bond. Choice A shows 8 electrons bonded to each carbon, making it a strong answer. Choices B and D can be eliminated because the second carbon makes five bonds, while choice C can be eliminated because the third carbon makes only three bonds.

147. D is the best answer. In order to have no overall charge, hydrogen would want one electron, carbon four electrons, and nitrogen five electrons. This gives a total of 10 electrons for the neutral molecule. Choices A and B both contain too many electrons, eliminating them as possible answer choices. Choice C has 10 electrons, but there is a formal charge of –2 on the carbon and +2 on the nitrogen. The electrons would most likely be distributed to have no formal charge. Choice C can be eliminated. Choice D contains 10 electrons and a neutral overall charge, making it the best answer.

148. A is the best answer. Atoms from the third period of higher in the periodic table may be able to hold more than 8 electrons due to vacant *d* orbitals available for hybridization. Choice A is a strong answer. The atom could be in period 3, but it could also be in higher periods. Choice B can be eliminated. It is the presence of *d* orbitals, not electronegativity, which allows the octet rule to be broken. Choices C and D can be eliminated. Choice A is the best answer.

149. A is the best answer. Formal charge = (# valence electrons) – (# bonds) – (# nonbonding electrons). Oxygen has 6 valence electrons, and nitrogen has 5 valence electrons. Oxygen A formal charge = 6 – 6 – 1 = –1. Nitrogen formal charge = 5 – 2 – 3 = 0. Oxygen B formal charge = 6 – 4 – 2 = 0.

150. A is the best answer. The formula for formal charge is:

Formal charge = group number of the atom – number of electrons in lone pairs – ½(number of electrons in bonding pairs)

In this case, the group number of nitrogen is 5. There are 2 electron in lone pairs and 6 in bonding pairs:

Formal charge = 5 – 2 – ½(6) = 0.

Choice A is the best answer.

151. C is the best answer. While the sum of formal charges determines the overall charge of the ion, the formal charge on a given atom does not represent an actual charge on that atom. Choice A can be eliminated. Determining the overall charge does not indicate individual atom electronegativity. Choice B can be eliminated. Determining the charge distribution requires knowledge of electronegativity differences between the atoms of the ion. Choice C is a strong answer. X-ray crystallography would determine the structure but would not determine electronegativity differences. Choice D can be eliminated, and choice C is the best answer.

152. C is the best answer. The sum of the individual atoms' formal charges represents the total charge on an ion or molecule. Formal charge = (# valence electrons) – (# bonds) – (# nonbonding electrons). All hydrogens have a formal charge of 0. Nitrogen formal charge = 5 – 4 – 0 = +1. Carbon formal charge = 4 – 4 – 0 = 0. Oxygen formal charge = 6 – 1 – 6 = –1. Sum of the formal charges is 0.

Bonds and Hybridization

153. B is the best answer. Only the double bonds contained in the ring system and the one double bond on the top of the ring structure are contained in the conjugated system. In order to be called a conjugated system, the bonds need to be alternating between single and double bonds, which gives a count of 11 in the chlorophyll-a molecule. Choice B is the best answer. The conjugated system is circled on the Chlorophyll-a molecule shown below.

154. D is the best answer. Atoms may form multiple bonds depending on the number of valence electrons they have. Period 15 atoms have 5 valence electrons. 3 extra electrons are needed to form an octet. These 3 electrons can be dispersed amongst 3 single bonds, 1 double bond and 1 single bond, or 1 triple bond. If more or less bonds are formed, this will result in a positive or negative atom, respectively.

155. A is the best answer. The pi bond is formed by the overlap of two p orbitals in the *x*, *y*, or *z* dimension of space. Choice A is the best answer. Both sp^2 and sp^3 orbitals are hybrid orbitals, eliminating choices B and C. The overlap of two *s* orbitals forms a sigma bond, eliminating choice D.

156. A is the best answer. The closer a bond is to the nucleus of the bonding atoms, the stronger the bond, because the electrons feel a stronger attractive force from the nucleus. A sigma bond is closer to the nucleus than a pi bond, making choice A a strong answer and eliminating choice B. The bonds between atoms are stronger than the bonds between molecules, eliminating choices C and D. Choice A is the best answer.

157. A is the best answer. Atoms that are bound together by a single bond rotate freely around that bond, which leads to fluctuation in the shape of the molecule. π bonds prevent free rotation, which locks the molecule into place. Choice A is the best answer as compound A possesses multiple double bonds in its molecular structure. Since these bonds would prevent the molecule from rotating freely, compound A would have the most rigidity in its structure. Compound B lacks double bonds and would rotate freely, allowing for the elimination of choices C and D.

158. D is the best answer. Atoms that are bound together by single bonds can rotate freely. π bonds prevent free rotation and lock molecules into place. Choices A and C can be eliminated as possession of π bonds in compound A leads to rigidity. Choice B can be eliminated as compound A possesses a double bond. Choice D is the best answer as compound B lacks double bonds and could rotate about any of its bonds.

159. B is the best answer. Estrogen is a hormone that is relatively nonpolar and is able to diffuse through the plasma membrane. Compounds must be relatively nonpolar and planar to pass through the lipid bilayer. The planar character gives rigidity in molecular structure that allows the compound to wedge through phospholipids. This likely makes options I and II components of the best answer. Charged functional groups increase the polarity of a compound and prevent it from passing through the membrane. Option III can be eliminated. Choice B is the best answer since it contains options I and II.

160. B is the best answer. T_3 is one of the thyroid hormones that had its receptor in the nucleus. In order to pass into the nucleus, it must be able to diffuse through both the plasma and nuclear membranes. Hydroxyl and carbonyl groups are polar, which would likely prevent the molecule from diffusing through the plasma membrane. Aromatic rings are nonpolar and lock a compound into a linear conformation, which would aid in allowing the molecule to pass through the membrane. Choice B is likely the best answer. Being highly flexible around a bond would mean the molecule was unlikely to be planar and unlikely to diffuse through the plasma membrane. F atoms are also highly polar, meaning they would likely prevent a molecule from diffusing through the membrane easily. Choice D can be eliminated.

161. B is the best answer. Adipose tissue is primarily composed of fat and is hydrophobic. A drug that would have a high V_D in fat tissue would also be hydrophobic. Aromatic rings are hydrophobic and importantly induce rigidity in molecular structure that allows hydrophobic compounds to associate with other nonpolar molecules. Option I is a component of the best answer. Hydroxyl side chains are polar. The scientist would be less likely to detect high concentrations of a hydroxylated drug, eliminating option II from the best answer. A prenyl group (3-methyl-but-2-en-1-yl) is a common modification to proteins that helps proteins interact with lipid membranes. Prenylation would allow a compound to be more hydrophobic, likely increasing the concentration the scientist would record. Option III is a component of the best answer.

162. B is the best answer. The sp^3 hybridized orbital has the combination of four orbitals, one s and three p orbitals, so one fourth (25%) is s character. Choice B is the best answer.

163. C is the best answer. In order to determine the hybridization, count the number of bonds. A carbon that contains a triple bond on one side and a single bond on the other has sp hybridization, eliminating choice A. A carbon that is in one double bond and two single bonds has sp^2 hybridization, eliminating choice B. Carbon 9 has four bonds, meaning it has one s and three p orbitals. These orbitals combine to form the bonds leading to sp^3 hybridization. Choice C is the best answer. Carbon cannot have more than four bonds, eliminating choice D.

164. C is the best answer. Nitrogen 8 uses four orbitals, including three of the orbitals for bonds and the other one for its lone pair of electrons. These four orbitals combine to lead to sp^3 hybridization, making choice C the best answer.

165. C is the best answer. The central atom in this bond is the oxygen atom, which has four orbitals. Two of the four orbitals are single bonds, while the other two orbitals are filled with the two lone pairs of electrons. Because there are four orbitals, the bond is sp^3 hybridized. An sp hybridized bond has angles of 180°, eliminating choice A, while an sp^2 hybridized bond has angles of 120°, eliminating choice B. An sp^3 hybridized bond has bond angles of 109°. Choice C is the best answer. An sp^3d hybridized bond has bond angles of 90°, eliminating choice D.

166. C is the best answer. Carbon 2 is sp^2 hybridized, which means that it has one s and two p orbitals that combine to form 3 sp^2 hybridized orbitals. Because one out of three orbitals is s, the hybridized orbital on C2 has one third (33.3%) is s character. Choice C is the best answer.

167. D is the best answer. Nitrogen 8 is sp^3 hybridized, so one s and three p orbitals combine to form four sp^3 hybridized orbitals. Because three out of the four orbitals are p, the hybridized orbital on the N8 nitrogen is three fourths (75%) p character. Choice D is the best answer.

168. C is the best answer. The structure of acetone is:

Acetone

The center carbon in acetone is sp^2 hybridized because it has two single bonds to the methyl groups and one double bond to the oxygen. This means that one s orbital and two p orbitals combine to form three sp^2 hybridized orbitals. Because two out of the three orbitals are p, two-thirds (66.6%) is p character. Choice C is the best answer.

169. C is the best answer. The sulfur atom in sulfur tetrafluoride has six electrons in its valence shell and is bonded to four fluorine atoms and has one lone pair of electrons. This gives it sp^3d hybridization. Tetrahedral geometry results from an sp^3 hybridized atom, while square planar results from an sp^3d^2 hybridized atom. Choices A and B can be eliminated. The lone pair of electrons in sp^3d repels the fluorine atoms to give seesaw geometry. Choice C is the best answer. The electronegativity of the sulfur and fluoride do not determine the geometry but rather the polarity of the bond. Choice D can be eliminated.

170. C is the best answer. The carbon is the central atom in the bond and has four groups attached to it. Carbons with four groups have sp^3 hybridization, which leads to bond angles of 109°. Choice C is the best answer.

171. B is the best answer. Carbon 5 is the central atom in the bond. It is connected to three other atoms through two single bonds and one double bond. This gives a carbon with sp^2 hybridization, which has bond angles of 120°. Choice B is the best answer.

172. C is the best answer. Nitrogen 8 is bonded to three other atoms and also contains a lone pair of electrons, as it has five electrons in its outer valence shell. This means the nitrogen has four groups attached to it, giving it sp^3 hybridization. sp^3 hybridized atoms have bond angles of 109°. Choice C is the best answer.

173. A is the best answer. The question stem notes that the nitrogen has sp^2 hybridization rather than sp^3 hybridization like most other nitrogen atoms. The two electrons on nitrogen can form a double bond with carbon, displacing an electron up on oxygen. This means that one of the resonance structures has a double bond, which would give sp^2 hybridization. Choice A is a strong answer choice. Nitrogen does not always have sp^2 hybridization, but it regularly has sp^3 hybridization. Choice B can be eliminated. The lone pair of electrons would give sp^3 hybridization, eliminating choice C. While the nitrogen does have three atoms attached, it also has a lone pair in one of the resonance structures. While choice D is a true statement, it is not as specific as choice A. Choice A is the best answer.

174. C is the best answer. The strongest bonds are intramolecular bonds found between atoms of the same molecule. The greater the number of sigma and pi bonds between two atoms, the stronger the bond, and the more energy that will be required to break the bond. A single bond contains one sigma bond, while a double bond contains one sigma bond and one pi bond, and a triple bond contains one sigma bond and two pi bonds. A triple bond has the greatest number of bonds, eliminating choices A and B, and making choice C a strong answer. Intramolecular bonds are stronger than intermolecular bonds and would require more energy to break. Choice D can be eliminated, as hydrogen bonds are intermolecular bonds. Choice C is the best answer.

175. D is the best answer. The delocalized electrons of benzene stabilize the molecule by creating shorter and stronger bonds between the carbons. While the aromatic ring is often depicted as alternating single and double bonds, in reality, all of the bonds have some single bond character and some double bond character. The bonds are not as long as the carbon-carbon bonds in an alkane, eliminating choice A. The carbon-carbon bonds are also not as short as those in an alkene, eliminating choice B. A triple bond would be shorter than the length of a carbon-carbon bond in an alkene. Because these bonds are a mix of single and double bonds, not triple bonds, choice C can be eliminated. These bonds contain some single bond character and some double bond character, making choice D the best answer.

176. D is the best answer. The delocalized electrons of benzene stabilize the molecule by creating shorter and stronger bonds between the carbons. While the aromatic ring is often depicted as alternating single and double bonds, in reality, all of the bonds have some single bond character and some double bond character. This means the C2-C3 bond that appears to be a double bond in the image is really a hybrid between a single bond and a double bond. The bonds are not as long as the carbon-carbon bonds in an alkane, eliminating choice A, while the carbon-carbon bonds are also not as short as those in an alkene, eliminating choice B. A triple bond would be shorter than the length of a carbon-carbon bond in an alkene. Because these bonds are a mix of single and double bonds, not triple bonds, choice C can be eliminated. These bonds contain some single bond character and some double bond character, making choice D the best answer.

177. B is the best answer. A sigma bond is also known as a single bond. The carbon-carbon single bond is a carbon-carbon sigma bond. The table shows that a carbon-carbon single bond is 83 kcal/mol, making choice B the best answer. Choice C is the energy for a sigma bond plus one pi bond, while choice D is the energy for a sigma bond plus two pi bonds. Choices C and D can be eliminated, making choice B the best answer.

178. A is the best answer. Remember that a single bond contains one sigma bond, while a double bond contains one sigma bond and one pi bond. The double bond has 146 kcal/mol and when the 83 kcal/mol for the sigma bond is subtracted, 63 kcal/mol are left. Choice A is the best answer. Choice B is the energy for one sigma bond, while choice C is the energy for one sigma bond plus one pi bond. Choice D is the energy for one sigma bond plus two pi bonds.

Resonance and Electron Delocalization

179. D is the best answer. Resonance structures are various arrangements of bonds within a molecule due to the movement of electrons. In order for a structure to count as a resonance structure, no atoms can be moved. No hydrogens are moved in choices A, B, and C, while choice D would require a hydrogen to be removed on the carbon that now has two double bonds to it. Choice D cannot be a resonance structure for this reason, making choice D the best answer.

180. D is the best answer. To have delocalized electrons, there must be more than one double bond in an alternating single-double bond carbon chain. This is called conjugation. Option I does not have two double bonds, eliminating it from the best answer. Both options II and III have double bonds separated by a single bond, making them part of the best answer. Choice D which contains both options II and III is the best answer.

181. D is the best answer. To have delocalized electrons, there must be more than one double bond in an alternating single-double bond carbon chain, also called conjugation. Options I and II do not contain two double bonds, meaning they do not have conjugation. Option III does contain two double bonds, but they are not separated by only one single bond. Option III does not have delocalized electrons. Choice D, which lists none of the options is the best answer.

182. D is the best answer. Resonance structures are various arrangements of bonds within a molecule due to the movement of electrons. In order for a structure to count as a resonance structure, no atoms can be moved. Choices A, B, and C only move electrons to create the resonance structures, eliminating them as best answers. Choice D cannot be a resonance structure because the carbon that is part of the carbonyl cannot have 5 bonds to it, only 4. Choice D is the best answer.

183. B is the best answer. A conjugated system contains alternating single and double bonds. Option I only contains one double bond, eliminating it as the best answer. Option II contains two double bonds, but they are not alternated by one single bond. Option II can be eliminated. Only option III has alternating single and double bonds, making it the best answer. Choice B contains only option III and is the best answer.

184. A is the best answer. The major resonance contributor structures minimize the formal charges on atoms. The formal charge on an atom is represented by a plus or minus sign next to the atom. Choice A has two charges, while choices B, C, and D have four, four, and five charges, respectively. Choice A has the fewest atoms with formal charges, meaning it will be a major resonance contributor. Choice A is the best answer.

185. C is the best answer. A resonance structure is formed by the movement of electrons within a molecule, without moving any atoms. Choices A, B, and D all move electrons only, eliminating them as best answers. Choice C moves a hydrogen atom in addition to the electrons, meaning it cannot be a resonance structure. Choice C is the best answer.

186. D is the best answer. A resonance structure is formed when electrons move within a structure, without the movement of other atoms. Choice A is not 2-pentanone, which does not contain an unsaturated hydrocarbon chain. Choice A can be eliminated. Both choices B and C involve moving a hydrogen onto the oxygen. Movement of atoms does not occur in resonance structures, eliminating choices B and C. Choice D shows that an electron has moved from the double bond to the oxygen, making choice D the best answer.

187. **D is the best answer.** The most minor resonance contributor is the structure at the highest energy level. Choice A displays no separation of charge and is most likely the major resonance contributor at the lowest energy level. Choice A can be eliminated. Atoms must not be moved when drawing resonance structures, only electrons. Choice B can be eliminated because a hydrogen atom was moved from nitrogen to the oxygen. Choices C and D both exhibit separation of charges, which would result in high energy levels, but carbon does not have an octet in choice D, making it at a higher energy level. Choice C can be eliminated. Choice D is the best answer.

188. **A is the best answer.** The resonance contributor with the greatest stability (or lowest energy level) makes up the greatest proportion of the actual structure. The lower the formal charges on most atoms, the more stable the structure. Choice A is a strong answer. A weighted sum of individual resonance structures depicts the actual molecule, not any single resonance structure. Choice B can be eliminated. Greater charge separation is indicative of a higher energy level. Choice C can be eliminated. Symmetry planes do not indicate resonance structure stability. Choice D can be eliminated, and choice A is the best answer.

189. **C is the best answer.** Resonance energy is the difference between the energy of the real molecule and the energy of the most stable Lewis structure. The most stable Lewis structure has the smallest resonance energy and likely minimizes the number of atoms with formal charges. Choice A has a +1 formal charge on oxygen (a very electronegative atom) and is likely unstable. Choice A can be eliminated. Choices B and C have −1 formal charges on nitrogen and oxygen, respectively, but choice C is at a lower energy level because oxygen is more electronegative. Choice B can be eliminated. Choice D overall charge of −2, while NCO^- has an overall charge of −1. Choice D can be eliminated, and choice C is the best answer.

190. **B is the best answer.** The resonance contributor with the greatest stability (or lowest energy level) makes up the greatest proportion of the actual structure. The lower the formal charges on most atoms, the more stable the structure. Having unpaired electrons does not indicate the stability of the molecule. Choice A can be eliminated. Structure D is likely less stable than structure A because it contributes less to the actual molecular structure. A greater separation of charge is indicative of less stability. Choice B is a strong answer. Individual resonance structures do not have delocalized electrons; the actual molecular structure does. Choice C can be eliminated. Structure D is likely less stable than structure B because it contributes less to the actual molecular structure. Less nonzero formal charges indicates greater stability. Choice D can be eliminated, and choice B is the best answer.

191. **C is the best answer.** Having the lowest absolute value heat of combustion would indicate the lowest energy level, but this does not explain the findings. Choice A can be eliminated. While a small degree of charge separation would result in a lower energy level, this finding does not compare the charge separation to the resonance structures. Choice B can be eliminated. The actual molecule is a weighted sum of its individual resonance contributors because this weighted sum allows the molecule to minimize its energy level (and maximize its stability). Choice C is a strong answer. Electron delocalization describes the ability for electrons to "spread out" and create additional resonance structures, but it does not allow for a comparison between the actual molecule and resonance structures. Choice D can be eliminated, and choice A is the best answer.

192. **D is the best answer.** The bonds between atoms result from the attraction of electrons in the bonds to the protons in the nuclei of the atoms. Remember that electrons are negatively charged and protons are positively charged. Dipole-dipole and hydrogen bonding are both intermolecular bonds that form between molecules, not intramolecular bonds that form between atoms. Choices A and B can be eliminated. Gravitational attraction plays an infinitesimally small role in the attraction between atoms due to their nearly negligible mass. Choice C is a possible answer, but it is probably not the best answer. Because the attraction involves negative and positive charges, the electrostatic force is the best answer. Choice D is the best answer.

193. **A is the best answer.** Competitive inhibitors increase K_M, also known as the Michaelis constant, which is defined as the concentration of substrate at with the velocity is $\frac{1}{2}V_{max}$. The most inhibited enzyme will have the highest K_M, which is logical because the inhibition means more substrate needs to be present to for the enzyme to work appropriately. The most inhibited enzyme should be the one with the most partially ionic bond. Bonds are partially ionic where there is a vast difference in electronegativities of atoms. Structure II has the greatest difference in electronegativities so it should have the highest K_M followed by structure I. So, Choice A is the best answer. No other answer choices have structure II as the highest K_M, so choices B, C, and D can be eliminated.

194. A is the best answer. Remember that electronegative atoms, like oxygen, tend to attract the electrons in bonds closer to their nuclei than less electronegative atoms. This means the oxygen will take on a slightly negative charge and the carbon will take on a slightly positive charge. The convention for writing the net dipole moment is to point the arrow towards the slightly negative portion of the molecule, meaning choice A is the best answer. The oxygen atom, not the methyl groups, will have an excess of negative charge, eliminating choices B and D. Choice C points the arrow in the opposite direction as the net dipole convention, eliminating it as the best answer.

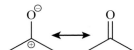

195. B is the best answer. Electronegative atoms tend to attract the electrons in a bond closer to their nuclei. The oxygen molecule has greater electronegativity than the carbon, meaning the net dipole moment is oriented towards the oxygen. Choice A orients the net dipole moment towards the electropositive carbon, which is the opposite of what is true. Choice A can be eliminated. Choice B is likely the best answer, as it orients the dipole moment towards the electronegative oxygen. There are no electronegative atoms to the left or right of the molecule, eliminating choices C and D.

196. C is the best answer. The question states that to be IR active the molecule must have a dipole moment. Dipole moments result when there are atoms with different electronegativities. Option I has an electronegative oxygen at the end of the molecule, making it part of the best answer. Benzene is aromatic, meaning it has no net dipole moment. Option II is not part of the best answer. Option III also has a net dipole moment due to the electronegative oxygen. Choice C is the best answer, as it contains options I and III but not II.

197. B is the best answer. A molecule contains a net dipole moment when it has atoms of varying electronegativities and the individual dipole moments of the bonds do not cancel out. All four of the bonds to the carbon in option I are hydrogens. While there is an electronegativity difference between carbon and hydrogen, the bonds are arranged in a manner that the net dipole moments of each bond will sum to cancel out. Option I can be eliminated. Similar to option I, option II contains four chlorine atoms attached to the carbon. While each individual bond will have a net dipole moment, the sum of the individual dipole moments cancel, eliminating option II. Option III contains three different bonds to the carbon. Because the $C-H$, $C-CH_3$, and $C-OH$ bonds will all have different dipole moments, the overall molecule will also have a net dipole moment. Choice B, which contains only option III, is the best answer.

198. A is the best answer. The dipole in ethanol results from the electronegativity difference between oxygen and carbon. Oxygen is more electronegative, so the partial positive charge is on the carbon, while the partial negative charge is on the oxygen. This means that the dipole vector points toward the oxygen, making choice A the best answer. The dipole vector does not point towards the oxygen in choices B, C, or D, eliminating them as the best answer.

Functional Groups and Their Features

199. A is the best answer. Haloalkanes are alkanes with halogens. Alkanes contain only carbon-carbon single bonds and the halogen atoms are found in Group 17 of the periodic table. Choice A contains chlorine, which is a halogen, and only carbon-carbon single bonds, making it a strong answer choice. None of choices B, C, or D contain halogens, eliminating them as the best answer. Choice A is the best answer.

200. B is the best answer. Alkanes contain only carbon-carbon single bonds. The only molecule that does not contain only carbon-carbon single bonds is choice B. Choice B contains a carbon-carbon double bond, which makes it an alkene, not an alkane. Choice B is the best answer.

201. B is the best answer. The term geminal refers to two of the same functional group attached to the same carbon. Remember that chlorine is also a halogen. While choice A contains two chlorines, they are each attached to separate carbons, eliminating choice A. Choice B shows two chlorines attached to the same carbon, meaning this is a geminal halide. Choice B is likely the best answer. Both choices C and D do not contain two halogens, eliminating them as best answers.

202. C is the best answer. First note that blood is largely composed of water. Water has a permanent dipole moment and is polar. The most soluble haloalkane will be the answer choice that has the strongest dipole moment and is the most polar. Fluorine is more electronegative than chlorine. 1-Fluorohexane will have a greater charge distribution between the halogen and terminal carbon than 1-chlorohexane. Choice A can be eliminated. Although fluorine is more electronegative than bromine, 1,1,1-tribromopropane has three electronegative atoms attached to the terminal carbon. This will generate a greater dipole moment than one electronegative atom. Choice B can be eliminated. The only difference between choices C and D is the length of the alkyl chain. Note that alkyl chains are non-polar. Propane is a shorter alkyl chain than pentane and minimizes the non-polarity of the molecule. Choice D can be eliminated. Choice C is the best answer.

203. D is the best answer. A double bond that is part of an alkene is slightly electronegative, meaning the more substitution around the double bond, the more stable the molecule will be. Larger functional groups, like methyl groups, provide more stability than smaller functional groups like hydrogens. Choice A only has one alkane as a substituent, while choice B has two. Choice C has three alkanes as substituents, while choice D has four. Because choice D is the most substituted, it will be the most stable and is the best answer.

204. A is the best answer. A geometric isomer exists when the substituents of a double bond are different, meaning they can be exchanged. This has the possibility of creating *cis* and *trans* isomers. In myrcene, all of the double bonds have two substituents on one end of the bond that are the same. Consequently, there is no possibility for geometric isomerism. Choice A is the best answer.

205. B is the best answer. Cations lack one or more electrons, which makes them unstable. Substituents that have electron density can help stabilize cations, meaning the most stable cations have the most substitution, while the least stable cations have the least substitution. The cation in choice A has carbons on either side to help donate some electron density, while the cation in group B on has one carbon attached. Choice B is less stable than choice A. Similar to choice A, choice C has two carbons, while choice D has three. Choice D is the most stable cation, while choice B is the least stable. Choice B is the best answer.

206. A is the best answer. The addition of sulfuric acid, a strong acid, most likely leads to the protonation of the hydroxyl to form water as a leaving group. This means the first step in the elimination reaction would be water leaving the molecule. This would form a carbocation, which could shift multiple places in the molecule via hydride shifts and methyl shifts. While the reaction would lead to some proportion of the product shown, many other products would also exist due to the shifting carbocation. Choice A is a strong answer choice. Dehydration can be acid catalyzed, eliminating choice B. Protonation of an alcohol to create a water leaving group can form an alkene, eliminating choice C. The alcohol required for the reaction could likely be synthesized to the needed quantity, eliminating choice D.

207. D is the best answer. Concentrated acid and heat would likely lead to protonation of nucleophilic groups in an alkene, not formation of an alcohol. Choice A can be eliminated. Use of hydrogen and a metal catalyst would reduce the alkene to an alkane via hydrogenation. Choice B can be eliminated. Use of ozone, O_3, leads to the addition of carbonyl groups, not alcohol groups, eliminating choice D. Dilute cold acid will promote hydration because the water in the acid is the source of the hydroxyl group. Choice D is the best answer.

208. C is the best answer. The hydroxyl group is a tertiary hydroxyl group in 2-methyl-2-butanol. Sulfuric acid will help protonate the hydroxyl group, allowing it to leave the molecule as water, forming a carbocation. The proton can leave from either side of the molecule, as shown in the mechanism below, leading to two possible products. If the hydrogen on C1 leaves as a proton, option I is formed, while if the hydrogen on C3 leaves as a proton, option II is formed. The methyl position would not move, eliminating option III. Choice C that includes only options I and II is the best answer.

209. C is the best answer. An electrophile "loves electrons", meaning it is usually positively charged or partially positively charged. Molecules that have excess electron density, such as oxygen and nitrogen, are often nucleophiles because they donate electrons. Choices A and B can be eliminated. Choice C contains a positive charge, so it is a strong answer choice. Choice D is likely neither a nucleophile nor an electrophile, eliminating it as the best answer. Choice C is the best answer.

210. A is the best answer. In the addition reaction, the bromine will add to the double bond. During the process of addition, a carbocation is formed. A carbocation is most stable when it is most substituted, and the bromine will then attack the carbocation. This leads to the bromine adding to the more substituted side of the double bond, which is on carbon two in this question. Choice A is a strong answer. Choice B can be eliminated because the bromine would add to the more substituted, not the less substituted side. The methyl group should not leave, eliminating choice C. Because this is an addition reaction, the double bond will be eliminated when the hydrogen and bromine add. Choice D, which describes an alkene, can be eliminated. The mechanism of the reaction is shown below.

211. D is the best answer. The alkene that forms the must stable carbocation would likely react the fastest with HBr, because the bromine ion could attack the carbocation to finish the reaction. Ethene has no substitution, while 1-Butene has substitution on one of the carbons of the double bond. 2-Butene also has only one substitution on each of the carbons that are part of the double bond. 2-Methyl-2-butene has two substitutions of one side of double bond, which would both provide electron density to stabilize the carbocation intermediate. Choice D is the best answer because it has a carbon with the must substitution.

212. B is the best answer. Aromatic rings are extremely stable and require excessive amounts of energy to disrupt their bonding. Benzene does have double bonds, eliminating choice A. Benzene does not undergo addition reactions because they would result in one double bond being converted to two single bonds, thus disrupting the aromaticity. This would be energetically unfavorable, making choice B the best answer. A substitution reaction does not disrupt aromaticity, eliminating choice A. While benzene is an alkene, choice D does not explain why benzene avoids substitution reactions.

213. C is the best answer. An aldehyde has a hydrogen attached directly to a carbonyl carbon. Choice A is a ketone, which does not have a hydrogen attached directly to the carbonyl carbon. Choice B is an ester, which has an −OR group attached to the carbonyl carbon. Choice C has a hydrogen attached to the carbonyl carbon, making it the best answer. Choice D is a carboxylic acid, as it has a hydroxyl attached to the carbonyl carbon.

214. B is the best answer. A ketal has two ether groups attached to a secondary carbon. Choice A shows two hydroxyl groups attached to the same carbon, making it a geminal diol. Choice B shows two −OR groups attached to the same carbon, making it the best answer. Choice C is a hemiacetal, while choice D is a hemiketal. Choices C and D can be eliminated, and choice B is the best answer.

215. C is the best answer. A hemiacetal has one ether group and one hydroxyl group attached to a primary carbon. The best way to identify a primary carbon is that it is only attached to one other carbon. Choice A is a geminal diol, while choice B is a ketal. Choice C has an ether group and a hydroxyl group attached to a primary carbon, making it the best answer. While choice D appears similar to choice B, the ether group and hydroxyl group are on a secondary carbon in choice D, making it a hemiketal.

216. D is the best answer. A hemiketal has one ether group and one hydroxyl group attached to a secondary carbon. Choice A is a geminal diol, while choice B is a ketal. Choice C is a hemiacetal, because it has the ether group and hydroxyl group attached to a primary carbon. Choice D shows the ether group and hydroxyl group attached to a secondary carbon, making choice D the best answer.

217. C is the best answer. Amine functional groups contain nitrogen attached to at least one other carbon. Each of the nitrogen atoms in the molecule are bonded to a carbon, meaning the best way to answer this question is by counting the number of nitrogens. There are 12 nitrogens in the molecule, each attached to at least one carbon, meaning all 12 nitrogens are contained in amine groups. Choice C is the best answer.

218. B is the best answer. Piperazine has nitrogen atoms with two alkyl groups attached. A primary amine only has one alkyl group attached, eliminating choice A. A secondary amine has two alkyl groups attached, making choice B a strong answer choice. A tertiary amine has three alkyl groups attached, eliminating choice C. A quaternary amine has four alkyl groups attached, eliminating choice D.

219. D is the best answer. The reaction favors the reactants indicating that the reactants are more stable. The basicity of the amines is unlikely to be the driving force behind the reaction, eliminating choices A and B. The aromaticity of the reactant stabilizes it, making it unlikely to be involved in a reaction that would eliminate the aromaticity. The lone pair of electrons on the neutral nitrogen atom plus the 4 electrons from the pi bonds meet the $(2n + 2)$ rule for aromaticity. The secondary amine in the products does not have two electrons on the nitrogen, meaning it is not aromatic. Choice C can be eliminated and choice D is the best answer.

220. A is the best answer. The lower pK_b value indicates that *p*-toluidine is more basic. An alkyl group also donates electrons, which makes an amine more electron-rich and better able to act as a base to attack free protons in solution. Choice A is a strong answer. The lower pK_b value indicates that *p*-toluidine is more basic, eliminating answers B and D. The alkyl group is electron-donating, not electron-withdrawing, eliminating choice C. Choice A is the best answer.

221. D is the best answer. A dipole moment is generated due to a difference in electronegativities between two atoms in a bond. The greater the difference in electronegativity, the greater the dipole moment. Since the carbon-chloride bond has the largest dipole moment, it has the greatest electronegativity difference. Choice D is the best answer.

222. B is the best answer. The electronegativity difference determines the distribution of electrons between bonded atoms. This distribution creates the polarity of the bond. Atomic size would contribute to the length of a bond, but not necessarily the polarity. Choice A can be eliminated. The difference in electronegativity between the two atoms determines the polarity. Choice B is a strong answer choice. The difference in number of protons or number of valence electrons may affect the bond length, but is less likely than the difference in electronegativity to affect the polarity. Choices C and D can be eliminated, and choice B is the best answer.

223. **C is the best answer.** The electrons in the $1s$ orbital are part of a sigma bond and are most likely covalent if the electrons are shared between two atoms. All of the molecules listed are covalently bonded, meaning the electrons are shared. Electronegative atoms attract electrons more, so the sharing is uneven within a bond. This concentrates negative charge around more electronegative atoms. Both F and Br are halogens that have much greater electronegativities than H. Choices A and B can be eliminated. A diatomic atom, like N_2, contains two atoms with the exact same electronegativity. The electrons should be equally shared, likely making choice C the best answer. There is still an electronegativity difference between B and H, eliminating choice D.

224. **D is the best answer.** Electronegativity is a measure of how strongly an element attracts electrons in a bond, while the dipole moment of a bond depends on whether the electrons are pulled to one side or other of the bond. In order to have a large dipole moment, one element must be pulling much harder than the other, meaning the electronegativity of one element must be much more than another. It is the difference in electronegativities between the two atoms, not whether they are both high, moderate, or low. Choices A, B, and C are weaker answer choices. If one atom has a high electronegativity, while another has low electronegativity, there will likely be a strong dipole moment. Choice D is the best answer.

225. **A is the best answer.** Electronegativity describes how strongly an element attracts electrons in a bond. Oxygen is more electronegative than hydrogen, meaning the electrons in the bond are found closer to oxygen than hydrogen. This gives oxygen a slightly negative charge, while the hydrogen gets a slightly positive charge. Choice A is a strong answer choice. While oxygen does have more valence electrons than hydrogen, it is the electrons in the bonds that determine the charge distribution. Choice B can be eliminated. While oxygen is sp^3 hybridized, this does not explain the electron distribution of the bond, eliminating choice C. Similarly, while the water molecule does have a bent shape, this also does not explain the electron distribution of the bond, eliminating choice D.

226. **D is the best answer.** Electronegativity differences between atoms create polar bonds. Carbon, chlorine, oxygen, and hydrogen all have electronegativity differences, meaning each bond is a polar bond. The only bonds that are completely nonpolar are ones between atoms that are identical. Options I, II, and III all have polar bonds, making choice D the best answer.

227. **B is the best answer.** Chlorine is very electronegative and carbon is not. Chlorine will hog the electrons, so choice A is not the best answer. There will be a dipole due to the differences in electronegativity, so choice B is a strong answer. The bond will be normal energy. All bonds have associated energies. There is no such thing as a zero energy bond, so choice C is not the best answer. A pi bond is a double bond, which is essentially impossible when carbon bonds a halogen because it would either expand chlorine's octet or put a positive charge on chlorine. These are unlikely to occur, so choice D is not the best answer.

228. **C is the best answer.** Electronegative groups hoard electrons; thus, they polarize a bond. Choice A is not the best answer. Electronegative leaving groups are generally great leaving groups because they are able to accept electrons to "leave" with. Choice B is not the best answer. Electronegative groups polarize the bond between them and carbon, which puts a partial positive charge on carbon. Electrophiles love electrons because they have a full or partial positive charge. Choice C is a strong answer. It is difficult to predict from electronegativities if a group will favor S_N1, S_N2, E1, or E2, so choice D is not the best answer.

229. **C is the best answer.** Choice A is not the best answer because ATP has 10 carbons. The molecular formula can be reduced to the lowest integer values by which all atoms are divisible. Since there is a prime number of N, O and P, the number of C and H cannot be reduced. Choice B is unlikely to be the best answer because there are 16 hydrogens on ATP. Remember not all hydrogens are drawn; always assume there are 4 bonds to carbon. Choice D is unlikely to be the best answer because there are not 12 carbons.

230. **D is the best answer.** The modified cysteine is called selenocysteine because it includes a Se atom in place of S. Notice that they are in the same group. Choices A and B are unlikely to be the best answer because they would not share similar properties to cysteine, so it would not be appropriate to call them a "modified cysteine." Choice C is serine which is not an "unusual amino acid." In fact, it is very common. UGA is the stop codon and serine is not encoded by the stop codon, it has its own codons. So, choice C can be eliminated, and choice D is the best answer.

Stereochemistry

231. D is the best answer. A chiral center is a carbon that is attached to four groups that are not chemically equivalent, meaning no two substituents are the same. The diagram below shows the three chiral centers. Remember that hydrogen atoms are not displayed on these drawings, but are still understood to be present. Because there are three chiral centers, choice D is the best answer.

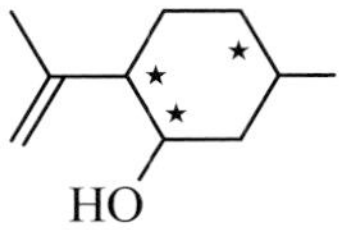

232. C is the best answer. Notice that the double bond has eliminated one of the chiral centers in the ring of isopulegols when forming pulegols. This means only the carbon attached to the hydroxyl and carbon six attached to the methyl group are now chiral centers because they are each attached to four different chemical groups. Choice C is the best answer.

233. B is the best answer. By convention, the intersection of two lines always represents a carbon atom in a Fischer projection. Choice B is the best answer.

234. C is the best answer is the best answer is the best answer. The Fischer projection shown is a shorthand representation of the structure shown below. In a Fischer projection, horizontal lines are oriented out of the page, while vertical lines are oriented into the page. This means that the hydroxide groups are hydroxyl groups are both coming out of the page.

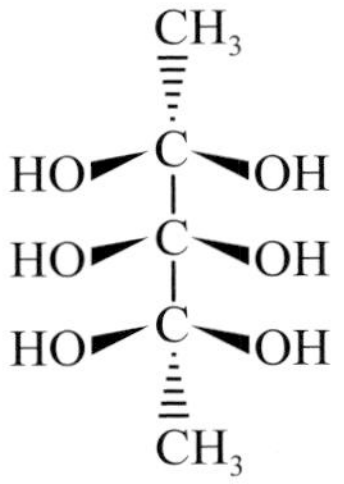

235. B is the best answer. A Newman projection represents a carbon-carbon single bond between two adjacent carbons. Assuming the carbon is neutral, all carbon atoms are the same size, eliminating choice A. The intersection of the three lines in the front of the projection represents carbon one, while the circle behind the intersecting lines represents carbon two. Choice B is a strong answer, and choice C can be eliminated. The radius of the bond is determined by the bond length; it is not described by a Newman projection. Choice D can be eliminated.

236. C is the best answer. A chiral molecule contains one or more chiral centers. A chiral center is where a carbon is attached to four different substituents. The carbon in choice A is bound to three hydrogens, while the carbons in choice B are bound to two or more hydrogens, eliminating them as chiral compounds. Carbon one of choice C is bound to four different groups: CH_3, H, CH_2CH_3, and Cl. Choice C contains a chiral carbon and is likely the best answer. Carbon one in choice D is bound to two methyl groups, eliminating it as the best answer.

237. C is the best answer. A chiral compound requires at least one chiral center, which occurs when a carbon is connected to four different groups. In 1,2-dibromopentane, carbons one and two have four different groups attached to them, but also notice that there is a plane of symmetry down the middle of the molecule. A meso compound has a plane of symmetry, even though there are chiral centers, meaning a meso compound is not a chiral compound. Choice A can be eliminated. An anomeric compound is one of two configurations of the ring form of a sugar. Because 1,2-dibromopentane is not a sugar, choice B can be eliminated. The plane of symmetry down the middle of the molecule makes choice C a strong answer choice. An enantiomer is one configuration of a chiral compound. Because 1,2-dibromopentane is not a chiral compound, choice D can be eliminated.

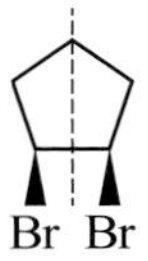

238. A is the best answer. A Fischer projection is a planar representation of a molecule. The horizontal lines come out of the board, while the vertical lines go into the board. Choices A and C show Fisher projections, making them possible answer choices, while choices B and D do not. Choices B and D can be eliminated. If the molecule is rotated as shown below, the hydroxyl group is oriented to the right, making choice A a better answer choice than choice C. Choice A is the best answer.

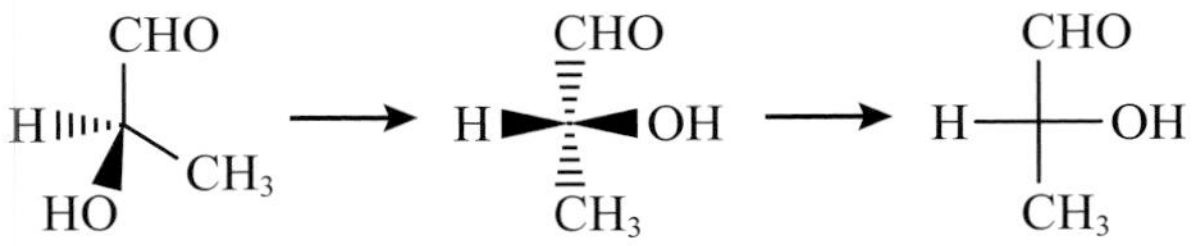

239. C is the best answer. Isomers are molecules that share the same chemical formula but are different compounds. Choice A is the same compound, just rotated. Choice A can be eliminated. The chemical formula is $C_6H_{11}OCl$. Choice B has 9 hydrogens and can be eliminated. Choice C has the same chemical formula but different bond-to-bond connectivity, representing a structural isomer. Choice C is a strong answer. Choice D has 13 hydrogens and can be eliminated. Choice C is the best answer.

240. C is the best answer. Isomers are molecules that share the same chemical formula but are different compounds. The molecular formula is $C_8H_{10}O$. All of the answer choices in fact have this molecular formula. Note, however, that choice C is actually the same molecule, just rotated. Choice C is the best answer.

241. C is the best answer. Geometric isomers have varying placements of groups around a double bond, such as *cis* and *trans* isomers. Choice A can be eliminated. Stereoisomers have the exact same connectivity but different chirality around one or more chiral carbons. Structures A and B do not contain chiral carbons, eliminating choice B. Tautomers are formed when a hydrogen is moved within a structure, such as the shifted hydrogen circled below. Choice C is likely the best answer. Because structures A and B are tautomers, choice D can be eliminated, and choice C is the best answer.

Structure A   Structure B

242. D is the best answer. Isomers are molecules that share the same chemical formula but are different compounds. The compound in question has an *R* absolute configuration. All else equal, having an *S* absolute configuration would the compound an enantiomer (a type of isomer), but choice A does not specify all else being equal. Choice A can be eliminated. Isomers must have the same number of atoms because they share the same chemical formula. Choice B can be eliminated. Because this molecule already as an *R* stereochemistry, choice C represents the same molecule, not an isomer. Choice C can be eliminated. Choice D states the correct molecular formula and displays an option with different bond-to-bond connectivity. This represents a structural isomer. Choice D is the best answer.

243. A is the best answer. Isomers are molecules that share the same chemical formula but are different compounds. The mass of the empirical formula is 14 grams. Divide the actual compound's molar mass by the empirical formula's mass to determine the scaling factor for the molecular formula. 56 g/14 g = 4. The molecular formula is C_4H_8. Choice A is the only answer choice with a molecular formula that matches this and is the best answer.

244. C is the best answer. Structural isomers are molecules with the same molecular formula but different bond-to-bond connectivity. Choice A is the same molecule; the double and single bonds on the first carbon have been drawn differently, but the connectivity is the same. Choice A can be eliminated. The actual molecule's molecular formula is $C_3H_6O_2$. Choice B has 4 hydrogens and can be eliminated. Choice C has the same molecular formula but different connectivity. Choice C is a strong answer. Choice D has 4 carbons and can be eliminated. Choice C is the best answer.

245. B is the best answer. Structural isomers are molecules with the same molecular formula but different bond-to-bond connectivity. First note that the molecular formula can be rewritten as $C_4H_{19}OH$, or 1-butanol. Moving the hydroxyl group to the second carbon generates 2-butanol. From 1-butanol, attaching carbon 4 to carbon 2 generates 2-methylpropan-1-ol. From 2-butanol, attaching carbon 4 to carbon 2 generates 2-methylpropan-2-ol. This sums to 4 structural isomers, making choice B the best answer.

1-butanol   2-butanol

2-methylpropan-1-ol   2-methylpropan-2-ol

246. C is the best answer. Conformers, or conformational isomers, have the same connectivity of atoms but varying degrees of rotations around single bonds. Because the connectivity of the two structures is not the same, choice A can be eliminated. Enantiomers have opposite chirality at all chiral centers. Neither structure contains a chiral carbon, eliminating choice B. Structural isomers have the same molecular formula but different connectivity, as is shown by the two molecules. Choice C is a strong answer choice. Geometric isomers have different *cis* or *trans* arrangements around one or more double bonds. Because no double bonds are present in the molecules, choice D can be eliminated, and choice C is the best answer.

247. C is the best answer. Conformers, or conformational isomers, have the same connectivity of atoms but varying degrees of rotations around single bonds. Because the connectivity of the two structures is not the same, choice A can be eliminated. Enantiomers have opposite chirality at all chiral centers. Neither structure contains a chiral carbon, eliminating choice B. Structural isomers have the same molecular formula but different connectivity, as is shown by the two molecules. Choice C is a strong answer choice. Geometric isomers have different *cis* or *trans* arrangements around one or more double bonds. Because no double bonds are present in the molecules, choice D can be eliminated, and choice C is the best answer.

248. D is the best answer. A meso compound contains a plane of symmetry within a molecule, which is not found for the first molecule. Choice A can be eliminated. Enantiomers are versions of chiral molecules. A chiral molecule requires at least one chiral center that would be connected to four different groups. Neither molecule has a chiral center, eliminating choice B. Epimers are different configurations of sugars in ring form. Because neither molecule is a sugar, choice C can be eliminated. Notice that the position of the double bond is different between the two molecules. A stereoisomer has the same bond connectivity but different rotation down a single bond. Choice D does not show different rotation but rather different placement of the double bond. Choice D is the best answer.

249. A is the best answer. Conformers, or conformational isomers, have the same connectivity but different rotation around a carbon-carbon single bond. This is shown by the projections in the question. Choice A is a strong answer. Enantiomers have opposite chirality at each chiral center. Because the connectivity is the same, the chirality is the same. Choice B can be eliminated. Structural isomers have different connectivity of the atoms. The connectivity of the atoms is the same for the two molecules because the second molecule is just rotated around the carbon-carbon single bond. Choice C can be eliminated. Geometric isomers have different *cis* or *trans* configuration around a double bond. These molecules do not contain double bonds, eliminating choice D.

250. B is the best answer. The degree to which groups overlap and have Van der Waals interactions determines which conformational isomer, or conformer, will have the greatest energy. The larger the size of each group that overlaps, the greater the Van der Waals interaction. Choice A shows the gauche conformation, which is staggered, but still would have some overlap between the methyl groups. Choice A is a possible answer. Choice B shows the eclipsed conformation, which has full overlap between the methyl groups. This would be higher energy than the gauche conformation, making choice B a better answer than choice A. Choice C shows the anti conformation, which would have the lowest energy. Choice C can be eliminated. Choice D shows overlap between the methyl groups and H but not the methyl groups directly. Choice D can be eliminated, as choice B shows direct overlap between the methyl groups.

251. B is the best answer. The conformer has the two largest groups staggered, but located next to each other. The antistaggered conformation would have the groups opposite one another, eliminating choice A. The conformational isomer that has staggered groups located next to each other is called the gauche conformation, making choice B a strong answer. The fully eclipsed conformation has the two largest groups directly on top of each other, which is not shown. Choice C can be eliminated. The eclipsed conformation has groups on top of each other, but the two largest groups do not have to be directly on top of one another. Choice D is not show, eliminating it as the best answer.

252. D is the best answer. The conformer has the atoms eclipsed, but the largest groups are not eclipsing each other. The antistaggered conformer has the two largest groups opposite one another, which is not shown. Choice A can be eliminated. The gauche conformation shows the two largest groups staggered but next to one another, which is also not shown. Choice B can be eliminated. The fully eclipsed conformation has the two largest groups eclipsing one another, which is not shown. Choice C can be eliminated. The eclipsed conformation has groups eclipsing one another, but the two largest groups are not. Choice D is the best answer, as this is most similar to the pictured conformer.

253. B is the best answer. A conformational isomer, or conformer, has varying rotation around a carbon-carbon single bond. A double bond cannot rotate. There are two carbon-carbon single bonds shown, making choice B the best answer.

254. B is the best answer. The Fisher projections of the two molecules show that the hydroxyl group is located on the opposite side in the second molecule. In a Fisher projection, this means that the molecule has the opposite chirality, or orientation around the chiral carbon. Conformers have varying degrees of rotation around a carbon-carbon single bond, which is not shown. Choice A can be eliminated. The opposite chirality at the single chiral center makes the two molecules non-superimposable mirror images, or enantiomers. Choice B is a strong answer. Structural isomers have different connectivity of the atoms, eliminating choice C. Geometric isomers have different *cis* or *trans* configuration around a double bond. The molecules do not have carbon-carbon double bonds, eliminating choice D.

255. B is the best answer. The (l), (d), (−), and (+) indicate the direction that a chiral molecule polarizes light. Both (l) and (−) indicate that a molecule rotates polarized light counterclockwise, while (d) and (+) indicate that a molecule rotates polarized light clockwise. Choices A and C can be eliminated, and choice B is likely the best answer. The *R* and *S* configurations of a chiral molecule do not indicate the direction plane polarized light rotates, eliminating choice D.

256. C is the best answer. An enantiomer is a non-superimposable mirror image of a chiral molecule. An enantiomer has the opposite configuration at each chiral center. Choice A is (L)-DOPA rotated around the carbon-carbon bond between the ring and the methine group, and choice B is also (L)-DOPA. Flipping choice C over the y-axis now makes the hydrogen come out of the board and the amine group go into the board. This is the opposite of (L)-DOPA, which has hydrogen going into the board and the amine group coming out of the board. Choice C is likely the best answer. Choice D is (L)-DOPA rotated around the carbon-carbon single bond between the methine group and the carbon attached to the amine and carboxylic acid. Choice D can be eliminated.

257. D is the best answer. Enantiomers and diastereomers are chiral molecules that have opposite stereochemical configurations at all or some of the chiral centers, respectively. There are no chiral centers in the two molecules, eliminating choices A and B. Epimers are diastereomers that differ in configuration around only one stereocenter. Because there are no stereocenters in these molecules, choice C can be eliminated. Geometric isomers have the same connectivity, but different spatial orientation. *cis* and *trans* isomers are examples of geometric isomers, making choice D a strong answer choice.

258. A is the best answer. Compared to the pyranose structure in the equilibrium, the structure shown in the question stem has the orientation of each of the groups flipped, which would give the opposite stereochemical configuration at each chiral center. Because the stereochemical configuration at each chiral center was switched, the two molecules are enantiomers, making choice A a strong answer choice. Structural isomers have the same chemical formula but different connectivity. The connectivity of the atoms is the same in both molecules, eliminating choice B. An epimer is a diastereomers that has the opposite stereochemical configuration at only one chiral center. Because all of the chiral centers have changed, choice C can be eliminated. Because the molecules are now enantiomers, or non-superimposable mirror images, they are not the same molecule. This eliminates choice D.

259. B is the best answer. The two molecules are non-superimposable mirror images of one another, likely making them enantiomers, not diastereomers. This eliminates choice A and makes choice B a strong answer choice. Also notice that the molecules have opposite rotation of plane polarized light, signified by the (+) and (−). Enantiomers have opposite rotation, further suggesting choice B is the best answer. Epimers are diastereomers that have opposite configuration at only one chiral center, eliminating choice C. Geometric isomers have different orientations around a double bond, which is not the case for these two molecules. Choice D can be eliminated.

260. B is the best answer. As signified by (+) and (−), the two compounds rotate plane polarized light in opposite directions. This suggests that they are enantiomers. Enantiomers have the exact same physical properties, including density and boiling point, eliminating options I and II. The only physical property that is different for enantiomers is the direction of rotation of plane polarized light, making option III a component of the best answer. Choice B, which includes only option III, is the best answer.

261. C is the best answer. The reduction reaction occurs with the addition of H_2 on a Pd catalyst to the carbon-nitrogen double bond, called an imine. Because a double bond is planar, the hydrogens can be added to the imine from either face, producing a 50:50 mixture of R and S enantiomers. Choices A and B can be eliminated. A 50:50 mix of enantiomers is called a racemic mixture, making choice C a strong answer. The individual products are chiral because 50% are the R configuration and 50% are the S configuration. While the overall mixture does not rotate plane polarized light, each molecule is chiral, eliminating choice D.

262. B is the best answer. To determine priority, first determine which atom connected to the central carbon has the highest atomic number. If there is a tie, then look at the next group. In this case, there are three carbon atoms connected to the central carbon. One of these carbons is connected to an oxygen that has the highest atomic number; thus, this group is the highest priority. This eliminates choice A. The ethyl group is a higher priority than the methyl group because its first carbon is attached to another carbon which has higher atomic number than the three hydrogens attached to the methyl carbon. Choice B is a strong answer choice, and choice C can be eliminated. The hydrogen is the lowest atomic number, giving it a priority of four. Choice D can be eliminated.

263. D is the best answer. The maximum number of stereoisomers is 2^n where n is the number of chiral centers. A carbon that has four different groups attached to it is a chiral center, and there are four chiral centers in glucose. Calculating the number of stereoisomers equals $2^4 = 16$. Choice D is the best answer.

264. A is the best answer. The most straightforward way to approach this question is to assign the priorities based on atomic weight then reverse the chirality, as the lowest priority group, hydrogen, is coming out of the board. Remember that by convention, the lowest priority group should be going into the board. The hydroxyl gets a priority of 1, while the carbon attached to the amine gets a priority of 2, followed by the aromatic ring that gets a priority of 3. This would give a counterclockwise arrangement, or the *S* configuration, but the hydrogen is coming out of the board, so the real configuration is *R*. Choice A is the best answer, and choice B can be eliminated. D and L do not refer to the stereochemical configuration, but rather the direction that a molecule rotates light. There is no direct relationship between D and L and *S* and *R*. Choices C and D can be eliminated.

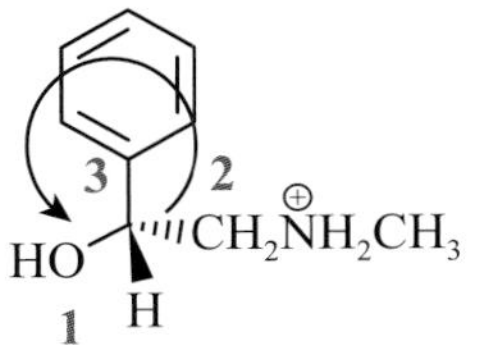

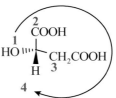

265. D is the best answer. The (+) and (−) indicate that the two molecules rotate light in opposite directions, meaning they are enantiomers. Enantiomers have the opposite stereochemical configuration at each chiral center, meaning they cannot be the same. Choices A and B can be eliminated. In (+)-1-phenylethanol, the hydroxyl receives a priority of 1, while the phenyl group gets a priority of 2, and the methyl group a priority of 3. This would give the counterclockwise configuration, or *S* configuration, but notice that the hydrogen is coming out of the page. Reverse the configuration to *R* to get the best answer. Because the two molecules are enantiomers, the (−) isomer will be *S*. Choice C can be eliminated, and choice D is the best answer.

266. A is the best answer. The (+) isoform of 1-phenylethanol has the *R* configuration, while the (−) isoform has the *S* configuration. The fact that there is some (+) rotation indicates that there must be more (+) isomer present. However, there is still a mixture because the rotation is not +42°, the amount of rotation of the pure enantiomer. Choice A is likely the best answer, and choice B is a weaker answer choice. A sample of pure *R* isomer would have a rotation of +42°, while a sample of pure *S* isomer would have a rotation of −42°. Choices C and D can be eliminated.

267. B is the best answer. The priorities are shown below. The priorities go clockwise, but the absolute configuration is *S* because H, the substituent with the lowest priority, is coming out of the page, and absolute configuration is determined when the lowest priority group is going into the page. Choice A can be eliminated, and choice B is the best answer. The D and L designations do not correspond to the *R* and *S* stereochemical configurations. Choices C and D can be eliminated.

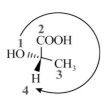

268. B is the best answer. The priorities are shown below. The priorities go clockwise, but the absolute configuration is *S* because H is coming out of the page. This eliminates choice A and makes choice B the best answer. The D and L designations correspond to the direction of rotation of plane polarized light and do not directly correspond to *R* or *S* configurations. Choices C and D can be eliminated.

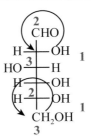

269. A is the best answer. The Fisher projection of D-glucose is shown. Remember that the horizontal lines indicate those atoms are coming out of the page. As shown below, both chiral centers have the priorities rotating counterclockwise, which would give the *S* configuration. However, because the hydrogens are on horizontal lines, they are coming out of the page, so both have an absolute configuration of *R*. Choice A is the best answer.

270. A is the best answer. Remember that Fisher projections represent atoms coming out of the page with horizontal lines, while stereochemistry is determined by orienting the lowest priority substituent into the board. On carbon two, the hydroxyl receives a priority of 1, while the carboxylic acid receives a priority of 2, followed by the chain with carbons three and four that receives a priority of 3. This would give a counterclockwise *S* configuration, but the hydrogen is coming out of the page, so the real configuration is *R*. Choices A and B are possible answers, eliminating choices C and D. For carbon three, the hydroxyl receives a priority of 1, followed by the carboxylic acid with a priority of 2, and the carbon chain with carbons one and two a priority of 3. This again would give a counterclockwise *S* configuration, but the hydrogen is coming out of the page, so the real configuration is *R*. Choice A is the best answer.

271. D is the best answer. On carbon 2, the hydroxyl has a priority of 1, the carboxylic acid has a priority of 2, and the carbon chain containing carbons three and four has a priority of 3. This would give the clockwise *R* configuration, but the hydrogen is coming out of the board, so the real configuration is *S*. Choices A and B can be eliminated. On carbon 3, the hydroxyl has a priority of 1, the carboxylic acid has a priority of 2, and the carbon chain containing carbons one and two has a priority of 3. This again would give the clockwise *R* configuration, but the hydrogen is coming out of the board, so the real configuration is *S*. Choice C can be eliminated, and choice D is the best answer.

272. A is the best answer. The structure shown in the figure is L-isoleucine, a nonpolar amino acid. There are two stereocenters in isoleucine, which are represented by the numbers in the parentheses in the answer choices. First, determine the stereochemistry at the C2 position. The $-NH_2$ receives highest priority, followed by the carboxyl group, then the alkane chain. Because hydrogen is pointed into the board, the priorities are counterclockwise, giving the *S* configuration. Next, determine the stereochemistry at the C3 position. The alkyl group containing the amine and carboxylic acid receives the highest priority, followed by the ethyl group, then the methyl group. This would give a clockwise priority order, but remember that the hydrogen is coming out of the board, so the configuration needs to be switched. C3 also is in the *S* configuration. By convention, the lower numbers are listed first, making choice A a better answer choice than choice B. C3 has the *S* configuration, eliminating choices C and D.

273. D is the best answer. Designation of absolute configuration requires a chiral carbon, which has 4 different substituents. While C1 carbon has 4 substituents, the substituents extending to the left and right (completing the cyclohexane ring) are identical. The C1 carbon only has 3 different substituents. It is not chiral and does not have an *R/S* designation. Choice D is the best answer.

274. B is the best answer. Addition of the ethyl substituent makes C1 carbon chiral. The lowest priority substituent about the C1 carbon (CH_3) is oriented into the page, and priority proceeds counterclockwise. C1 carbon absolute configuration is *S*. Priority proceeds clockwise about C2 carbon, but the lowest priority is oriented out of the page. C2 carbon absolute configuration is *S*. Note in the supplement below that C1 carbon priorities are labeled in circles, while C2 carbon priorities are labeled in squares.

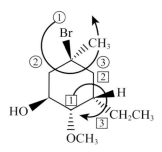

275. C is the best answer. Lateral (extending left/right) substituents in Fischer projections are oriented out of the page. For all chiral centers, the lowest priority group is a hydrogen substituent extending laterally. Looking at choice C, C2 carbon priorities proceed counterclockwise, but this must be flipped from normal convention. C2 carbon is *R*. C3 carbon priorities proceed clockwise, but this must be flipped from normal convention. C3 carbon is *S*. Looking at choice C, C4 carbon priorities proceed counterclockwise, but this must be flipped from normal convention. C4 carbon is *R*.

276. C is the best answer. A neat solution is one without water, so in this case it would be pure 1-phenylethanol. Compounds that are optically active have the ability to rotate plane polarized light because the molecules are chiral. Both molecular weight and boiling point would not explain why one species is optically active and one is not, eliminating choices A and B. Because 1-phenylethanol is optically active, it is chiral, while the non-optically active 2-phenylethanol species is achiral because it does not rotate light. Choice C is the best answer, and choice D can be eliminated.

277. C is the best answer. By definition, chiral molecules are able to rotate plane polarized light. If a solution contains 50% of one enantiomer and 50% of the other enantiomer, called a racemic mixture, half of the solution will rotate plane polarized light in one direction and the other half of the solution in the opposite direction. This means that the overall solution has a net rotation of zero. Option I is a possible answer. A meso compound has a plane of symmetry within the molecule and also does not rotate plane polarized light. Option II is part of the best answer. Chiral molecules do rotate plane polarized light, eliminating option III. Choice C is the best answer, as it contains only options I and II.

278. C is the best answer. Priority is determined by the atomic weight of the substituents on the double bond. On the left side of the double bond, the long alkane chain takes higher priority than the alkane chain that contains the hydroxyl. Similarly, on the right side of the double bond, the long alkane chain takes priority over the hydrogen. Because the higher priority groups are on the same side of the double bond, it is a *cis* or *Z* isomer. Because the highest priority substituents are not on opposite sides of the double bond, choices A and B can be eliminated. A *Z* isomer is also known as a *cis* isomer and has the highest priority groups on the same side of the bond. Choice C is the best answer. Because the isomer can be determined, choice D can be eliminated.

279. A is the best answer. Linoleic acid is a doubly unsaturated fatty acid, often called an omega-6 fatty acid. Notice that it has two double bonds that are in the *cis* configuration. This means the two highest priority groups, determined by the highest molecular weight of the substitutions on the double bond, are on the same side of the bond. *Cis* is also known as *Z*, while *trans* is also known as *E*. Because both are *cis*, choice A is the best answer.

Substitution Reactions of Alkanes

280. D is the best answer. A substitution reaction exchanges one substituent that is in a single bond to a molecule with a new substituent that is also in a single bond to a molecule. Loss of two sigma bonds to form one pi bond is an elimination reaction, eliminating choice A. A sigma bond cannot be converted to two pi bonds, eliminating choice B. Substitution reactions exchange one sigma bond for another sigma bond, eliminating choice C and making choice D the best answer.

281. C is the best answer. A S_N1 reaction forms a carbocation in the first step of the mechanism when a good leaving group leaves the molecule. This makes option I a part of the best answer. The rate determining step is how quickly the leaving group can leave to form the carbocation, which is a unimolecular, not bimolecular, set. Option II can be eliminated. In the second step, a nucleophile attacks the carbocation to complete the reaction. Thus, option III is part of the best answer. Choice C contains only options I and III is the best answer.

282. C is the best answer. An S_N2 reaction occurs all in one step when the nucleophile attacks the electrophile, displacing the leaving group. Because the rate of the reaction will depend on how often the nucleophile and electrophile interact, the reaction is bimolecular. In a bimolecular reaction, the concentrations of both the nucleophile and the electrophile control the rate of the reaction, eliminating choices A and B, and making choice C a strong answer choice. A bimolecular reaction depends on the concentrations of the reactants, eliminating choice D.

283. B is the best answer. Notice that the leaving group leaves in Step I to form a carbocation intermediate that is then attacked by a nucleophile in Step II. This means this is an S_N1 reaction. In an S_N1 reaction, the slow step is the formation of the carbocation, shown in Step I. Choice A can be eliminated, and choice B is a strong answer choice. Because the formation of the carbocation is much slower than the attack of the nucleophile, choices C and D can be eliminated.

284. C is the best answer. The iodine leaving group is constant between both reactions, so it is unlikely it becomes a worse or better leaving group, eliminating choices A and B. Both methanol and methoxide are nucleophiles, but methoxide is a stronger nucleophile than methanol due to the extra electron density that gives methoxide its negative charge. Reactions favor an S_N2 mechanism in the presence of a strong nucleophile and an S_N1 mechanism in the presence of a weaker nucleophile. Choice D can be eliminated, and choice C is the best answer.

285. C is the best answer. According to the question, the reaction occurs by S_N1 chemistry in the presence of methanol. S_N1 reactions have a carbocation intermediate, which is planar. When the nucleophile attacks, it can attack from the top or from the bottom, giving a racemic mixture of 50% *R* and 50% *S*. This means options I and II are part of the best answer. Because S_N1 is a substitution reaction, the iodine will leave in order for the methanol to add. Option III can be eliminated, because the methanol nucleophile would attack the carbocation intermediate. Choice C, which contains only options I and II, is the best answer.

286. **C is the best answer.** Alkanes that contain a halide on the terminal end likely proceed by S_N2 chemistry because formation of a carbocation by bromine leaving would create a highly unstable primary carbocation via S_N1 chemistry. S_N2 reactions depend on the concentrations of both reactions, likely explaining why the rate of the reaction increases as more NaI is added. Alkanes that contain a halide on a tertiary carbon likely undergo S_N1 substitution reactions, because the departure of the halide creates a well-stabilized tertiary carbocation. S_N1 reactions only depend on the concentration of one of the reactants, the one forming the carbocation. As 2-chloro-2-methylpropane creates the carbocation, increasing the concentration of NaI in an S_N1 reaction would not increase the reaction rate. Both bromine and chlorine are good leaving groups due to their large size. Choices A and B are not the most likely contributors to the difference in reaction rates between the two reactions. Since 1-bromobutane proceeds by a S_N2 mechanism the rate depends on the concentration of the nucleophile. However, the 2-chloro-2methylpropane reaction proceeds by S_N1, so the rate only depends on the concentration of the electrophile and not the nucleophile (I^-). Choice C is a strong answer choice. Choice D, which states the opposite, can be eliminated.

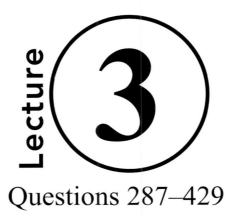

Lecture **3**

Questions 287–429

Oxygen Containing Reactions

ANSWERS & EXPLANATIONS

ANSWER KEY										
287. A	300. C	313. D	326. A	339. B	352. A	365. B	378. B	391. B	404. A	417. A
288. C	301. C	314. B	327. C	340. B	353. A	366. C	379. A	392. A	405. B	418. A
289. A	302. A	315. A	328. B	341. B	354. D	367. D	380. B	393. A	406. C	419. C
290. B	303. D	316. C	329. A	342. C	355. C	368. A	381. C	394. B	407. A	420. D
291. A	304. A	317. A	330. B	343. D	356. C	369. B	382. C	395. D	408. C	421. A
292. A	305. B	318. C	331. A	344. A	357. C	370. A	383. B	396. C	409. A	422. D
293. C	306. D	319. B	332. C	345. B	358. A	371. B	384. C	397. C	410. A	423. B
294. B	307. A	320. B	333. B	346. D	359. B	372. C	385. A	398. A	411. B	424. D
295. A	308. D	321. A	334. A	347. B	360. B	373. B	386. D	399. C	412. A	425. C
296. C	309. A	322. C	335. C	348. B	361. D	374. B	387. B	400. B	413. D	426. B
297. A	310. D	323. B	336. A	349. B	362. C	375. A	388. A	401. B	414. C	427. D
298. D	311. B	324. C	337. C	350. C	363. A	376. C	389. A	402. A	415. C	428. C
299. C	312. D	325. C	338. B	351. D	364. C	377. A	390. A	403. A	416. A	429. D

The Attackers: Nucleophiles

287. **A is the best answer.** Primary alcohols are compounds in which the alcohol is bonded to a carbon with one or fewer bonds to another carbon molecule (RCH_2OH). Methanol, which only has a single carbon atom, is a primary alcohol. Sulfur is similar to oxygen, so the thiol is most similar to methanol, which makes choice A a strong answer. Secondary alcohols occur when the alcohol is bonded to a carbon atom with two additional carbon atom bonds, while a tertiary alcohol has three carbon atoms bonded to the central carbon. This eliminates choices B and C. Quaternary alcohols are not possible as they would violate the octet rule for the central carbon atom, eliminating choice D.

288. **C is the best answer.** The structure is shown below. An alcohol with one carbon attached to the carbon with hydroxyl group is a primary alcohol, while a molecule with two carbon atoms attached to the carbon with the hydroxyl group is a secondary alcohol. This eliminates choices A and B. There are three carbons attached to the carbon with the hydroxyl group. This matches the description for a tertiary alcohol, so choice C is the best answer. Quaternary alcohols would have four carbon atoms attached to the hydroxyl carbon, which would require the formation of five bonds to the carbon atoms, so choice D can be eliminated.

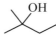

289. **A is the best answer.** The answer must contain a syn (same side) diol. This eliminates choices B and D. Choice A is a strong answer because it contains the two new alcohol groups produced in the reaction plus a third alcohol group that was present in the starting material.

290. **B is the best answer.** The first step in naming a molecule with IUPAC nomenclature is identifying the longest chain of continuous carbon molecules. The longest chain in this molecule is eight carbons long, so the name of the molecule will have octane at its root which eliminates choices C and D. The next step is to identify the correct numbering of the molecule. The carbon atoms are numbered along the continuous chain in a way that ensures the alcohol substituent has the lowest number. Choice A results from initiating the numbering on the wrong side of the molecule, which would cause the alcohol group to have a higher number. Choice B is a better answer because it accurately numbers the carbon atoms so that the alcohol group has the lowest number.

291. **A is the best answer.** According to the table, primary alcohols are the slowest to react, and 1-pentanol is the only primary alcohol. Choice A is a strong answer. 2-Methyl-3-pentanol is a secondary alcohol, which will react faster than primary alcohols, so choice B can be eliminated. 2-Methyl-2-pentanol is a tertiary alcohol, which will react the fastest, and choice C can be eliminated. 2-Hexanol is also a secondary alcohol, so choice D can be eliminated.

292. **A is the best answer.** When determining solubility, a classic rule of thumb is "like dissolves like". This refers to molecules that are polar being soluble in polar solvents and insoluble in nonpolar solvents. Short chain alcohols are polar molecules due to the strong polarity in their hydroxyl group and the lack of large, nonpolar alkyl chains. This means ethanol will likely be miscible with water, so choice A is a strong answer. Bonds between carbon and hydrogen atoms are essentially nonpolar, so large hydrocarbons are most likely to be nonpolar. Cyclohexane is a cyclic hydrocarbon molecule, 2-butene is a nonpolar alkene, and hexane is a 6-carbon alkane that is also nonpolar. Choices B, C, and D can be eliminated.

293. **C is the best answer.** The boiling and melting point of a molecule is largely determined by the intermolecular forces. The stronger the intermolecular forces a molecule experiences, the higher its melting and boiling point. London dispersion forces are the weakest intermolecular forces. They arise from random interactions between the electrons of adjacent atoms. Since cyclohexane and cyclohexanol are similar with the exception of one substituent, their London dispersion forces are unlikely to vary greatly. This eliminates choices A and B. Additionally, if a molecule has greater London dispersion forces, it is more likely to be a solid at room temperature. Hydrogen bonding is one of the strongest intermolecular forces and arises between molecules with a hydrogen atom bonded to either a fluorine, oxygen, or nitrogen atom that interact with one another. Cyclohexanol has a hydrogen atom bonded to an oxygen atom, while cyclohexane does not. The hydrogen bonding in cyclohexanol raises its melting point causing it to be a solid at room temperature. This eliminates choice D and makes choice C the best answer.

294. **B is the best answer.** 1-Butanol will have a boiling point in the middle of 1-propanol and 1-pentanol. As the alkyl chain of molecules increases, the London dispersion forces between the alky chains increase. This increases the boiling point of the molecule when compared to the smaller molecule. Choice A represents an increase in the boiling point from 1-propanol while not exceeding the boiling point of 1-pentanol, making it a possible answer, but it is still important to evaluate the other choices. Choice B is right in the middle of the boiling points of 1-propanol and 1-pentanol, making it a better answer than choice A. The boiling point of 1-butanol will be lower than that of 1-pentanol, so choices C and D can be eliminated.

295. A is the best answer. The ethanol molecule's oxygen acts as a nucleophile attacking the sulfur atom while displacing the chloride ion. Choice A is a strong answer. The electrophile or atom that accepts the electrons is the sulfur molecule, so choice B can be eliminated. This reaction does not process through a radical, so choice C can be eliminated. While reducing agents donate electrons, they do so in a relatively permanent way. In contrast, the nucleophile in this reaction is donating electrons to form a new bond with the electrophile. This makes choice D a weaker answer. Choice A is the best answer.

296. C is the best answer. The molecule that will displace the alcohol group is the nucleophile, while the carbon molecule of the alcohol acts as the electrophile. The OH group in the alcohol does not act as a nucleophile or an electrophile in the substitution reaction, so choices A and B can be eliminated. Hydroxide is not a good leaving group; however, water is a good leaving group. A general rule for determining the relative strength of a nucleophile is that weak bases are good leaving groups. Weak bases are stable molecules, which explains why they do not participate as readily in acid-base reactions. This also means they are more likely to leave the original molecule in a substitution reaction since they are more stable. Water is a weaker base than hydroxide, which is a strong base. By protonating the alcohol, OH is converted to water which is a better leaving group. This makes choice C the best answer.

297. A is the best answer. The reaction described requires a proton to protonate the ether and form a leaving group. So the question is really asking to identify the compound that can act as a proton donator, or acid. Only choice A is an acid. HCl is one of the strong acids and is the best answer. Cl_2 can be used to halogenate alkenes. $SOCl_2$ can convert alcohols into alky chloride molecules. $AlCl_3$ can be used to halogenate aromatic compounds. Choices B, C, and D can be eliminated.

298. D is the best answer. The loss of a peak within the 3200 cm^{-1} region implies loss of a hydroxyl group. The hydroxyl group was likely attacked by a nucleophile during the reaction. The best way to protect a hydroxyl group is through utilization of protective groups. Choices A and B can be eliminated as they would lead to the formation of an acetal or a ketal respectively. Acetals and ketals are used for protecting groups in carbonyl reactions. Choice C would create an alkyl halide and can be eliminated as the hydroxyl group would be lost from the formation of the alkyl halide. Choice D is the best answer as a tosylate would prevent the alcohol from reacting. Upon completion of the procedure, the hydroxyl group could be restored by removing the tosylate.

299. C is the best answer. The above synthesis step did not produce adequate product because −OH is not a good leaving group. −OH must be made into a better leaving group in order for the reaction to proceed. NaOH would dissociate into Na^+ and OH^- after addition to the reaction vessel. OH^- would likely perform an acid/base reaction with the hydroxyl group of the reactant. This would make the substitution reaction harder to proceed, as −O^- is a worse leaving group than −OH. Choice A can be eliminated. Diethyl ether (Choice B) would not react with the reactant. Choice B can be eliminated. Note that diethyl ether is a common solvent because of its general lack of reactivity. Alcohols can be converted to a type of ester called a sulfonate to become better leaving groups. The hydroxyl oxygen of the reactant will nucleophilically attack the sulfur in choice C. Cl^- will function as a leaving group, ultimately forming a bond with the hydrogen of the hydroxyl group. At this point, the hydroxyl group has been converted to a particular type of sulfonate called a tosylate. Tosylates are strong leaving groups because sulfur can make many bonds with its empty d orbitals, allowing any negative charge to be well-distributed. CN^- will then be able to displace the tosyl group in an S_N2 reaction. See below. Choice C is a strong answer. Choice D is unlikely to react with the reactant in any productive way. At most, the oxygen bound to the methyl group with form a bond with the hydrogen of the hydroxyl group. Choice D can be eliminated. Choice C is the best answer.

300. C is the best answer. The question states that THF is an ether. An ether is a compound with an oxygen atom bonded to two alkyl groups. Choice A is an amide and can be eliminated. Choice B contains an ester since the oxygen molecule is bonded to a carbonyl in addition to an alky group. It also has an aldehyde group. Choice B is a weaker answer and can be eliminated. Choice C is the only ether and is a strong answer. Choice D is a primary alcohol and can be eliminated.

The Targets: Electrophiles

301. C is the best answer. Both ketones and aldehydes exhibit sp^2 hybridized planar geometry. Choices A and B can be eliminated. Steric hindrance is when substituent groups physically block a molecule's ability to undergo a nucleophilic attack. Bulky nucleophiles are particularly affected by steric hindrance. In both ketones and aldehydes, the site of nucleophilic attack by a base would be at the carbonyl carbon. As opposed to ketones, aldehydes have a hydrogen substituent attached to the carbonyl carbon. This minimizes steric hindrance, making the reaction occur more quickly than it would with a ketone. Choice D can be eliminated, and choice C is the best answer.

302. A is the best answer. $LiAlH_4$ is a strong reducing agent, meaning a free hydride will attack the carbonyl carbon. The chlorine atom will then leave as chloride and the resulting molecule will be a substituted aldehyde. The molecule with the least steric hindrance will be the one that is the smallest in size. Hydrogen is the smallest atom, making choice A the best answer.

303. D is the best answer. Carbonyls can be made more or less reactive via substituents. Substituents influence reactivity by either withdrawing or donating electron density. Withdrawing groups increase reactivity, while donating groups decrease reactivity. Choice A is not the best answer as the addition of HCl would form an acyl chloride, which is an electron withdrawing substituent. Out of all of the choices presented, formation of an acyl chloride would produce the most reactive product. Choices B and C, while tempting, are not the best answers. Choice B would lead to the formation of an acid anhydride, which is slightly more reactive than the carboxylic acid that would be formed from choice C. Choice D is the best answer as forming an amide would make the compound much less reactive than either an anhydride or a carboxylic acid.

304. A is the best answer. Compound A is a ketone while compound B is an aldehyde. The additional R group on ketones tends to be somewhat donating which lowers the electrophilicity of ketones. Aldehydes are more electrophilic than ketones. Since aldehydes are more electrophilic, their carbonyl is more vulnerable to attack. Choice A is a strong answer as it accurately describes the reactivity of compound A.

305. B is the best answer. The reactivity series of carbonyls is as follows: acid halide > acid anhydride > aldehydes and ketones > carboxylic acids > esters. The MCAT® requires knowledge of carbonyl structure from the chemical formula, and choice A is an acid anhydride, choice B is an acid halide, choice C is a ketone, and choice D is a carboxylic acid. Choice B is the best answer

306. D is the best answer. The IR indicates that compound A has a carbonyl bond somewhere in it and compound B has both and C–O bond and a C=O bond. The susceptibility of carbonyls to nucleophilic attack is such that acid anhydrides are more reactive than aldehydes and ketones, which are in turn more reactive than esters. Based on the information given, compound A is probably an aldehyde or ketone, while compound B could be either an acid anhydride or an ester. It is difficult to tell from this information alone, so choice D is the best answer.

307. A is the best answer. A carbonyl is defined as a carbon double bonded to oxygen. Carbonyls are associated with planar stereochemistry and certain polarities. The carbon tends to possess a partial positive charge while the oxygen exhibits a partial negative charge. The planar stereochemistry allows for low steric hindrance while the partial charges make the carbonyl carbon more susceptible to attack. Choice A is a strong answer as it best describes the criteria that make a carbonyl so reactive. Choice B can be eliminated as the expected charges are reversed in the answer choice. Choices C and D can also be eliminated as carbonyls do not exhibit nonpolar stereochemistry.

308. D is the best answer. Acetyl chloride is an acid halide and can undergo nucleophilic substitution at the carbonyl carbon. The fastest reaction will occur with the nucleophile that is least stable alone in solution. Once it reacts with the acid halide to become a carboxylic acid derivative, it is unlikely to revert back to an acid halide. The carboxylic acid would form an anhydride. Anhydrides have carboxylate ion leaving groups, which are stable due to resonance. Choice A is not the best answer. While the ethoxide and methoxide leaving groups in choices B and C are unlikely to leave once reacted with an acetyl chloride, amide anion leaving groups are the least stable of all the answer choices in solution, as nitrogen-containing groups serve as good nucleophiles. Choice D is the best answer.

309. A is the best answer. Acyl chlorides must be formed with a very strong nucleophile in order to force the hydroxide ion off the carbonyl in a carboxylic acid. In solution, HCl breaks apart into H^+ and Cl^-. The chloride ion is a poor nucleophile in this format, likely making choice A the best answer. The chloride ion in choices B, C, and D is more nucleophilic and reacts via nucleophilic substitution with the carboxylic acid for form the acyl chloride.

310. D is the best answer. The same product is formed in each reaction, so choices A and B can be eliminated. Acyl chlorides are more reactive the carboxylic acids, so they do not require a catalyst. The reactivity of carboxylic acid derivatives is determined by the quality of the leaving group. Halides are better leaving groups than hydroxide ions, so acyl halides will react faster than carboxylic acids. Choice D is a better answer than choice C.

311. B is the best answer. The anhydride is formed because it is more reactive than the acid, which increases the rate of reaction with hydrazine. Carboxylic acids are less reactive than anhydrides, so choice A can be eliminated. This makes choice B a strong answer. While smaller rings can be more reactive due to the increased ring strain, three and four carbon rings are more likely to experience this ring strain rather than five membered rings. The carbon atoms in a five membered ring have similar bond angles to molecules with a tetrahedral configuration and are relatively stable. This eliminates choices C and D.

Substitution Reactions: Carboxylic Acids and Their Derivatives

312. D is the best answer. A carboxylic acid has a carboxyl group that contains a carbon double bonded to oxygen and single bonded to a hydroxyl. Because the carbon and oxygen have different electronegativities and are both non-metals, the bond is polar covalent, making option I part of the best answer. A double bond is sp^2 hybridized, while a single bond is sp^3 hybridized. This makes options II and III part of the best answer. Choice D, which contains all three options, is the best answer.

313. D is the best answer. Carboxylic acids are more acidic than aldehydes because the negative charge of the conjugate base can be stabilized through resonance. Choice A can be eliminated. The functional groups of both glutamate and aspartate contain a terminal carboxylic acid, eliminating choice B. Carboxylic acids can undergo substitution reactions at the carbonyl, eliminating choice C. Hydrogen bonding can occur between two points of a carboxylic acid—the OH and the carbonyl. Having two hydrogen bonds increases the intermolecular forces between the acids, giving the solution a higher, not lower, boiling point. Choice D is the best answer.

314. B is the best answer. The carbon attached to the double bonded oxygen and alcohol group in a carboxylic acid are counted as the first carbon on the chain. Choice A is a strong answer as it utilizes priority properly in naming the compound, and choice B can be eliminated as "bi" is not the proper IUPAC prefix. Choices C and D can be eliminated as they would only be correct if the carbon attached to the carbonyl were considered the fifth carbon in the chain. Note that the prefix "bis" is used in naming coordination compounds and complex ions and would not be utilized in the nomenclature of a carboxylic acid.

315. A is the best answer. The conversion of (L)-DOPA to dopamine requires the loss of the COOH groups, which is called a decarboxylation reaction. Choice A is a strong answer. An amide is a carboxylic acid derivative where the bond to the hydroxyl group is replaced by a bond to a nitrogen atom. There is no amide present in (L)-DOPA, so choices B and C can be eliminated. Carboxylation reactions result in the substitution of a carboxylic acid for another substituent. This is the reverse of the reaction described in the figure, so choice D can be eliminated.

316. C is the best answer. The solubility of a compound largely depends on the polarity of that compound and the polarity of the solvent. As a general rule, solutes with a similar polarity as the solvent will dissolve well. For organic acids with similar substituents, the longer the hydrocarbon chain, the more nonpolar a molecule is. Since water is a polar solvent, the compound in the list that has the shortest chain will be the most soluble. Lauric acid has the shortest chain (hydrophobic region), so it will be the most soluble in water, making choice C the best answer.

317. A is the best answer. Room temperature is roughly 25°C. If the melting point of a substance is lower than temperature of its surrounding, it will be in the liquid form. Oleic acid is the only fatty acid in the list with a melting point lower than room temperature; therefore, it is the only oil. Choice A is the best answer. Choices B, C, and D all have melting points that are higher than room temperature, so they will remain solid.

318. C is the best answer. Choice A is the main benzoic acid compound, so it can be eliminated. Choice B is a phenol group, which is not part of the starting material, choice B can be eliminated. The name indicates that the benzoyl group is a 2 substituent on benzoic acid. The group is circled below. Choice C is a strong answer. While there are benzene rings in the compound, a benzoyl group is a benzene ring with a carbonyl attached, so choice D can be eliminated.

319. B is the best answer. Electrophiles are atoms that are capable of accepting electron density. If a molecule has a slightly positive charge, it will more easily accept a nucleophilic attack. Nucleophiles are electron-dense atoms that are willing to donate their electron density and form a new bond. For this reaction, the double bond of the aromatic carbon will act as a nucleophile, so choice A can be eliminated. The carbonyl has a slightly positive charge due to the oxygen atom's strong electronegativity, which makes it a better electrophile. Choice B is a strong answer. The reaction rate can be increased by protonating the leaving group, which is the hydroxyl group, to make it more stable. The sulfuric acid achieves this and is a catalyst, so choice C can be eliminated. An oxidation reaction involves the transfer of electrons, but does not usually result in the formation of new bonds. This particular reaction is a nucleophilic substitution reaction, so choice D can be eliminated.

320. B is the best answer. Decarboxylation reactions occur when a COOH group is removed from a molecule in the form of CO_2. To achieve this spontaneously, the resulting carbanion needs to be relatively stable. The only molecule of the listed options is choice B. Beta keto esters are subject to decarboxylation reactions because the temporary carbanion that is formed can be stabilized by resonance with the carbonyl located at the beta position. Choices A, C, and D would all require a significant amount of heat to undergo a decarboxylation reaction and would be unlikely to do so at room temperature, so they can be eliminated. Choice B is the only beta keto ester and is the best answer.

321. A is the best answer. Alcohols are oxidized to carboxylic acids. Ethanoic acid is the carboxylic acid that results from the oxidation of ethanol, so choice A is a strong answer. Diethyl ether can be synthesized via a dehydration reaction between two molecules of ethyl alcohol. This requires an acid catalyst and heat, so choice B can be eliminated. Ethyl alcohol and ethanol are the same molecule, so choice C can be eliminated. Converting ethyl alcohol to ethane is a multistep reaction that requires the use of a reducing agent, rather than an oxidant. This eliminates choice D and makes choice A the best answer.

322. C is the best answer. 3-Oxo-pentanoic acid is a beta keto carboxylic acid. Beta keto carboxylic acids can undergo decarboxylation reactions, which release CO_2. This makes choice C the best answer.

323. B is the best answer. Isomerization reactions are the rearrangement of a molecule into a new molecule that has the same chemical formula, but with a different arrangement. The reaction described in the scheme does not have the same chemical formula since a water molecule has been added to maleic anhydride, so choice A can be eliminated. The addition of water to a molecule to break a bond is called a hydrolysis reaction. The conversion of an anhydride to a carboxylic acid is an example of this, so choice B is a strong answer. A carboxylation reaction occurs when a new carboxylic acid substituent is added to a molecule. While a carboxylic acid is created, this is the result of the addition of water to the anhydride, so choice B is better than choice C. A carboxylic acid is not eliminated from the original molecule, so a decarboxylation reaction has not occurred. Choice D can be eliminated.

324. C is the best answer. Amino acids have both a carboxylic acid end and an amino group. The nitrogen of the amino group can attack the carbonyl of the carboxyl end to link two amino acids together in a growing peptide. This type of bond between amino acids is called a peptide bond, making option I a component of the best answer. Because the bond that forms is between carbon and nitrogen, which are both non-metals, it is a covalent bond. Option II is a component of the best answer. Van der Waals interactions are intermolecular, not intramolecular interactions. Option III is not part of the best answer. Choice C contains only options I and II and is the best answer.

325. C is the best answer. Carboxylic acid derivatives, like anhydrides, can be hydrolyzed to form carboxylic acids when they are reacted with water. The lone pair of electrons on the oxygen attacks the electrophilic carbonyl carbon. A catalyst increases the rate of the reaction but is not consumed by the reaction. The hydrolysis reaction can be catalyzed by an acid, which protonates the carbonyl, and the final product is deprotonated, which regenerates the acidic proton. Since the water molecule is consumed in the reaction, choice A can be eliminated. The water molecule donates electrons to form a new bond with the carbonyl, which would allow it to be classified as Lewis base, not as an acid, so choice B can be eliminated. In the reaction, the water molecule acts as a nucleophile and attacks the carbonyl. Choice C is a strong answer. The carbonyl acts as an electrophile in this reaction by accepting the electron density from the attacking water molecule. This eliminates choice D.

326. A is the best answer. An acyl chloride is more reactive than an ester, so the alcohol will react with the acyl chloride to form an ester by displacing the chloride atom. An ester is composed of a carbonyl with an alkoxide group bonded to the carbonyl carbon, so choice A is a strong answer. An ether can be formed by a reaction between two alcohol molecules, so choice B can be eliminated. An amide group is a carbonyl with an amino group bonded to it. There is no nitrogen source in the reaction proposed, so choice C can be eliminated. An imide is similar to an amide, but the nitrogen atom is bonded to two carbonyl groups. Choice D can be eliminated.

327. C is the best answer. Similar to the alcohol formation of an ester, an amine reacts with a carboxylic acid to form an amide. An ester is formed from the reaction of alcohol with a carboxylic acid, so choice A can be eliminated. An ether is formed by reacting two molecules of alcohol with high temperatures. Choice B can be eliminated. The lone pair of the nitrogen group forms a bond to the carbonyl carbon via a nucleophilic attack. Since water is a weaker base than an amine, it is a better leaving group. After the carbonyl reforms its double bond, the water molecule is kicked off, which results in the formation of an amide, so choice C is a strong answer. While technically, the amide could form an imide via a second substitution reaction on a different molecule of carboxylic acid, this is less likely to occur, making choice D a weaker answer.

328. B is the best answer. All of the answer choices are carboxylic acid derivatives. To answer this question quickly, ignore the rest of the molecule and only look at the carbonyls to determine the best answer. An amide is a molecule with an amine group attached to a carbonyl. This molecule does not contain any nitrogen atoms, so choice A can be eliminated. The oxygen atoms next to the carbonyls are attached to alkyl groups. This makes choice B a strong answer. Acyl chlorides are molecules with chloride atoms attached to the carbonyl carbon. While this molecule contains multiple chloride molecules, none of them are attached to the carbonyl, so choice C can be eliminated. The carbonyl molecules do not have hydroxyl groups attached to them, so they are not carboxylic acids, eliminating choice D.

329. A is the best answer. In this reaction, the hydrogen is removed from the phenol to make an electron rich anion that can attack the electrophilic carbonyl. Since it is attacking the carbonyl, it is acting like a nucleophile, so choice A is a strong answer. The carbonyl is accepting the electrons from the nucleophile, so it is acting as the electrophile, eliminated choice B. Nucleophiles donate electrons, which make them Lewis bases, so choice C is a weaker answer. While reducing agents also donate electrons, they do not form new bonds, but rather change the oxidation state of the molecules with which they are reacting, making choice D a weaker answer.

330. B is the best answer. Decarboxylation indicates that the reactant loses CO_2. Since the structure of choices A and C still contain a carbonyl group, they can be eliminated. According to the question, the product is a Z alkene, so the phenyl groups need to be on the same side of the double bond. Choice B satisfies this requirement and is a strong answer. Choice D represents the E isomer since the phenyl groups are on opposite sides of the double bond, so choice D can be eliminated.

331. A is the best answer. This question can be solved by using the different relative reactivity of carboxylic acid derivatives. Acyl halides are the most reactive carboxylic acid derivative, and the acetate ion will successfully substitute for the chloride of acetyl chloride to generate acetic anhydride. Choice A is a strong answer. Carboxylic acids, esters and amides are more stable than the anhydride. This is because their substituents are worse leaving groups that the acetate ion, so even if the acetate ion successfully attacks the carbonyl, it will be kicked off. This will result in no net reaction, so choices B, C, and D can be eliminated.

332. C is the best answer. Chlorine (Cl_2) will not react with butanoic acid, so choice A can be eliminated. HCl is a strong acid and is capable of protonating the butanoic acid. This can convert the hydroxyl group into a better leaving group and help catalyze the nucleophilic attack of a chloride ion, so choice B is a possible answer. Thionyl chloride ($SOCl_2$) is a reagent that can convert butanoic acid to butyl chloride. The first step in the reaction is converting the hydroxyl group into a sulfur containing group that can act as a better leaving group. Thionyl chloride also provides chloride ions, which can then perform a nucleophilic attack on the carbonyl and generate an acyl chloride. This makes choice C a stronger answer than choice B. $LiAlH_4$ is a reducing agent that can reduce carboxylic acids to alcohols, so choice D can be eliminated.

333. B is the best answer. Decarboxylase enzymes produce CO_2. Pyruvate is a reactant, so choice A is not the best answer. HCO_3^- is bicarbonate which is how CO_2 is transported in the blood. However, this conversion happens through another enzyme, and bicarbonate is not the product of pyruvate decarboxylase and choice C can be eliminated. H_2O is produced in many reactions but not in decarboxylation reactions, so choice D is not the best answer.

334. A is the best answer. Decarboxylations produce CO_2 which is a gas. Gases like CO_2 are only minimally soluble in solutions, so they dissolve out. The CO_2 that leaves pulls the reaction towards the products side due to Le Châtelier's principle that describes the equilibrium between reactions, so choice A is a strong answer. The Bohr effect does relate to CO_2 but only in terms of hemoglobin and oxygen saturation, so choice B is not the best answer. Hund's rule refers to electron configuration, so choice C is not the best answer. Michaelis-Menten kinetics describe the kinetics that govern enzymatic reactions. They do not relate to this non-enzymatic question, so choice D is not the best answer.

335. C is the best answer. The first step in the formation of an acid chloride with $SOCl_2$ is converting the hydroxyl group into a better leaving group by reacting with a $SOCl_2$ molecule. This first step also generates a chloride ion, which can then attack the carbonyl and generate an acid chloride. An elimination reaction occurs when two molecules are removed from an atom, and a new double bond is formed. Since the end product has a chloride substituted for a hydroxyl and no new double bond, choice A can be eliminated. A conjugate addition occurs when an alkene that is adjacent to a carbonyl undergoes a nucleophilic attack. This eliminates choice B. A nucleophilic substitution occurs when a carbonyl with a good leaving group is attacked by a nucleophile. The carbonyl will reform and displace the good leaving group, which results in a final product with the nucleophile "substituted" for the original leaving group. If the carbonyl is unable to reform because it does not have a good leaving group, the reaction is a nucleophilic addition since the nucleophile did not replace the original substituents. This makes choice C a stronger answer than choice D.

336. A is the best answer. The first step of the reaction scheme is necessary to activate the electrophile by creating a more reactive species. By creating a more reactive species, the next step in the reaction can proceed more quickly. Acid chlorides are more reactive than carboxylic acids since their leaving group is a chloride ion rather than a hydroxide ion. This is because chloride ions are weaker bases than hydroxide ions and are more stable. Choice A is a strong answer, and choice B can be eliminated. Carbonyl carbons are electrophilic, not nucleophilic, so choice C can be eliminated. The acid chloride is consumed in the formation of the anilide, so by definition it is not a catalyst, eliminating choice D.

337. C is the best answer. The only difference between the answer choices is the substituent on the alpha carbon. Electron withdrawing groups on the alpha carbon increase the partial positive charge on the carbonyl carbon, thus rendering the molecule more reactive to nucleophilic attack. Alkyl groups are electron donating, so choice A would be less reactive and can be eliminated. Hydroxide is an electron withdrawing group, so choice B is a strong answer, but bromine is also an electron withdrawing group. The bromine group is will withdraw more electron density than the hydroxyl substituent as can be seen in the analogous situation where acyl halides are more reactive than carboxylic acids. The increased electron withdrawing effect of the halide results in a slightly larger partial positive charge on the atom to which the halide is bonded. Choice C is a better answer. Choice D is the acid without any substituents which would be less reactive than choices B and C, so it can be eliminated. Choice C is the best answer.

338. B is the best answer. An ether is a compound with an oxygen molecule is bonded to two alkyl or aromatic groups. While this molecule contains an oxygen bonded to two carbon atoms, one of those carbon atoms is bonded to a carbonyl. This is better defined as an ester, so choice A can be eliminated, and choice B is a strong answer. The ester group in isoamylacetate is circled below.

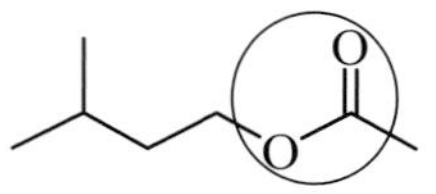

The molecule contains an ester, which is a carboxylic acid derivative, but since the substituent on the carbonyl carbon is not a hydroxide, it is not a carboxylic acid. Choice C can be eliminated. There is no alcohol group present, so choice D can be eliminated.

339. B is the best answer. An amide is functional group with an amine substituent bonded to a carbonyl group. The amide groups are circled in the structure below. There are four nitrogen atoms, so there is a possibility of 4 amide groups. Since there are only two carbonyl molecules, there can be a maximum of 2 amides. The two carbonyl compounds are bonded to amine groups, so there are two amides in this molecule. Choice B is the best answer.

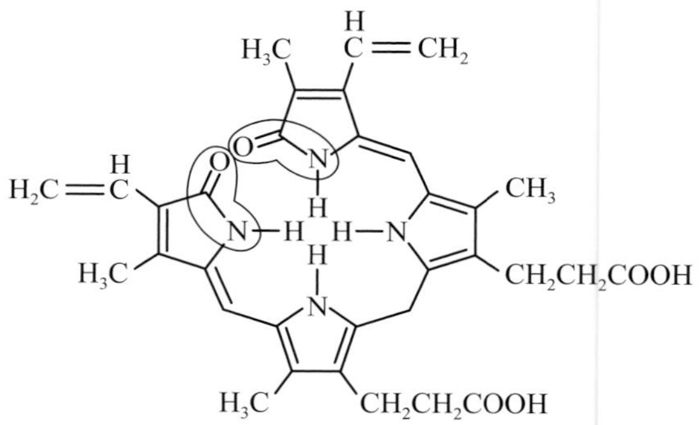

340. B is the best answer. An ether is a functional group with an oxygen atom bonded to two alkyl or aryl groups. The oxygen atom bonded to the phenyl groups is also bonded to a carboxylic acid. Since it is bonded to a carboxylic acid, it is classified as an ester. Choice A and choice D can be eliminated. The functional groups are indicated below and include an ester, phenyl group, and carboxylic acid, so choice B is a strong answer. While the aromatic ring contains multiple double bonds, there is not an isolated alkene in the molecules, so choice D can be eliminated.

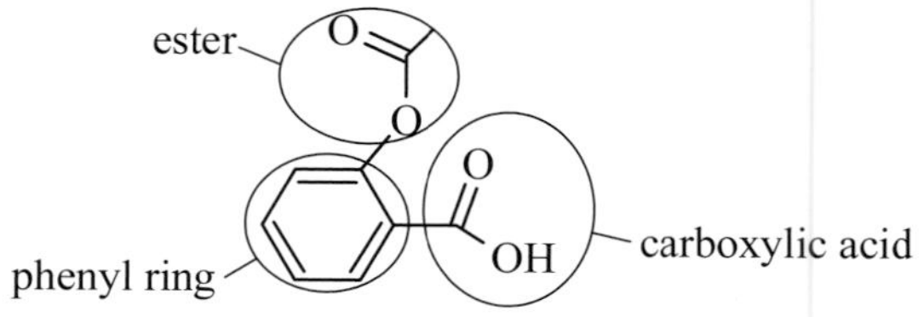

341. B is the best answer. While there are more than one chloride molecules, this is not the purpose of including bis at the beginning of the molecule. Choice A can be eliminated. The name indicates the plane of symmetry that is in the middle of the molecule. By including the bis at the beginning of the name, the 2,4,6-trichlorophenyl group can be named once as a complex substituent and understood to mean that it is present on both sides of the oxalate molecule. The naming of a molecule is never reflective of a particular reaction and is a reflection of the specific atoms of a molecule and their arrangement, so choice C can be eliminated. When using a prefix for the number of atoms, "di" is used for two molecules, not "bis', so choice D can be eliminated.

342. C is the best answer. Large hydrocarbons contain many nonpolar bonds and are thus considered nonpolar molecules. Nonpolar molecules are hydrophobic since water is a polar solvent. Carboxylic acids contain polar bonds and are hydrophilic. Section 1 is the long alkane chain, so it is nonpolar and hydrophobic, while section 2 is a carboxylic acid, so it is polar and hydrophilic. This makes choice C the best answer.

343. D is the best answer. The nitro groups are electron withdrawing, so they activate the electrophilic carbonyl carbon by withdrawing electron density. This eliminates choice A. Since they withdraw electron density from the carbonyl, they increase its partial positive charge. This increases its electrophilicity and reactivity, making choice B a weaker answer. Since the carbonyl is an electrophile, not a nucleophile, choice C can be eliminated. Choice D is the best answer.

344. A is the best answer. The acid protonates the carbonyl oxygen of the propionic anhydride. Carbonyls are activated by protonation of the oxygen and the anhydride is the electrophile. Choice A is a strong answer. Since isoamyl alcohol is a nucleophile in this reaction, choices B and C can be eliminated. Protonating the isoamyl alcohol would make it a weaker nucleophile or deactivate it, so choice D can be eliminated.

345. B is the best answer. To answer this question, simply take the ketoacid shown in the question stem, and replace the carbonyl group with an amine. The R-group will remain the same, and the table can be used to determine which amino acid would be formed. Glycine has a hydrogen atom as its R-group, but the original ketoacid has an isopropyl R-group, so choice A can be eliminated. The side chain (circled below) matches valine's side chain, so choice B is a strong answer. The R-group for aspartic acid and lysine are not present in the original ketoacid, so choices C and D can be eliminated.

346. D is the best answer. To answer this question, simply take the ketoacid shown in the question stem, and replace the carbonyl group with an amine. The R-group will remain the same, and the table can be used to determine which amino acid would be formed. The side chain is not a single hydrogen atom, so choice A can be eliminated. Serine has a hydroxyl in its R-group, so choice B can be eliminated. The R-group for aspartic acid contains a carboxylic acid, so choice C can be eliminated. The side chain (circled below) matches asparagine's side chain, so choice D is the best answer.

347. B is the best answer. The final product is an amide with two ethyl groups attached, so using simple ammonia would not yield the correct product. Choices A and D can be eliminated. Choices B and C use diethyl amine, which would yield a amide with two ethyl groups. Comparing these two answers, the reaction that utilizes the acid chloride will be more reactive than the carboxylic acid, so choice B is a stronger answer than choice C.

348. B is the best answer. This molecule on the left is tosylate, which is used to protect alcohols. This occurs through an S_N1 reaction where the alcohol is the nucleophile and the halide is the leaving group. So, choice B is the best answer. To make an aldehyde, the alcohol would have to be oxidized. There is no oxidizing agent (such as $KMnO_4$) present, so choice A is not the best answer. Of note, the carbonyls on the tosylate cannot be called aldehydes because they are not bound directly to carbon. A carboxylic acid would also be produced through oxidation or alternatively through carboxylation, so choice C is not the best answer. Alkynes are produced through specialized reactions often via $NaNH_2$ so choice D is not the best answer.

349. B is the best answer. Carbon is a poor nucleophile, so choice A can be eliminated. Nitrogen is a great nucleophile because of its lone pair of electrons, so choice B is a strong answer. Oxygen can act as a nucleophile but not when it is a carbonyl. Biotin only contains carbonyls, so choice C is not the best answer. Sulfur can be a nucleophile, but the sulfur in biotin is sterically hindered, so choice D is not as strong as choice B. The mechanism of biotin reactions is not required for the MCAT® but nitrogen is the nucleophile which can be deduced by process of elimination. The mechanism for this nucleophilic substitution is shown below.

350. C is the best answer. An electrophile attracts electrons. ATP is cleaved to ADP and P_i when attacked by a nucleophile, so ATP is an electrophile and choice A is not the best answer. NAD^+ is reduced to NADH by addition of an H^-. The H^- is the nucleophile, so NAD^+ is the electrophile, and choice B is not the best answer. NADH is already reduced, so it cannot continue to act as an electrophile, making choice C is a strong answer. FAD is a molecule with similar function as NAD^+. It is reduced to $FADH_2$ through addition of H^+ and H^-. H^- is the nucleophile, so FAD is an electrophile, and choice D is not the best answer.

351. D is the best answer. The reactant (R)-3-methyl-3-bromohexane is a substituted halogenated hydrocarbon that will favor S_N1 or E1 reactions. S_N2 or E2 can only occur on a tertiary carbon like this one if the nucleophile is very strong. Water is only a moderately strong nucleophile, so S_N1 and E1 would be favored. Any time S_N1 occurs, E1 is also occurring. E1 is favored in the presence of a base. Water is not a very good base so the S_N1 reaction will be favored and choice A can be eliminated. S_N1 produces racemic mixtures, so the best answer must list the R and S forms in the same proportions, so choices B and C can be eliminated. Of note with choice C, the 2-hexene product would be produced in the same proportion as the 3-hexene product because either carbon 2 or carbon 3 could be attacked by the base to donate electrons for the alkene. Choice D is the best answer because the S_N1 products are favored equally, and the E1 products are less favored but still equal.

352. A is the best answer. The acetate ion is electron rich, so it is more likely to be a nucleophile than an electrophile. Choice A is stronger than choice B. A catalyst is a compound that is added to a reaction to increase the rate of the reaction. By definition, a catalyst is regenerated and thus not consumed by the reaction. The acetate ion is consumed in the reaction, so choice C can be eliminated. Generally the solvent of a reaction is written under the reaction arrow, but this is not always the case. Since there is no obvious specification of the solvent for this reaction, choice D is a weaker answer than choice A.

353. A is the best answer. A chiral molecule will be optically active. The ester formation occurs via an S_N2 reaction mechanism, so it will result in the inversion of stereochemistry and formation of an optically active molecule. Choice A is a stronger answer than choice B. A secondary alkyl halide will still participate in the reaction with acetate, but it will do so at a slower rate since it is more sterically hindered. This eliminates choices C and D.

354. D is the best answer. Increasing the concentration of alcohol increases the concentration of a reactant. The increased reactant concentration will drive the reaction to the right and result in a greater production of ester. Option I is true, so choice B can be eliminated. Anhydrides are more reactive than carboxylic acids, so substituting the anhydride for the carboxylic acid will lead to more product. Option II is true, so choice D is the best answer. Acid catalyzes the reaction and increases the rate, so more product will be produced in a given amount of time. While the effect of option III is a little vague, but since options I and II are true, choice D is the best answer.

355. C is the best answer. The acid protonates the hydroxyl of the carboxylic acid, converting it to water, which is a good leaving group. Option I is true, so choice B can be eliminated. The acid catalyst does not protonate the nucleophile. If this occurred, the nucleophile would be much weaker and the reaction rate would decrease. Option II is false, so choice D can be eliminated. The acid catalyst also activates the electrophile by protonating the carbonyl oxygen, which makes the carbonyl carbon more electron deficient. Option III is true, so choice C is the best answer.

356. C is the best answer. The reaction occurs via a nucleophilic attack by the amine on the alkyl halide. There is no water molecule released from the reaction, so a dehydration reaction has not occurred. Choice A can be eliminated. Similarly, a water molecule is not consumed by the reactions, so choice B can be eliminated. An addition of an alkyl group to an amine is called an alkylation, so choice C is a strong answer. Dehydrohalogenation reactions occur when a hydrogen atom and halide are eliminated from a molecule and usually produce alkenes. While the reaction does eliminate a halide, a hydrogen atom is not removed, so choice D can be eliminated.

357. C is the best answer. Only tertiary amines form amine picrates. Choice A is a primary amine, so choice A can be eliminated. Choice B is a secondary amine and can be eliminated. Choice C is the only tertiary amine and is the best answer. Choice D is a quaternary amine, so it is a weaker answer.

358. A is the best answer. Protein primary structure is the string of amino acids linked via peptide bonds. Peptide bonds are an example of an amide bond, wherein a carboxyl carbon is linked to a nitrogen group. Amide bonds can be broken via hydrolysis, which is only possible under extreme chemical conditions (high temperature, strong acid) that are unlikely to occur in biological systems. Choice A is a strong answer. Low temperature environments are conducive to hydrolysis. Choice B can be eliminated. Once an amide bond is formed, electronic interactions do not factor into stability of primary structure; these many for secondary, tertiary, and quaternary structure. Choice C can be eliminated. Primary structure can be disrupted in a low pH, high temperature environment, not just via genetic mutation. Choice D can be eliminated. Choice A is the best answer.

359. B is the best answer. The intermediate is a peroxide with two oxygen atoms linked in a sigma bond. Peroxides can be unstable, especially at higher temperatures. Intermediates are usually unstable and difficult to isolate, so choice A is a weaker answer. The presence of the extra oxygen indicates a higher oxidation state than the reactant, so choice B is a stronger answer than choice C. Transition states are high energy configurations that occur prior to new bond formation or bond breakage, whereas an intermediate is a molecule that is formed after the new bonds are created. Choice D is not a strong answer.

360. B is the best answer. Sodium hydroxide dissociates into Na^+ and OH^- in solution. OH^- is a strong base than will undergo nucleophilic attack of the carbonyl carbon. Note that the carbonyl bond is polarized due to the electronegativity of oxygen: partial positive charge on carbon, and partial negative charge on oxygen. Substituents that donate electron density will reduce this positive charge, whereas substituents that withdraw electron density will increase this positive charge. Reaction rate will be maximized if the partial positive charge on charge is as large as possible, because this facilitates a favorable electronic interaction. CH_3 is weakly donating. Choice A can be eliminated. CCl_3 is strongly withdrawing due to the highly electronegative Cl atoms. Choice B is a strong answer. OCH_3 is moderately donating. Choice C can be eliminated. Br is weakly withdrawing. Choice D can be eliminated in favor of choice B.

361. D is the best answer. The least amount of ring strain occurs in the chair confirmation. That is why this confirmation is preferred by glucose. Planar has the most strain and the boat forms have intermediate strain.

362. C is the best answer. Choice A is glucose. With its six-membered ring, its bonds are 120° which is ideal for a sp^3 bond. Additionally, glucose enters the chair confirmation to reduce strain even further. Glucose has the least strain, so choice A is not the best answer. Choice B is uracil. It has more strain than glucose because the double bond prevents entering into the chair confirmation. However, with a six-membered ring, choice B is not the best answer. Choice C is penicillin. It has a four-membered ring that experiences significant strain. Choice C is a strong answer. Choice D is morphine. It has a six-membered ring coming out of the page that experiences some strain but not nearly as much as the four-membered ring in penicillin. Choice C is a better answer choice than choice D.

363. A is the best answer. Penicillin has a four-membered ring that is at risk for reactivity due to the high energy bonds created through ring strain. Choice A is likely the best answer. Choice B is not the best answer because the dimethyl site would be sterically protected and not reactive. Choice C is not the best answer because the carbonyl oxygen is not very reactive (although the carbonyl carbon is). Choice D is not the best answer because sulfur is relatively stable in most organic compounds. Carbonyls, oxygen and nitrogen are more reactive.

Addition Reactions: Aldehydes and Ketones

364. C is the best answer. Ketones are functional groups with a carbonyl bonded to two alkyl groups. Choice A does not contain a carbonyl and is an alcohol, so it can be eliminated. An amide is a carbonyl with an amine group, so choice B can be eliminated. The ketone functional group is circled in the compound below. Choice C is a strong answer. Choice D is a carboxylic acid and can be eliminated.

365. B is the best answer. The reaction involves two hydrogen atoms replaced by a carbonyl making the transformation an alkane to a ketone. An aldehyde is a carbonyl that is bonded to an alkyl group and a hydrogen atom. Since the product contains a ketone, not an aldehyde, choice A can be eliminated. Since the ketone is in a cyclic ring, choice B is a strong answer. The product is a ketone, not an alkane, so choice C can be eliminated. An ether is an oxygen atom bonded to two alkyl groups, so choice D can be eliminated.

366. C is the best answer. A beta hydrogen is bonded to the carbon that is two carbons away from the carbonyl carbon. The hydrogen atom labeled 1 is bonded directly to the carbonyl carbon, so choice A is a weak answer. Hydrogen two is bonded to the alpha carbon, which is the carbon bonded to the carbonyl. Choice B can be eliminated. Hydrogen three is bonded to the beta carbon, so choice C is a strong answer. A carbon that is three bonds away from the carbonyl is a gamma carbon, so choice D can be eliminated.

367. D is the best answer. The ring in the question stem is a five membered ring. Carbohydrates that are six membered rings are called pyranoses, while five membered rings are called furanoses. Since the structure in the question stem is a five carbon ring, so choices A and B can be eliminated. To determine if the sugar is a ketose or an aldose, look at the anomeric carbon. If it is bonded to a hydroxyl and hydrogen atom, then it is an aldose, whereas if it is bonded to a hydrogen atom and a carbon, then it is a ketose. The R replaces the OH group, which indicates that the furanose (five membered ring) is of an aldose because the anomeric carbon is bonded to a hydrogen atom and the equivalent of an OH group. Choice D is a better answer than choice C.

368. A is the best answer. When determining the solubility of a compound in a particular solvent, the simple principle of "like dissolves like" is useful. This means that polar molecules will dissolve in polar solvents. Since water is a polar solvent, the best answer will be the molecule with the greatest polarity. 1-Heptanol is an alcohol, which are polar molecules due to the polar bond of the hydroxyl group, so choice A is a strong answer. Alkanes are nonpolar molecules, so choice B can be eliminated. Ketones (choice C) and aldehydes (choice D) have polar bonds between the carbonyl oxygen and carbon, but they are less soluble in water because they are unable to participate in hydrogen bonding, so choices C and D can be eliminated.

369. B is the best answer. The electrophilic nature of a molecule is improved if it has a larger partial positive charge. An electrophile can be improved if it is bonded to an electron withdrawing group. Carbon 1 has an OCH_3 bonded to it which is electron withdrawing. Carbonyls have the ability to resonate, so the carbon is a stronger electrophile. This makes choice B a stronger answer than choice A. Carbon 3 does not have an electron withdrawing group bonded to it, so choice C can be eliminated. Carbon 4 has two electron withdrawing groups, so choice D is a stronger electrophile than choice A, but since the carbonyl has the ability to resonate, choice D can be eliminated, and choice B is the best answer.

370. A is the best answer. The boiling point of a molecule is largely determined by its intermolecular forces. The stronger the intermolecular force, the higher a boiling point will be. Alcohols have higher boiling points due to hydrogen bonding. Choice A is a strong answer. London dispersion forces are the primary intermolecular forces of alkanes. The boiling point of different alkanes is largely determined by the size of the alkane, with larger alkanes having a higher boiling point. Alkanes will have lower boiling points than alcohols, so choice B can be eliminated. Although ketones and aldehydes can hydrogen bond with water, they do not hydrogen bond with themselves, so choices C and D can be eliminated.

371. B is the best answer. A carbonyl is a carbon atom that has a double bond to an oxygen atom. The first step in the reaction scheme results in the addition of an alkene to the carbonyl. Next, the alkene is converted to a carbonyl by reacting it with O_3. Product C is shown below. It contains one carbonyl. Choice B is the best answer.

372. C is the best answer. The excess of vinyl lithium will initially proceed through the same reaction as depicted in the reaction scheme. The acidic condition of the reaction will protonate the hydroxide and create a water molecule, which is a better leaving group. A second molecule of vinyl lithium will attack the carbon and the water molecule will leave. After ozonolysis of the two alkenes, two carbonyls will remain. Choice C is the best answer. The new product is shown below.

373. B is the best answer. Ozonolysis of an alkene (Product A to Product C) will produce an aldehyde in place of the alkene. The reactant for this reaction also contained an alcohol group in addition to the alkene. The reaction that converts Product C to Product D uses sulfuric acid and heat. Aldehydes are relatively inert to these reactants, so the main functional group that will participate is the alcohol. Under these conditions, the OH will be protonated and eventually kicked off as an alkene is created. This release of water is a dehydration reaction, so choice A can be eliminated, and choice B is a strong answer. An aldol condensation would result in a much larger molecule since it would involve combining two aldols in to one molecules, so choice C can be eliminated. A hydrogenation reaction would result in the creation of an alkane, not an alkene, so choice D can be eliminated.

374. B is the best answer. The oxygen atom in 3-pentanone becomes a hydroxyl group after the carbonyl undergoes a nucleophilic attack by the vinyllithium. This oxygen eventually leaves with the water molecule in the conversion of Product C to Product D. The oxygen comes from the ozonolysis of the alkene. This oxygen comes from O_3. There is no reaction that adds water to one of the products, so the oxygen atom can not come from a water molecules. Choice C can be eliminated. The oxygen atom of the OH group in Product C eventually leaves as a water molecule to form Product D, so choice D can be eliminated.

375. A is the best answer. The addition of OH and H to a double bond is called hydration. One simple way to remember this is that a water molecule is actually being added across the double bond. Choice A is a strong answer. Dehydration reactions result in the loss of a water molecule from a compound, so choice B can be eliminated. Hydrogenation reactions add two atoms of hydrogen to a molecule. Since only one atom of hydrogen is added along with a hydroxyl group, choice C can be eliminated. Nucleophilic substitution reactions are most often seen with carbonyl compounds. With these reactions, a nucleophile attacks the carbonyl. When the carbonyl reforms, a leaving group is kicked off and the final product is a carbonyl with a new functional group. Choice D can be eliminated.

376. C is the best answer. The product is formed by moving a single hydrogen atom from the alcohol to the alkene to form a ketone. Since there is no change in the oxidation state of the atoms, it is neither an oxidation nor reduction. Choices A and B can be eliminated. Tautomerization is the interconversion of constitutional isomers. A classic example is the keto-enol tautomerization. Step two is an example of a keto-enol tautomerization, so choice C is a strong answer. The hydrogen atom does not add via a nucleophilic attack, which is the first step of a nucleophilic substitution, so choice D can be eliminated.

377. A is the best answer. The hydration of the alkyne will always place the hydroxyl group on the most substituted carbon (Markovnikov). Since the alcohol product tautomerizes to form a ketone, an aldehyde cannot be formed. Choice A is a strong answer. The anti-Markovnikov alcohol product would result in a terminal alcohol, so choice B can be eliminated. While it is true that aldehydes are more unstable and more acidic than ketones, neither of these properties answer the question of why the reaction only results in the production of a methyl ketone. Choices C and D are weaker answers, so choice A is the best answer.

378. B is the best answer. The oxidation of a primary alcohol to aldehyde requires a mild oxidant. If K_2CrO_4 is used, it will oxidize the alcohol to a carboxylic acid. Choice A can be eliminated. PCC is a mild oxidant, so choice B is a strong answer. $LiAlH_4$ is a reducing agent that will not react with a primary alcohol, so choice C can be eliminated. O_3 is primarily used to break alkene bonds, so choice D can be eliminated.

379. A is the best answer. The formation of benzalacetone proceeds through an aldol condensation reaction. The first step of this reaction is the generation of an enolate via deprotonation of an alpha hydrogen. Acetone is the only carbonyl with an alpha hydrogen, so it forms the enolate ion and acts as the nucleophile. Choice A is a strong answer. The electrophile is the carbonyl that is attacked by the enolate, so choice B can be eliminated. The acetone is deprotonated, so it is acting as an acid, making choice C a weaker answer. There is no change in the oxidation state of the reactants, so acetone is neither an oxidant nor a reductant, eliminating choice D.

380. B is the best answer. The formation of benzalacetone proceeds through an aldol condensation reaction. The first step of this reaction is the generation of an enolate via deprotonation of an alpha hydrogen. Benzaldehyde is not a nucleophile because it has no alpha hydrogen to form the enolate ion. Choice A can be eliminated. Instead, it is attacked by the enolate ion of acetone, making it an electrophile. Choice B is a strong answer. Since it is accepting electron density, it is acting more like a Lewis acid, eliminating choice C. There is no change in the oxidation state of the reactants, so acetone is neither an oxidant nor a reductant, eliminating choice D.

381. C is the best answer. The reactions of a carbonyl and alkene that are capable of resonating are similar to the addition reactions of dienes. Molecules that are able to stabilize electron density via resonance are more likely to act as electrophiles. Both the carbonyl (1,2 addition) and the terminal carbon of the alkene (1,4 addition) can act as electrophiles since they are able to delocalize the new electron density. Choice A can be eliminated since it only includes carbon 1. Carbon 2 is less capable of resonating if it accepts electron density, so it is less likely to act as an electrophile. Choices B and D can be eliminated.

382. C is the best answer. Tautomerization is the interconversion of constitutional isomers. A classic example is the keto-enol tautomerization which involves the rearrangement of bonds to switch between and ketone and an enol. While hydroxide can often act as a nucleophile, it does not attack the carbonyl in this reaction, so choice A can be eliminated. The intermediate results from the deprotonation of the alpha carbon and creation of the enolate ion. This does not process through an electrophilic addition, so choice B can be eliminated. The intermediate is the enolate ion of the original ketone which results from tautomerization and then deprotonation. Choice C is a strong answer. Since the intermediate is generated by deprotonation, it is not in resonance with cyclohexanone. Choice D can be eliminated.

383. B is the best answer. Reacting 1-butanol with methanal will result in a molecule with two, 4-membered ether chains. Choice A can be eliminated. Methanol, a nucleophile, will attack the carbonyl of butanal to form a hemiacetal. A second methanol molecule will attack the hemiacetal to form the acetal. Choice B is a strong answer. 1,1-Dibutanol and water will not result in a net reaction since diols are not reactive to neutral water, so choice C can be eliminated. A reaction of propanal with methanol will result in a final molecule with a three-carbon chain instead of the four carbon chain seen in the question stem. Choice D can be eliminated.

384. C is the best answer. The reaction in the question stem proceeds through a nucleophilic addition mechanism. The carbonyl carbon is attacked by nucleophile. Since the carbonyl carbon is an electrophile, choice A can be eliminated. The carbonyl oxygen in formaldehyde is relatively inert in the base catalyzed reaction. At the conclusion of the reaction, it will be protonated to form one of the hydroxide groups, but it is not the primary nucleophile, so choice B is a weaker answer. Hydroxide is a much stronger nucleophile than water. This explains the need for the basic conditions, as it creates the hydroxide ion that can then act as a nucleophile. Choice C is a stronger answer than choice D.

385. A is the best answer. The acid protonates the oxygen of the carbonyl, which draws more electron density away from the carbonyl carbon. This carbon becomes more electrophilic as it becomes more electron deficient, so choice A is a strong answer. The nucleophile is the water molecule, which is not affected by the protonation of the carbonyl oxygen. Choice B can be eliminated. Since the water molecule is a nucleophile, choice C can be eliminated. Protonation of the oxygen of water would weaken its ability to act as a nucleophile by decreasing its ability to donate electron density. Choice D can be eliminated.

386. D is the best answer. The carbonyl carbon, like any carbonyl reaction acts as an electrophile since it has a partial positive charge due to its double bond to the highly electronegative oxygen atom. Choice A can be eliminated. The hydrogen ion supplied by the acidic conditions protonates the carbonyl oxygen. In this reaction, it technically acts as an electrophile, so choice B can be eliminated. In an acidic solution, hydroxide ion is not present. Therefore, water functions as the nucleophile and attacks the activated electrophile. Choice C is a weaker answer than choice D, which is the best answer.

387. B is the best answer. An acetal is a compound that has a carbon with two ether groups. Since the pyranose from only has one ether attached to it, choice A can be eliminated. There is a hydroxyl group and an ether attached to the same carbon forming a hemiacetal. Choice B is a strong answer. An ester is a functional group formed by a carbonyl with an ether bond. There is not a carbonyl in the pyranose form, so choice C can be eliminated. While technically there is one ether molecule in the pyranose form, that carbon also is attached to a hydroxyl group, so it is more specifically a hemiacetal. Choice D is a weaker answer.

388. A is the best answer. The anomeric carbon is the carbon in the ring that was originally a carbonyl before being attacked by the hydroxyl group of another carbon. To locate the anomeric carbon, first identify the oxygen in the ring. One of the two carbon atoms bonded to this oxygen is the anomeric carbon since this oxygen atom is the one that performed the nucleophilic attack. Choices B and D can be eliminated. The carbon that is directly bonded to a hydroxyl group is the anomeric carbon. Since C5 is bonded to a CH_2OH group, choice D can be eliminated. C1 is bonded to the ring oxygen and another hydroxyl group, so choice A is the best answer.

389. A is the best answer. The carbon is attached to two ethers and a hydrogen atom. By definition this makes it an acetal. Choice A is a strong answer. If one of the ethers was a hydroxyl group, then it would be a hemiacetal. Choice B can be eliminated. An ester is a functional group formed by a carbonyl with an ether bond. There is not a carbonyl at the anomeric carbon, so choice C can be eliminated. While technically there is one ether molecule at the anomeric carbon, that carbon is also attached to a second ether group, so it is more specifically an acetal. Choice D is a weaker answer.

390. A is the best answer. This is classic example of the formation of imines and enamines via amines. The substrate for this reaction is any aldehyde or ketone. Of these choices, the only that contains both is choice A. The expulsion of ketones, which have a sweet odor, from the breath is indication of a condition called diabetic ketoacidosis, but knowing that is not required for answering this question.

391. B is the best answer. The product is the result of the nucleophile attacking the alkene and forming an enol that tautomerizes back to a ketone. The first step is the lone pair of electrons on the molecule with two ketones attacking the terminal end of the alkene. This molecule is capable of resonating and creates an enolate ion. If the other carbon of the original alkene was protonated, then the reaction would be a 1,2 addition, so choice A can be eliminated. The oxygen of the enolate ion is protonated, so the reaction proceeds via a 1,4 conjugate addition. Choice B is a strong answer. An electrophilic addition reaction results from a π bond being broken and two new σ bonds being formed. Since a pi bond is not broken in this reaction, choice C can be eliminated. While the alkene undergoes nucleophilic attack by the lone pair of electrons, there is not a suitable leaving group, so the reaction is not a substitution. Choice D can be eliminated.

392. A is the best answer. To answer this question, look at the intermediate product to determine which carbonyl undergoes a nucleophilic attack. The ring is formed by a new sigma bond between carbon 1 and carbon 3. Since carbon 3 is a carbonyl, carbon 1 has to act as the nucleophile. This makes the α hydrogens of carbon 1 likely candidates for removal to create the enolate. Choice A is a strong answer. Carbons 2 and 3 do not have any hydrogen atoms, so choices B and C can be eliminated. Carbon 4 has α hydrogens, but creation of an enolate that would then attack carbon 2 would result in a ring without a methyl group attached, so choice D can be eliminated.

393. A is the best answer. (S)-3-methyl-2-heptanone would lose its chirality because the chiral carbon is the alpha carbon. It is the configuration of the alpha carbon that is affected by tautomerization since it goes from an sp^3 to an sp^2 carbon which cannot have an R or S configuration. Choice A is a strong answer. The carbon that determines the chirality for (R)-4-methyl-2-heptanone is carbon 4, which is not affected by tautomerization, so choice B can be eliminated. The molecules in choices C and D both have their chirality determined by carbon 3, but carbon 2 is the carbon molecule that is affected by tautomerization, so they can be eliminated.

394. B is the best answer. Hydrogen atoms of aldehydes are not acidic since deprotonation of an aldehyde would create a more positive carbonyl carbon which would be more unstable. Choice A can be eliminated. The hydrogen attached to the α carbon is the most acidic due to the ability of the carbonyl to resonance stabilize the anion. Choice B is a strong answer. Compared to the alpha carbon, the hydrogen atoms on the beta and gamma carbons are less acidic because they are further away from the carbonyl carbon. Choices C and D can be eliminated.

395. D is the best answer. The hydrogen atoms on alkanes and alkenes are not strongly acidic, particularly when compared to the hydrogen atoms of a ketone or aldehyde. Choices A and B can be eliminated. Pentanal is the most acidic because it is an aldehyde. The hydrogen attached to the α carbon is more acidic than other hydrogen atoms. Aldehydes are more acidic than ketones, so choice C can be eliminated, but both are less acidic than alcohols. It is important to note that the acidic hydrogen is attached to the alpha carbon and not the carbonyl carbon. Choice D is the best answer.

396. C is the best answer. The hydrogen atom labeled number 1 is bonded to a beta carbon, so it is less acidic than hydrogen 2 which is bonded to an alpha carbon. Choice A can be eliminated. Hydrogen 3 is also bonded to an alpha carbon, but it is located between two carbonyls, so it has the most resonance stabilization of the conjugate base anion. Increased stability of a conjugate base leads to increased acidity. See the resonance structures below. This makes choice C a strong answer. Hydrogen 4 would be expected to have a similar acidity as hydrogen 2 since it is also bonded to an alpha carbon, but less acidity than carbon 3, so choice D can be eliminated.

397. C is the best answer. While the oxygen of the ketone is capable of hydrogen bonding due to their highly polar bonds with water molecules, this does not explain the increased acidity since the hydrogen bonding is not the major source of stabilization of the conjugate base. Choice A can be eliminated. The oxygen of the ketone withdraws electron density from the base, so choice B can be eliminated. If a compound is more acidic, it must be due to stabilization of the conjugate base anion. The double bond in the ketone allows resonance stabilization of the alpha carbon. See the resonance structures in answer 396. Choice D can be eliminated, and choice C is the best answer.

398. A is the best answer. The reaction is the reverse of oxidation (reduction), so the reducing agent $NaBH_4$ will achieve the conversion. Choice A is a strong answer. PBr_3 is a reagent used to brominate an alcohol, so choice B can be eliminated. $Na_2Cr_2O_7$ is an oxidizing agent and can be used to create camphor from borneol as in the forward reaction, but the question is asking for the reagent needed to perform the reverse reaction, so choice C can be eliminated. O_3 is used to break apart an alkene and create an aldehyde or ketone, so choice D can be eliminated.

399. C is the best answer. The treatment of product D with LiAlH$_4$ will produce a diol that can form a ketal when reacted with a ketone. Choices A and C are the only answers that are ketals, so choices B and D can be eliminated. Choice A would result from a three carbon diol, while choice C would result from a reaction with a five carbon diol. Since Product D is a five membered diol, choice C is a better answer than choice A.

400. B is the best answer. The first step of the reaction protects the ketone from nucleophilic attack by decreasing the electrophilicity of the carbonyl carbon. If this step is not performed, the vinyl lithium, which is a strong nucleophile, will attack the carbonyl and add a new alkene bond to the molecule at the carbonyl carbon. Choice A can be eliminated, and choice B is a strong answer. Since this new bond would be formed, the same final product will not be obtained, so choice C can be eliminated. There is no way to tell what effect skipping the first step will have on the rate. It is possible that it will actually proceed at a faster rate given the additional reaction site that is available after not performing the first step, so choice D can be eliminated.

401. B is the best answer. The nucleophile must contain a CN group eliminating choices C and D. HCN is too weak of a nucleophile for a reaction to take place, so choice A can be eliminated. CN$^-$ is a strong enough nucleophile to attack 2-Hexanone and produce the final product shown in the question stem. Choice B is the best answer.

402. A is the best answer. The question states that the addition of HBr with hydrogen peroxide creates the anti-Markovnikov product; the Br adds to the less substituted carbon. Choice A is a strong answer. Choice B is the Markovnikov product since the Br is added to the most substituted carbon of the alkene, so it can be eliminated. Choice C is the original reactant, so it can be eliminated. 2-Isopropylbutane would be the expected product if the reactant underwent a reduction reaction, so choice D can be eliminated.

Oxidation and Reduction of Oxygen Containing Compounds

403. A is the best answer. The product is an aldehyde, which is more oxidized than an alcohol. PCC must be an oxidizing agent. Choice A is a strong answer, and choice B can be eliminated. An acid-base reaction is not taking place in the conversion of citronellol to citronellal, so choices C and D can be eliminated.

404. A is the best answer. 3-Hexanol is a lower oxidation state than 3-Hexanone, and only choice A is a reducing agent. Choices B and C are both oxidizing agents and can be eliminated. AlCl$_3$ is an important reagent for many aromatic reactions, so choice D can be eliminated.

405. B is the best answer. An aldehyde is a higher oxidation state than an alcohol. The oxidation has to be done carefully so that the aldehyde is not oxidized all the way to a carboxylic acid. This requires a milder oxidizing agent. LiAlH$_4$ is a reducing agent, so choice A can be eliminated. Choices B and C are both oxidizing agents, but K$_2$CrO$_4$ is a stronger oxidizing agent and will convert the alcohol to a carboxylic acid while dilute cold KMnO$_4$ will stop the oxidation at the aldehyde. Choice B is a stronger answer than choice C. Ozone will break apart double bonds, so choice D can be eliminated.

406. C is the best answer. The carbon atom of a carboxylic acid is at a higher oxidation state than the carbon atom in either an alcohol or an aldehyde. LiAlH$_4$ is a reducing agent, so choice A can be eliminated. Dilute cold KMnO$_4$ will oxidize the primary alcohol, but it is a weaker oxidizing agent and will stop the oxidation reaction at an aldehyde. Potassium chromate is a strong oxidant, and the reaction will completely oxidize the product to a carboxylic acid. Choice C is a stronger answer than choice B. Although ozone produces an oxidized product, it only works on alkenes. Choice D can be eliminated.

407. A is the best answer. The hydrolysis of the ester forms an alcohol and a carboxylic acid that is deprotonated by the base. Choice A is a strong answer. Dehydration reactions result in the loss of a water molecule. In this reaction, one net molecule of hydroxide is added to the molecule, so choice B can be eliminated. There are no molecules of hydrogen added to the molecule, so choice C can be eliminated. A decarboxylation reaction results in the loss of a molecule of carbon dioxide, so choice D can be eliminated.

408. C is the best answer. Acetic anhydride is more reactive than acetic acid and will not successfully react with acetic acid. Choice A can be eliminated. Acetic acid will not undergo a net reaction when reacted with itself, so choice B can be eliminated. Ethanol will react to displace the OH and form the ethyl ester. An alcohol and an acid combine to form an ester. Ethyl chloride can undergo an S$_N$2 reaction with a good nucleophile, but since acetic acid is not a strong nucleophile, it is unlikely that a reaction will occur. Choice D can be eliminated.

409. A is the best answer. Carboxylic acids can be reduced to either alcohols or aldehydes depending on the strength of the reduction agent. Random error describes unpredictable error, while systematic error tends to arise from improper use of measurement tools. Choice A is the strongest answer as the addition of a reduction agent such as LiAlH$_4$ to a carboxylic acid would produce an alcohol. The mislabeling of the reagent would be attributed to random error.

410. A is the best answer. D-glucose is the only aldehyde listed. α-D-glucopyranose contains a hemiacetal instead of the aldehyde that is normally present in glucose, so choice B can be eliminated. D-fructose contains a ketone, so it would not react with bromine water. Choice C can be eliminated. α-D-fructofuranose contains a hemiketal, but no aldehyde, so choice D can be eliminated.

411. B is the best answer. Since there would be no water molecules to hydrate the formaldehyde if methanol was used instead of water, choice A can be eliminated. Two molecules of methanol would add to the formaldehyde forming an acetal. Choice B is a strong answer. A ketal is a molecule with two ether bonds, and two alkyl groups. If the original reactant was a ketone rather than an aldehyde, a ketal would be formed, so choice C can be eliminated. As described above, a reaction would occur, so choice D can be eliminated.

412. A is the best answer. Based on the question, the 2-butanone is less reactive which means it is less electrophilic (electron deficient). To account for the difference in reactivity, alkyl groups must be electron donating making 2-butanone's carbonyl carbon less electrophilic. Choice A is a stronger answer than choice B. Formaldehyde is less sterically hindered than butanone since it has hydrogen atoms bonded to the carbonyl carbon instead of alkyl groups. Choice C can be eliminated. Aldehydes and ketones are not acting as nucleophiles in this reaction, so the difference in reactivity between the two compounds is not due to a different in their nucleophilicity. Choice D can be eliminated.

Carbonyls as Nucleophiles: Aldol Condensation

413. D is the best answer. An aldol reaction occurs when an enolate ion attacks the carbonyl carbon of another molecule. The carbonyl carbon is an electrophile, so choice A can be eliminated. While the carbonyl oxygen can technically act as a nucleophile when it undergoes protonation, this is step does not always occur in an aldol reaction and often occurs in the final workup of the product, so choice B is a possible answer, but the other choices should still be evaluated. A hydroxide ion deprotonates the alpha carbon to generate an enolate ion, but the nucleophilic attack on the carbonyl carbon is performed by the enolate ion. The enolate ion is the nucleophile because it is the electron rich substance. Choice D is a stronger answer than choices B and C.

414. C is the best answer. In an aldol addition, one of the carbonyls is converted to an enolate ion and the alpha carbon of the enolate ion attacks the other carbonyl carbon. The attacked carbonyl becomes an alcohol and the enolate carbonyl remains a carbonyl. Choices A and B can be eliminated, and choice C is a strong answer. An alkene bond is generated when the alpha carbon is deprotonated, but the electrons in this double bond are used for the addition reaction, so the final product does not contain an alkene. Choice D can be eliminated.

415. C is the best answer. Because the reaction is base catalyzed, the first step cannot be protonation, eliminating choices A and B. The deprotonation forms the enolate ion, which is the nucleophile. Choice C is a better answer than choice D.

416. A is the best answer. In an acid catalyzed reaction, the acid will protonate the carbonyl oxygen making the carbonyl carbon more electron deficient, thus activating the electrophile. In a base catalyzed reaction, the base deprotonates the alpha carbon, which activates the enolate nucleophile. Choice A is a strong answer. Choice B states the opposite and can be eliminated. Since one set of conditions acts on the electrophile, while the other acts on the nucleophile, choices C and D can be eliminated.

Bonding and Reactions of Biological Molecules

417. A is the best answer. In order to separate monosaccharides from a chain, water must be added, so choices C and D can be ruled out. Starch is a 1-6 bonded polysaccharide, so choice A is the best answer.

418. A is the best answer. In order to undergo hydrolysis of a glycosidic bond, a monosaccharide must be attached to another molecule such as another sugar or nucleic acid. Of the above, lactose is a disaccharide and may undergo hydrolysis, and glycogen is also a polysaccharide and will also undergo hydrolysis via glycogenolysis. Uridine is a nucleoside, which means it contains a sugar and can also undergo hydrolysis. Hypoxanthine (also found as 6-hydroxypurine) is a purine base found in RNA, and does not contain a sugar, and is therefore not susceptible to hydrolysis.

419. C is the best answer. Hydrolysis will break all ester bonds—if DNA or ATP is hydrolyzed, the only pieces that remain are monosaccharides, purines, pyrimidines, and phosphates, none heavy enough to be over 250 g/mol. The hydrolysis of glycogen produces only monosaccharides, which are also not heavy enough. Phospholipid hydrolysis would yield free fatty acid tails, which may be many carbons long and heavier than 250 g/mol, so choice C is the best answer.

420. D is the best answer. The mechanism above depicts a polysaccharide being broken down into monosaccharides via hydrolysis. The hydrolysis of sucrose produces glucose and fructose monosaccharides. The product to the left of the addition sign, glucose, is a pyranose. As mannose is also a pyranose, choice B is the best answer. It is important to note that ribose would resemble the second sugar, fructose, as they are both furanoses.

421. A is the best answer. In the first step of a hydrolysis reaction under acidic conditions, the oxygen linking the sugars would likely be protonated by a hydronium ion. Protonation of oxygen A would lead to the creation of a highly resonance-stabilized intermediate. Choice A is the best answer, as a hydronium ion would be present under acidic conditions. A hydroxide ion is unlikely to be found in acidic conditions, which allows for the elimination of choices B and D.

422. D is the best answer. To answer this question, it is important to realize that the reaction depicted is the hydrolysis of sucrose. Sucrose is composed of a glyosidic linkage between glucose and fructose that is alpha with respect to glucose and beta with respect to fructose. While choice B is a true statement, choice D is the better answer. The anomeric carbon on fructose is numbered 2, unlike glucose. Due to this, choice D is the best answer.

423. B is the best answer. The simple way to answer this question is to recognize that only phenol has both an alcohol and alkene present. The science behind this answer is that usually the keto form is much more stable than the enol form. However, a few exceptions exist, primarily when there is aromatic stabilization and also more mildly in the case of beta carbonyl. In this case, acetone and glucose fit neither criteria. Acetoacetic acid does have a stabilizing carbonyl, however this effect is relatively mild compared to phenol, an aromatic compound, which will be much more strongly stabilized and will favor the enol, making choice B the best answer.

424. D is the best answer. In keto-enol tautomerization, a strong base is used to move a double bond from a carbonyl to the carbon backbone, resulting alkene hydroxyl. To shift fructose towards glucose, the double bond must be moved towards the end of the chain, since glucose is an aldose sugar. Keto-enol tautomerization will cause the double bond to move to the more substituted carbon in thermodynamically favorable conditions (high heat and time), while the double bond will move towards the less substituted carbon in kinetic conditions (low heat and time). Since shifting towards the end of the carbon chain moves the double bond towards a less substituted carbon, this is a kinetic reaction condition, making choice D the best answer.

425. C is the best answer. In keto-enol tautomerization of diketones, an aprotic solvent is favored as a protic solvent will result in hydrogen bonding and pseudo-ring formation between the two ketone groups. Of these solvents, methanol is the only protic solvent which would inhibit tautomerization, so choice C is the best answer.

426. B is the best answer. In hydrolysis, water is added as a reactant break apart another molecule. A catalyst is a compound that is not consumed by the reaction, but acts to facilitate the reaction and increase the rate. Since water is added to the reactant, it is not a catalyst and choice A can be eliminated. Choice B is a strong answer. Water is not produced by the reaction, so choice C can be eliminated. A spectator ion is an ion that appears on both sides of a reaction in an unchanged form. Since a water molecule is consumed, and it is not an ion, choice D can be eliminated.

427. D is the best answer. Hydrolysis is breaking a bond with the addition of water. In dipeptides and other longer amino acid chains, this occurs on a peptide bond. While acidic conditions would denature a protein, a dipeptide contains too few amino acids to be considered a protein. Choice A can be eliminated. Hydrolysis will break the peptide bond, resulting in two amino acid products. Choice B can be eliminated. Hydrolysis includes the addition of water, not water as a product. Choice C can be eliminated, and choice D is the best answer.

428. C is the best answer. Hydrolysis of proteins involves using water to cleave a peptide bond. This question is more-or-less asking to identify the peptide bond in the protein segment. A peptide bond is the biological term for an amide bond, which is formed when the amine on one amino acid acts as a nucleophile to attack the carbonyl of the carboxylic acid on another amino acid. The resulting bond is between a carbonyl carbon and nitrogen, labeled as bond 3. Choice C is the best answer.

429. **D is the best answer.** The reaction shown in the question stem is an example of saponification. The conversion of fatty acids to soaps is achieved vial ester hydrolysis through the reaction with a strong base at high temperatures. Hydrogen peroxide (H_2O_2) will not react with fatty acids, so choice A can be eliminated. Acid-catalyzed hydrolysis of esters can occur, but the question stem asks about the production of stearate which is the conjugate base of stearic acid. This will not be produced in acidic conditions, so choice B can be eliminated. NADH is a reducing agent, so choice C can be eliminated. Sodium hydroxide will achieve ester hydrolysis and produce the desired conjugate base, so choice D is the best answer.

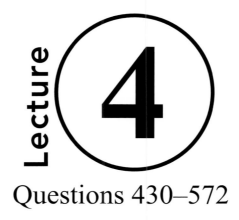

Lecture

(4)

Questions 430–572

Thermodynamics and Kinetics

ANSWERS & EXPLANATIONS

ANSWER KEY										
430. D	443. C	456. A	469. A	482. B	495. D	508. B	521. B	534. C	547. D	560. D
431. A	444. B	457. B	470. A	483. C	496. A	509. A	522. C	535. D	548. B	561. D
432. C	445. D	458. A	471. D	484. B	497. B	510. A	523. C	536. D	549. D	562. B
433. D	446. B	459. A	472. C	485. B	498. D	511. C	524. C	537. B	550. A	563. D
434. A	447. B	460. A	473. C	486. B	499. A	512. B	525. B	538. D	551. D	564. C
435. B	448. B	461. B	474. B	487. A	500. C	513. A	526. C	539. C	552. C	565. A
436. C	449. C	462. C	475. A	488. C	501. D	514. B	527. C	540. D	553. D	566. B
437. C	450. D	463. A	476. C	489. B	502. C	515. D	528. A	541. B	554. C	567. B
438. D	451. B	464. A	477. C	490. D	503. B	516. C	529. D	542. B	555. C	568. A
439. D	452. A	465. B	478. D	491. C	504. A	517. C	530. A	543. A	556. C	569. B
440. C	453. D	466. D	479. C	492. C	505. D	518. C	531. C	544. C	557. C	570. A
441. C	454. D	467. C	480. D	493. C	506. B	519. B	532. B	545. B	558. A	571. A
442. B	455. B	468. B	481. B	494. A	507. A	520. C	533. B	546. D	559. A	572. B

Physical Properties of Systems and Surroundings

430. D is the best answer. By definition, neither matter nor energy can be exchanged between an isolated system and its surroundings, so choice D is the best answer.

431. A is the best answer. By definition, only energy can be exchanged between a closed system and its surroundings, so choice A is the best answer.

432. C is the best answer. By definition, both matter and energy can be exchanged between an open system and its surroundings, so choice C is the best answer.

433. D is the best answer. First note that 46°C does not correspond to a doubled absolute temperature. This is because the Celsius scale does not have its absolute zero at zero°C. In order to double absolute temperature, °C (an interval scale) must first be converted to Kelvin (a ratio scale). K = °C + 273. A starting temperature of 23 °C equates to 296 K. Doubling 296 K results in 592 K. Choice D is the best answer.

434. A is the best answer. The Boltzmann constant can be calculated by dividing the gas constant, R, by Avogadro's constant: $k = \dfrac{R}{N_A}$. It has the units of $\dfrac{J}{K}$. This allows the energy of a gas, in J, to be related to the changes in temperature, making choices A and B better answer choices than choices C and D. The kinetic energy, not the potential energy, of a gas is related to temperature. Choice A is the best answer.

435. B is the best answer. The kinetic energy of a gas at a given temperature is related by the equation $KE = \dfrac{1}{2}kT$, where k is the Boltzmann constant and T is the temperature of a gas in Kelvin. Notice that number of moles of gas is not relevant to the problem, as it is not a variable in the equation. Rearranging the equation, Boltzmann's constant can be solved for by $k = \dfrac{2\,(KE)}{T}$. This gives a value close to 1.4×10^{-23} J/K. Choice A results from failing to multiply by two. Choice B most closely matches the calculated answer and is the best answer. Choice C results from using 1.7 instead of 2 and not multiplying by the kinetic energy. Choice D results from not multiplying by the kinetic energy.

436. C is the best answer. Boltzmann's constant relates the changes in the energy of a gas to the change in temperature of a gas. It has the units of J/K. The internal energy of a gas is described by the rotational and translational kinetic energy of a gas. Correlating these values with either an increase or decrease in temperature would allow for the quantification of Boltzmann's constant. Options I and II are components of the best answer. The heat released from or absorbed by a gas does not describe the internal energy of a gas, eliminating option III from the best answer. Choice C that contains options I and II is the best answer.

Chemical Kinetics

437. C is the best answer. Write the balanced reaction: $C_2H_6O + 3O_2 \rightarrow 2CO_2 + 3H_2O$. Since carbon dioxide is produced at twice the rate at which ethanol is consumed, choice C is the best answer.

438. D is the best answer. The rate of a reaction depends on the temperature of the reaction, the availability of reactants including the surface area, and if a catalyst is present so options I, II and III should all be included. Choice D is the best answer. Do not confuse the rate with the rate constant. The rate constant is affected by temperature and by the presence of a catalyst only.

439. D is the best answer. Rate constants depend on temperature, so choice A can be eliminated. Catalysts often work by optimizing the mechanism of a reaction, so choice B can be eliminated. Furthermore, answer choices that use absolute terms like "never" are usually false. Rate laws are based on the fact that product formation is predictable under maintained conditions, so choice C can be eliminated. Collisions must have sufficient energy and the correct spatial orientation in order to create a reaction, so a large number of collisions do not result in product formation. Choice D is the best answer.

440. C is the best answer. Each answer choice starts with a molecular collision so that part can be ignored. For the second part of each answer, the energy of the collision is more important than the temperature. The reason the temperature changes a reaction rate is because temperature increases velocity of molecules and thus the energy of collisions. So, choices A and B can be eliminated. Between spatial orientation and duration of contact, the orientation is more important, so choice C is the best answer.

441. C is the best answer. The Arrhenius equation states that $k = Ze^{E_a/RT}$ which can be rearranged to eliminate the exponent to be $\ln k = \dfrac{E_a}{R}\left[\dfrac{1}{T}\right] + \ln Z$. This takes the form of a $y = mx + b$ plot, where the slope of the line is equal to $-E_a/R$. The slope of the line is -10 in the graph. This means that activation energy can be solved for by the equation $-10 = -E_a/R$. $E_a = 10R = 10 \times (8.314$ J/mol K$) = 83.14$ J. The activation energy cannot be negative, eliminating choice A. Choice B results from forgetting to multiply by the slope. Choice C best matches the calculated answer and is likely the best answer. Choice D results from determining that the slope is -100 rather than -10.

442. B is the best answer. Enzymes lower the activation energy of an equation, which is the distance from I to II. More specifically, they lower the peak that is marked as II. They have no effect on the overall ΔG of the reaction, which is the distance from I to III and could be modified by lowering I or III. So, choices A, C and D can be ruled out, and choice B is the best answer.

443. C is the best answer. Competitions between kinetic and thermodynamic reactions have predictable outcomes. Kinetic products tend to be less stable as they require less activation energy, while thermodynamic products tend to be more stable as they require higher activation energy. Choices A and B are not the best answer, as the kinetic reaction would not form the most stable product. Choices C is a strong answer, while choice D can be eliminated as thermodynamic reactions do not have lower activation energies.

444. B is the best answer. An enolate is formed when a ketone encounters basic conditions. Asymmetric ketones tend to form two different enolates. Low activation energy tends to favor kinetic products. Furthermore, low temperature conditions also encourage the formation of a kinetic product. As the question stem produces conditions that would favor a kinetic product, choice B is the best answer. It is possible to replace "most substituted enolate" with "the thermodynamic product" and "least substituted enolate" with the "kinetic product" within the question stem in order to address this question.

445. D is the best answer. The balanced reaction is $C_6H_{12}O_6 + 6O_2 \leftrightarrow 6CO_2 + 6H_2O$. So, the rate law should be sixth order with respect to oxygen, making choice D the best answer. This is true only of elementary reactions. Otherwise, the rate law must be experimentally determined.

446. B is the best answer. The reaction rate is equal to $k[A]^a[B]^b[C]^c$ for the equation $aA + bB + cC \rightarrow$ Products. This question is asking what the number in front of A is in the balanced equations which can be figured out from the data in the table. In real life, a, b, and c do not have to be integers but they will almost certainly be integers on the MCAT® for ease of calculation. Between row 2 and row 3, the rate changes by a factor of 12. The concentration of C changes by a factor of 3. If C was second order, the change in rate would be $3^2 = 9$ but this can be ruled out because the concentration of A also changed by a factor of 2, which means the rate would have to change by a factor of 18, which it did not. So, the only option is that A is second order, and C is first order, making a and c 2 and 1 respectively. For B, look at rows 2 and 4 in the table. Between those rows, the rate changed by a factor of 8. The concentration of A and B both doubled. Since A is second order, it changed the rate by a factor of $2^2 = 4$, and B must be first order to change the rate by the additional $2^1 = 2$. This means the balanced equation is $2A + 1B + 1C \rightarrow$ Products. This means that if 1 mole of each B and C are added, 2 moles of A will be needed for the reaction to go to completion, making choice B is the best answer. Choice A is a trick. To solve these problems, do not simply read a row from the table.

447. B is the best answer. Remember, rate laws cannot be determined from the balanced equation unless the reaction is known to take place in a single step. For this reaction, use the table provided. When the concentration is doubled, the rate quadruples. Since four is two squared, this suggests the rate law is second order, which makes choice B the best answer.

448. B is the best answer. Comparing the first two lines, doubling the hydrogen concentration doubles the rate. Since $2^1 = 2$, the reaction is first order to hydrogen. Comparing line 2 to line 4, tripling the NO concentration increases the rate by about nine times. Since $3^2 = 9$, the reaction is second order to NO, so choice B is the best answer.

449. C is the best answer. All reactions proceed more rapidly toward equilibrium at higher temperatures regardless of whether they are exothermic or endothermic, so choices A and B can be eliminated. Temperature increases the velocity and thus frequency and energy of collisions, so choice C is a strong answer. If endothermic, a reaction will favor the products at higher temperature whereas if exothermic, a reaction will favor the reactants at higher temperature. So, the equilibrium constant is only greater at higher temperatures for endothermic reactions. Since choice D is not universally true, it can be eliminated.

450. D is the best answer. All reactions increase in rate when the temperature is increased, which means choices A and B can be eliminated. Choice C would imply that rate and temperature are directly proportional. The Arrhenius equation reveals this is not the case, so choice C can be eliminated, and choice D is the best answer.

451. B is the best answer. Recall that for gases, partial pressures can be used as a concentration term because $PV = nRT$. This is just a plug and chug problem. Use the equation:

$$\log[A]t = -kt/2.303 + \log[A]0.$$
$$\log[A]0 = \log[100] = 2$$
$$-kt/2.303 = -5 \times 10^{-5} \times 46,000/2.3 = -1$$

Thus $\log[A]t = 1$ or $[A]t = 10$.

452. A is the best answer. The rate constant for a given reaction varies with temperature, so option I is a strong answer. A reaction rate depends on the concentration of products and reactants but this question asked for the rate constant, so options II and III can be eliminated. This makes choice A the best answer.

453. D is the best answer. The most common way to determine the rate law is via option I, so choices B and C can be eliminated. This information could also be displayed in a graph, so option II is a strong answer. Knowing the mechanism of a reaction is another less common method but is often utilized in organic chemistry, so option III should be included, and choice D is the best answer.

454. D is the best answer. Choice A would describe a reaction with Rate = $k[A][B]^2$ so this is not the best answer. Choice B would describe a reaction with Rate = $k[A]^2[B]$ so this is not the best answer. Choice C is a bit vague but is probably saying the same thing as choice A and can be eliminated for the same reason. Any single step reaction has a rate law in which the powers are the number of molecules of a given type which collide. Half of a molecule cannot collide, so there is no way this reaction takes place in a single step, and choice D is the best answer.

455. B is the best answer. Reactants appear on the left side of reactions, so choice A can be eliminated. Iodide appears only on the right of the reaction, so it is a product and choice B is a strong answer. Intermediates are unstable molecule, between the reactants and products, so choice C can be eliminated. Catalysts facilitate reactions and are not consumed or produced by the reaction, so choice D can be eliminated.

456. A is the best answer. More than one mechanism can generate the same rate law, so scientist A cannot be sure his or her mechanism is correct based on just the experimental rate law. So, choices B and C can be eliminated. However, if the mechanism is correct then the experimental rate law must also be correct because a mechanism only produces one possible rate law. Choice A is the best answer, and choice D can be eliminated.

457. B is the best answer. To determine reaction order, add the exponents. $1 + 2 = 3$, so choice B is the best answer.

458. A is the best answer. Just use the exponent on [A] because that is all the question asks. So choice A is the best answer.

459. A is the best answer. Reagents that do not affect the rate are said to be of order 0 so choice A is the best answer. Consider also that $[B]^0 = 1$, so 0 is also the exponent used for B is the reaction.

460. A is the best answer. Add the two reactions and cancel $NOBr_2$ since it appears on both sides. So, the overall reaction should be the one without $NOBr_2$. On this basis, choices C and D can be eliminated. Choice B can be eliminated because neither equation includes $Br(g)$. So, choice A is the best answer.

461. B is the best answer. The slow step is the rate determining step of a reaction. According to the reactions, step 2 is the slow step and thus the rate determining step. So, choices A and C can be eliminated. A reaction proceeds at the rate of the rate determining step, so choice B is the best answer. Choice D would only be true if both reactions were slow.

462. C is the best answer. Choice A can be eliminated because a rate law with reactants at zero concentration would be zero. Choice B can be eliminated because step 1 will not run to completion until step 2 begins. Step 2 will remove product from step 1 and drive step 1 forward via Le Châtelier's principle. Whenever the fast step precedes the slow step, the fast step is assumed to reach equilibrium and the equilibrium concentrations are used for the rate law of the slow step, so choice C is a strong answer. Choice D can be eliminated because step 1 being the fast step allows for the prediction of the rate law for step 2. If step 1 were the slow step, choice D would be a strong answer.

463. A is the best answer. Catalysts are consumed and then regenerated. The bromine consumed in step 1 is regenerated in step 2 so choice A is the best answer. H_2O_2 is a reactant in both steps so choice B can be eliminated. H^+ is a product in step 1 and a reactant in step 2, so it is the opposite of a catalyst, and choice C can be eliminated. O_2 is a product in step 2, so choice D can be eliminated.

464. A is the best answer. A catalyst increases the rate by lowering the energy of activation. Option I is part of the best answer, while option II can be eliminated. A catalyst cannot change the equilibrium position, only the kinetics of the reaction. Option III can be eliminated. Choice A contains only option I and is the best answer.

465. B is the best answer. A catalyst changes the pathway of a reaction. From the Arrhenius equation, $k = Ae - E_a/RT$, the rate constant depends upon the activation energy E_a. A catalyst lowers the activation energy, and thus changes the rate constant and rate, so options I and II are components of the best answer. Option III can be eliminated because a catalyst has no effect on the equilibrium of a reaction, just the rate at which it arrives at equilibrium.

466. D is the best answer. Catalysts do not change overall kinetic energy, so choices A, B and C can be eliminated. A catalyst changes the energy of activation, so choice D is the best answer.

467. C is the best answer. An enzyme cannot change any of the thermodynamic properties of a reaction, only the kinetic properties. The free energy of the reactants and products is not changed by the addition of an enzyme catalyst. Choices A and B can be eliminated. Enzymes help reactions to occur by lowering the activation energy of the reaction, $\Delta G\ddagger$. Choice C is likely the best answer. The overall free energy change of a reaction is also not affected by the addition of a catalyst. Choice D can be eliminated.

468. B is the best answer. Catalysts do not change the stability of a certain set of products, but they are actively involved with reactions (because they change the transition state). So, choice A can be eliminated on the basis of incorrectly defining a catalyst. Choice B is a reasonable answer because it provides an explanation to the question. Choice C can be eliminated because although manganese dioxide results in different product formation, it could be a catalyst in a second reaction. Choice C can be eliminated. Similarly, choice D can be eliminated because affecting the reverse reaction would have nothing to do with a second reaction forming new products. Although catalysts do lower the activation energy of reverse reactions, the fact that the reverse reaction involved oxygen gas would result in very little product being formed. Choice D can be eliminated, and choice B is the best answer.

State and Path Functions: Internal Energy, Heat, and Work

469. A is the best answer. Work and heat relate to the change in energy of a system when it goes from one state to another. They thus depend on how a system changes between states and are not themselves state functions, so options II and III cannot be part of the best answer. Temperature is a state function, so choice A is the best answer.

470. A is the best answer. When the enthalpy of a system goes down, the enthalpy of the environment generally goes up. By increasing enthalpy, the energy and entropy of the surroundings also increase, so choice A is the best answer.

471. D is the best answer. State functions do not directly relate to conservation of energy so choices A and B can be eliminated. Pressure, volume and temperature are state function but there are others, so the Helmholtz function may depend on other variables, and choice C can be eliminated. A state function is defined as an equation that does not depend on the path taken by a system to a state. They depend only on the final state. So, choice D is the best answer.

472. C is the best answer. The exchange of temperature between two objects in direct contact is mediated by the zeroth law of thermodynamics. Over time, the temperature of both objects will become equal. The new temperature reached is generally in between the original temperatures of the objects. On the MCAT®, answers leaning to one "extreme" tend to not be the best answer. Since Choices A and B both state the temperature would "directly match the original" they are not likely to be the best answer. Choice C is a strong answer as it best describes the conditions defined by the zeroth law. Choice D can be eliminated as this is not a likely occurrence.

473. C is the best answer. Choice A is the first law. Choice C is the zeroth law. Choices B and D are the second and third law respectively. Do not confuse these with Newton's laws, which are similar.

474. B is the best answer. The Zeroth Law of Thermodynamics states that if two thermodynamic systems are each in thermal equilibrium with a third, then they are in thermal equilibrium with each other. Chamber 2 is in thermal equilibrium with both chambers one and three, because no net heat exchange occurs between the chambers. Heat flows whenever there are temperature differences. If no heat exchange is occurring, the temperature must be equal. This eliminates all answer choices but choice B, meaning the temperature of chamber two will also be 52 K. Choice B is the best answer.

475. A is the best answer. Air and vacuum are the best insulators so choice A is a strong answer. Storm windows and thermoses utilize this phenomenon. Choice B can be eliminated because the air in the hollow walls cannot spontaneously generate heat. Choice C can be eliminated because the walls do not need to be hollow to trap air so this does not answer the question. Choice D can be eliminated for the same reason as choice B—there is no reason to believe the air between the walls is undergoing any reaction.

476. C is the best answer. The question is a restatement of the Zeroth Law of Thermodynamics: no object can reach absolute zero. If it did, it could no longer radiate heat. If choice A were true, objects would all eventually reach absolute zero, so choice A can be eliminated. Heat can be transferred by conduction, convection or radiation so choice B is not entirely true and can be eliminated. Choice C restates the Zeroth Law, so it is a strong answer. Choice D can be eliminated because the question is referring to the Zeroth Law. The First Law is the law of conservation of energy, which does apply to radiation, so choice D is not the best answer.

477. C is the best answer. Conduction is due to molecular collisions. When molecules are far apart, there are fewer collisions and there is greater resistance to conduction. The molecules are farthest apart in a gas so choice C is the best answer.

478. D is the best answer. Like fluid flow or electric current, the rate of heat flow through a slab is constant and independent of slab thickness. So, choice D is the best answer.

479. C is the best answer. From the formula, the temperature difference is directly proportional to the length and inversely proportional to the cross-sectional area. This means that the temperature difference is proportional to the ratio L/A. The passage says that the cross-sections of the slabs are square, so to find the cross-sectional area of a slab, square its height. The ratio L/A for slabs 2, 3, and 4 respectively are: $\frac{1}{6}$, $\frac{1}{2}$, and 1. Slab 4 has the greatest ratio, and thus the greatest temperature difference. So, choice C is the best answer.

480. **D is the best answer.** From the formula, k is proportional to L/A. So, the slab with the greatest L/A ratio has the greatest k. The L/A ratios for slabs 2, 3, 4, and 5 respectively are $\frac{1}{6}$, $\frac{1}{2}$, 1, and 2. Slab 5 must have the greatest k, and choice D is the best answer.

481. **B is the best answer.** The formula for linear expansion is: $\Delta L = \alpha L_0 \Delta T$. The change in length can be calculated from the numbers provided in the question stem and the change in temperature.

$$\Delta L = (17 \times 10^{-6} °C^{-1})(0.5\ m)(17°C) = 1.4 \times 10^{-4}\ m$$

Choice A results from forgetting to multiply by the change in temperature. Choice B most matches the calculated answer and is the best answer. Choice C results from forgetting to multiply by the linear coefficient of expansion. Choice D results from forgetting to multiply by both the linear coefficient of expansion and the original length of the stainless steel instrument.

482. **B is the best answer.** In general, molecules increase in size following a temperature increase due to greater bond vibration resulting from the increased kinetic energy. The coefficient of thermal expansion quantifies the relationship between the increase in temperature and size. Expansion along three dimensions is quantified as the coefficient of volumetric thermal expansion, β. β can be utilized in the following equation: $\Delta V/V = \beta \Delta T$, where V = initial volume and T = temperature. Note that the question stem indicates cubic expansion; volume can be calculated simply by multiplying all three dimensions together. For simplicity, round each value in the table to the nearest whole number.

$V_0 = (2. \times 10^{-9})(4 \times 10^{-9})(5 \times 10^{-9}) = 40 \times 10^{-27} = 4 \times 10^{-26}$.

$V_{final} = (3 \times 10^{-9})(4 \times 10^{-9})(1 \times 10^{-8}) = 12 \times 10^{-26}$.

Solving the left side of the equation:

$(12 \times 10^{-26} - 4 \times 10^{-26})/(4 \times 10^{-26}) = 2. \ 2/(30^{-25}) = \frac{2}{5} = 0.40$.

Choice B is the best answer.

483. **C is the best answer.** Since the gas is kept at constant pressure, calculate work with $P\Delta V$. The volume of the gas is decreased, so work is done on the gas, so choices A and B can automatically be eliminated. Count the squares beneath the function because this gives the change in pressure-volume. There are 16 squares and each square having sides of 50 Pa and 0.5 m³ is 25 joules. $16 \times 25 = 400$, so choice C is the best answer.

484. **B is the best answer.** There is no volume change, so no work is done, and choice B is the best answer.

485. **B is the best answer.** The volume is increased, so work is done on the surroundings meaning negative work done on the gas. So, choice D can automatically be eliminated. The squares beneath the path represent the work done. There are 24 squares. Each square is worth 25 J. $24 \times 25 = 600$ J, so choice B is the best answer.

486. **B is the best answer.** From A to C work on the gas is negative because the gas is expanding. From C to D no work is done. From D to A work on the gas is positive because the gas is being compressed. Count the squares inside the loop to find the work done. There are 38 squares times 25 J/square equals 950 J. The upper path represents more work and is negative so the net work is negative, and choice B is the best answer.

487. **A is the best answer.** Work done *by* a gas is just the negative of the work done on the gas so choice A is the best answer. Choice B can be eliminated because work was done by the gas. Choices C and D are based on adding or subtracting the heat exchanged. The heat exchanged is not a factor in the calculation for work, only for energy, so choices C and D can be eliminated.

488. **C is the best answer.** Use the First Law of thermodynamics. One way of writing it is $q_{in} + w_{on} = \Delta E$. So, $55 - 23 = 32$ J, and choice C is the best answer. Choice A is the work done by the gas but does not account for the heat, so choice A can be eliminated. Choice B has no mathematical basis and can be eliminated. Choice D results from using the incorrect sign for the heat.

489. **B is the best answer.** The first law is a statement of conservation of energy. Option I is a typical example of the conservation of energy, with kinetic and potential interchanging indefinitely. So option I is not a violation and should not be included in the best answer, which eliminates choices A, C and D. Option II violates the first law because a battery transfers energy to whatever circuit it is connected to, which means it should eventually die. So, option II is a component of the best answer. Option III violates the second law of thermodynamics but not the first, so it should not be included in the best answer.

490. **D is the best answer.** The gas does work on the surroundings, lowering its energy and thus its temperature so option I is a component of the best answer. Based on the formula, $K.E. = \frac{3}{2}RT$. So, option II is a component of the best answer. As for option III, a force is exerted on the piston over the distance through which is moves based on the formula $W = Fd$. So option III should be included, and choice D is the best answer.

491. **C is the best answer.** Since the cylinder is held at constant volume, there is not work done and choice A can be eliminated. If volume was not held constant, the gas would expand when heat is added. However, the question states this does not occur, so choice B can be eliminated. Heat added to a gas would be utilized as kinetic energy since work cannot be done by the constant volume system. Kinetic energy is proportional to temperature and pressure so both would increase as well, and choice C is a strong answer. Since pressure is energy per unit volume, increasing the energy of the gas will increase the pressure, so choice D can be eliminated.

492. C is the best answer. According to the ideal gas law, if the volume increases and the pressure is constant, the temperature must increase. If temperature increases, not all the energy is doing work, so choice A can be eliminated. Likewise, since the gas is expanding, work is being done so not all the energy is used to raise the temperature of the gas, so choice B can be eliminated. Choice C combines choices A and B and is a strong answer. Choice D can be eliminated because the cylinder can be heated at constant pressure as long as volume can change.

Enthalpy and Entropy

493. C is the best answer. Heat, q, is related to enthalpy, H, but is not equivalent to enthalpy, so choice A can be eliminated. Enthalpy is defined exactly as $U + PV$, so choices B and D can be eliminated, and choice C is the best answer.

494. A is the best answer. Enthalpy change is an extensive property, so when the coefficients triple, so does the enthalpy change. Admittedly, the kJ/mol notation used in such cases is a bit confusing, but it really means kJ per number of moles shown in the equation. So, choice A is the best answer. Choices B and D result from not taking into account the coefficients. Choice C results from dividing by instead of multiplying by the coefficient.

495. D is the best answer. Since this is just the reverse of the given reaction, just change the sign of the enthalpy. So choice D is the best answer.

496. A is the best answer. Bond energies are generally defined in terms of the energy required to break a bond. The energy required to form a bond is thus the negative of the bond energy. Calculate heats of reaction by products – reactants: $2\,[(2(-464)] - [(2(-436)) + (-496)] = -488$ kJ/mol. So, choice A is the best answer.

497. B is the best answer. Reverse the reaction of the formation of NaCl from its gaseous ions and change the sign of its enthalpy change. Then add this to the reaction for the heat of hydration.

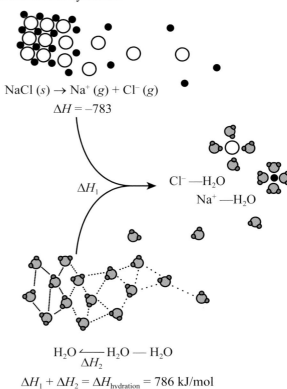

$NaCl\,(s) \rightarrow Na^+\,(g) + Cl^-\,(g)$
$\Delta H = -783$

ΔH_1

$Cl^- - H_2O$
$Na^+ - H_2O$

$H_2O \xleftarrow{\Delta H_2} H_2O - H_2O$

$\Delta H_1 + \Delta H_2 = \Delta H_{hydration} = 786$ kJ/mol

$H_2O\,\Delta H_1 \Delta H_1 + \Delta H_2 = \Delta H_{hydration} = 786$ kJ/mol $- 783$ kJ/mol $+ 786$ kJ/mol $= 3$ kJ/mol, so choice B is the best answer.

498. D is the best answer. The heat of hydration is the sum of the endothermic breaking of the hydrogen bonds of between water molecules and the exothermic formation of the bonds between water molecules and ions. Since the heat of hydration is negative, the energy released by the formation of water-ion bonds must have a greater magnitude than the energy absorbed by the breaking of hydrogen bonds. So, choice D is a strong answer, and choices A and B can be eliminated. Choice C can be eliminated because water-ion bonds are not true ionic bonds.

499. A is the best answer. Bond strengths are not all that different from each other; they differ by maybe a factor of 2. However, the question asks about the amount of heat per gram so the species that is the lightest will give off the most heat. Hydrogen is much lighter than the others, so choice A is the best answer. This is part of the reason that fuel cells, which use hydrogen, are thought of as a possible future source of energy for automobiles.

500. C is the best answer. The energy contained in the covalent bonds of a molecule likely relate to the heats of formation of the particular bonds. The heat of formation of taxane can be determined by measuring the energy put into the reaction, when the bonds are broken, and the energy that comes out of a reaction, when the new bonds are formed. A scientist would likely measure both in order to determine the heat of formation. Options I and II are likely components of the best answer. Changes in entropy of the reactants do not provide information about the heats of formation, eliminating option III. Choice C is the best answer because it includes only options I and II.

501. D is the best answer. Heat of formation requires measurements of the thermal properties of a compound, allowing choices B and C to be eliminated. A bomb calorimeter cannot be used to measure the properties of a non-flammable compound, while choice D can measure any reaction that can be contained in an insulated vessel.

502. C is the best answer. The bond dissociation energy is the energy that must be put into a reaction in order to break the bonds within the reactants. The heats of formation also describe the energy contained in the bonds within the reactants, making the bond dissociation energy equal to the heat of formation. As the bond dissociation energy equals the heat of formation of the reactants, choices A, B, and D can be eliminated, and choice C is the best answer.

503. B is the best answer. The heat of formation of $O_2(g)$ is zero, because oxygen is most stable under standard conditions in the diatomic form so choice A can be eliminated. Choice B corresponds to the reaction:

$$1/2 O_2(g) \rightarrow O(g)$$

Doubling this does indeed give the energy needed to break an oxygen-oxygen double bond, so this is a strong answer. Choice C can be eliminated because there are no oxygen-oxygen double bonds present in CO_2. Choice D is also not the best answer because double bonds do not, in general, have twice the energy of single bonds.

504. A is the best answer. Nucleotides found in their triphosphate form, such as ATP and GTP, have three phosphates on them. The terminal phosphate that is typically cleaved is the γ phosphate. The β phosphate is the middle phosphate of the three, while the α phosphate is the one attached to the nucleotide. Choices A and B are more likely than choices C and D to be the best answer. When a phosphate is released, energy is also released. This is one of the main driving principles behind many biological reactions. A reaction where energy is released is an exothermic reaction, not an endothermic reaction. Choice A is a better answer choice than choice B.

505. D is the best answer. If the scientist must cool the solution as dextrose is dissolved, this suggests that the solution gives off heat during the process. This would make the reaction exothermic, making option I a component of the best answer. An endergonic reaction is a reaction that has a positive ΔG. If a reaction is exothermic, this likely implies that the ΔG would be negative, likely making option III part of the best answer and eliminating option II. In general, a solution increases entropy, as compounds break apart into ions. If the ΔH is negative and ΔS is positive, the ΔG must be negative by the following equation: $\Delta G = \Delta H - T\Delta S$. Choice D, which has both options I and III, is likely the best answer.

506. B is the best answer. Deal with entropy, ΔS, first because it is the most straightforward. The reaction increases the number of molecules present which increases disorder, so entropy must increase and ΔS is positive. This rules out choice A. The reaction releases heat so enthalpy, ΔH, must be negative. This rules out choice C. The Gibbs free energy, ΔG, must also be negative because $\Delta G = \Delta H - T\Delta S$. If ΔH is negative, and ΔS is positive, then ΔG must be negative. Choice B is the best answer.

507. A is the best answer. Enthalpy can be described with the formula $\Delta H = \Delta U + P\Delta V$, so the best answer is choice A. Internal energy can be thought of as potential energy but choices B, C and D all incorrectly define the second variable. Experimentally, a coffee cup calorimeter is a constant pressure calorimeter and measures the heat of a reaction. A bomb calorimeter is a constant volume calorimeter and measures the change in internal energy of a reaction.

508. B is the best answer. Endothermic reactions require heat and thus they feel cold. This makes choice B the best answer. Work is defined by $W = P\Delta V$. Positive work arises when the change in volume is positive, which occurs in exothermic, not endothermic reactions. Choice A can be eliminated. Exothermic reactions are often more dangerous than endothermic reactions.

509. A is the best answer. Bond formation decreases the number of molecules present so entropy must decrease so choices B and D can be eliminated. Bond formation also requires enthalpy, which is associated with a negative sign, so choice A is the best answer, and choice C can be eliminated.

510. A is the best answer. By convention, a substance at 0 K has an entropy of zero, so choice A is the best answer. Choices B and C would have measurable (non zero) entropy so they can be eliminated. Entropy does depend on temperature, so choice D can be eliminated.

511. C is the best answer. The blocks became more ordered, so they decreased in entropy, so option I and choice D can be eliminated. By stacking the blocks, the man experienced an increase in entropy. The macromolecules in his body were combusted and released gas and water to increase entropy. So option II is a component of the best answer, and choice B can be eliminated. Universal entropy was increased because the man's increase in entropy while stacking the blocks was greater than the decrease of entropy experienced by the blocks, systems always tend toward disorder. So, option III should be included, and choice C is the best answer.

512. B is the best answer. The chemical bond energy of the nutrients within the man went into increasing the potential energy of the blocks and to energy lost as heat. The part that became the potential energy of the blocks retained or increased its potential to do work, but the part that became heat lost much of its potential. So, choice A can be eliminated and choice B is a strong answer. Choice C is not as strong as choice B because some of the chemical energy in the man retained ability to do work, so choice C be eliminated. Choice D is a distractor that is unrelated to the system in question and can be eliminated.

513. A is the best answer. Consider the white and black marbles as different entities. Two black marbles are the same thing and two white marbles are the same thing. Having two different marbles on each side is more disordered than having two of the same marbles on each side. So, choice A is a strong answer, and choice D can be eliminated. Having less than two marbles on one side decreases the disorder on that side, so choices B and C can be eliminated, and choice A is the best answer.

514. B is the best answer. Option I is a typical example of the conservation of energy, with kinetic and potential interchanging indefinitely. It does not violate the first or second law, so option I and choices A, C and D can be eliminated. The never dying battery disobeys the first law of thermodynamics because it would have to be creating energy to not die, so option II can be eliminated. The second law of thermodynamics is that entropy must increase in isolated systems. Entropy is the energy that cannot do work, since it must increase, there is no system in which all energy can be converted into work so option III violates the second law, and choice B is the best answer.

515. D is the best answer. The second law of thermodynamics is that entropy must always increase, so choices A and B can be eliminated. Choice C incorrectly pairs this notion with the first law, which is that energy can neither be created nor destroyed. So, choice D is the best answer.

516. C is the best answer. An aqueous solution has more entropy than a solution with precipitate only so in the reaction, entropy decreases. So, choices A and B can be eliminated. From the second law of thermodynamics, entropy must always increase, so choice D can be eliminated. This leaves choice C as the best answer.

517. C is the best answer. Gases have much higher entropy than other phases, so choice C is the best answer. Choice A has the least entropy. Choices B and C have an intermediate amount of entropy.

518. C is the best answer. Gases have the highest entropy, so the correct answer must have the gas sample listed last. Choices A and D can be eliminated. Solutions have higher entropy than pure phases of a similar type, since the species are mixed. So, choice C is the best answer.

519. B is the best answer. Entropy in relation to phase composition is as follows: gas > liquid > solid. Choices A and D can be eliminated. Larger, more complex molecules have greater entropy than smaller, less complex molecules because there are more electron orbitals to spread energy across. CH_4 is smaller than C_5H_{12}. Choice C can be eliminated in favor of choice B. Choice B is the best answer.

520. C is the best answer. Entropy generally follows the trend: gas > liquid > solid. Sublimation is a phase transition from solid to gas. This indicates an increase in entropy. Option I is true, and choice B can be eliminated. Condensation is a phase transition from gas to liquid. This indicates a decrease in entropy. Option II is not true, and choice D can be eliminated. Hydrocarbons and $O_2(g)$ combine to form $H_2O(g)$ and $CO_2(g)$ in combustion reactions. Because the products are always gases, combustion reactions generally result in an increase in energy. Option III is true, and choice A can be eliminated. Choice C is the best answer.

Accounting for Energy: Gibbs Free Energy and Hess's law

521. B is the best answer. In the formula, it is T, not ΔT, so the temperature must be constant, and choice C can be eliminated. Pressure and volume can both change to independently change ΔH and ΔS. So, choice B is the best answer.

522. C is the best answer. Gibbs free energy of the universe is decreased with each reaction, so it does not follow the conservation of energy law. This is because for a reaction to occur it must have a negative ΔG or it must be paired with a reaction that has a negative ΔG. So, the Gibbs free energy of the universe is always decreasing meaning energy is being lost. This eliminates option I and means option III must be a component of the best answer, so choice C should be selected.

523. C is the best answer. Free energies and entropies can be manipulated in the same way as enthalpies.

$$H_2(g) + \frac{1}{2}O_2(g) \rightarrow H_2O(g) \quad \Delta G° = -229 \text{ kJ/mol}$$

$$H_2(g) + \frac{1}{2}O_2(g) \rightarrow H_2O(l) \quad \Delta G° = -237 \text{ kJ/mol}$$

The desired reaction is:

$$H_2O(l) \rightarrow H_2O(g)$$

Reverse the second reaction and then adding the two reactions: −229 kJ/mol − (−237 kJ/mol) = +8 kJ/mol. So choice C is the best answer.

524. C is the best answer. The reaction with the most positive ΔG will be the least spontaneous. The nonpolar gases are the ones prior to formation of the gas in the table. So, the gas that will least spontaneously form will result have the greatest proportion of nonpolar gases in the container. So, choice C is the best answer.

525. B is the best answer. In order to be spontaneous at all temperatures, both terms on the right side of $\Delta G = \Delta H - T\Delta S$ must be negative meaning ΔH must be negative meaning the reaction is exothermic, and ΔS must be positive. So, choice B is the best answer.

526. C is the best answer. NaCl is typically soluble in water due to the large increase in entropy. The change in entropy occurs because one molecule of NaCl splits into Na^+ and Cl^- in water. A spontaneous reaction has a negative ΔG, which can be calculated from the formula $\Delta G = \Delta H - T\Delta S$. Choices A and B indicate that spontaneity depends upon enthalpy change only, making these weak answer choices. Because the overall ΔG depends on the temperature, choice C is likely the best answer. Although the change in enthalpy changes slightly with temperature, for MCAT®, assume that the change in enthalpy for a reaction remains constant with temperature change. Choice C is the best answer.

527. C is the best answer. Recall that T is in Kelvin so it will always be a nonzero positive number. If enthalpy and entropy change are negative, when entropy or temperature are very large, or enthalpy is very small, the Gibbs free energy will be positive, so choice A can be eliminated. When entropy and enthalpy are positive, if enthalpy is very large or entropy and temperature very small, the Gibbs free energy will be positive, so choice B can be eliminated. If enthalpy is negative and entropy is positive, then Gibbs energy change must be negative and the reaction must be spontaneous, so choice C is the best answer. When enthalpy is positive and entropy is negative, Gibbs free energy will always be positive, so choice D can be eliminated.

528. A is the best answer. Choices C and D can be immediately eliminated because pressure is not a variable in the formula. In the formula $\Delta G = \Delta H - T\Delta S$, when a reaction is exothermic, ΔH is negative. When entropy decreases, the second term, $T\Delta S$ is negative. ΔH needs to remain larger than $T\Delta S$ for ΔG to be negative. This occurs only at low temperature, so choice A is the best answer.

529. D is the best answer. Nonspontaneous reactions occur so choices A and B can be eliminated. Nonspontaneous reactions have a positive change in Gibbs free energy, so regardless of the temperature, they are still not spontaneous. Choice C can be eliminated. Nonspontaneous reactions can occur by coupling them to a more spontaneous reaction, so that the total free energy change is negative. So, choice D is the best answer.

530. A is the best answer. According to the second law of thermodynamics, the entropy gain of the universe must always be positive. The entropy of a system, however, can be negative, as long as the surroundings experience an increase in entropy that exceeds the negative entropy change experienced by the system, so choice A is a strong answer. Choice B does not make sense, being endothermic is independent of entropy change, so choice B can be eliminated. Choices C and D can be eliminated because reactions that decrease entropy of a system occur as long as the entropy of the environment increases reciprocally.

531. C is the best answer. Since the reaction forms a liquid from gases, the entropy of the system must decrease when the reaction is run. So, choice A can be eliminated. Presence of a catalyst is independent of the spontaneity of a reaction. Catalysts change the activation energy, also known as $\Delta G\ddagger$ but not the overall ΔG. So, choice B can be eliminated. Since entropy decreases, according to $\Delta G = \Delta H - T\Delta S$, such a reaction must be exothermic in order to be spontaneous, so choice C is a strong answer, and choice D can be eliminated.

532. B is the best answer. Choice A is a reasonable statement that does not answer the question. Endothermic reactions can be coupled to exothermic reactions but this does not relate to the scientists claim, so choice A can be eliminated. Catalysts have no effect on spontaneity, they only affect rate via decreasing the $\Delta G\ddagger$, which is not the same as the ΔG. So if an endothermic reaction is spontaneous with a catalyst, it is spontaneous without the catalyst. Choice B challenges the scientist's statement and is a strong answer. Choice C directly agrees with the scientist's statement, so it can be eliminated. Choice D neither supports nor refutes the scientist's statement, so it can be eliminated.

533. B is the best answer. An intermediate is a molecule that is created in one step of an overall reaction and used in a later step. NO(g) is the reactant in step 1, not a product of any of the steps. It cannot be an intermediate, eliminating choice A. Step 1 results in the formation of $N_2O_2(g)$, which is then used as a reactant in step 2. Because $N_2O_2(g)$ is created then used, it is an intermediate. Choice B is a strong answer. $O_2(g)$ is a reactant of step 2 and is not created then used. Choice C can be eliminated. $NO_2(g)$ is the product of step 2, not an intermediate. Choice D can be eliminated.

534. C is the best answer. Hess's Law of Heat Summation states that "The sum of the enthalpy changes for each step is equal to the total enthalpy change regardless of the path chosen." Reactions 1, 2, and 3 must be added in such a way that sums to the reaction indicated as the first step in the synthesis. First note that reaction 1 must be reversed in order for $CO(g)$ to be on the right side. $\Delta H_1 = 283$ kJ. Next note that reaction 2 must be reversed and multiplied by 3 in order for the correct number of $H_2(g)$ to appear on the right side. $\Delta H_2 = 726$ kJ. At this point, reaction 3 can remain as is in order to balance out the rest of the equation. $\Delta H_3 = -803$ kJ. Summing $\Delta H_1 + \Delta H_2 + \Delta H_3 = 283$ kJ + 726 kJ – 803 kJ = 206 kJ. Choice C is the best answer. Note that if one simply added $\Delta H_1 + \Delta H_2 + \Delta H_3$ without any rearrangements, choice A would be a promising answer. Also note that choice B could be obtained by reversing reaction 2 but keeping reactions 1 and 3 the same. This would equate to summing $\Delta H_1 - \Delta H_2 + \Delta H_3$. Further, note that reversing reaction 1 (283 kJ), reversing and multiplying reaction 2 by 3 (726 kJ), and dividing reaction 3 by 2 (401.5 kJ) would result in 608 kJ, or choice D.

535. D is the best answer. Hess's Law of Heat Summation states that "The sum of the enthalpy changes for each step is equal to the total enthalpy change regardless of the path chosen." Reactions 1, 2, and 3 must be added in such a way that sums to the reaction generates HCN from CH_4 and NH_3. First note that reaction 3 must be halved in order to obtain 1 mole of HCN. Halving reaction 3 also halves the change in enthalpy: $\Delta H_3 = 135$ kJ. Next note that reaction 2 must be reversed in order to put the CH_4 on the left side. $\Delta H_2 = \sim 75$ kJ. Next note that reaction 1 must be reversed in order to put NH_3 on the left side, and it must be halved in order to balance out the N_2. $\Delta H_1 = \sim 46$ kJ. Summing $\Delta H_1 + \Delta H_2 + \Delta H_3 = 135 + 75$ kJ + 46 kJ = 256 kJ, which is closest to choice D. Choice D is the best answer.

536. D is the best answer. The activated complex is also known as the transition state. It is the highest energy species in a reaction that is transiently formed by the breaking of bonds in the reactants and the forming of bonds in the products. The activated complex cannot have a free energy lower than any of the other compounds in a reaction, making choice D the best answer.

537. B is the best answer. The transition state of a reaction is often the highest energy state of a reaction, as this is the point in which all bonds are being broken and formed simultaneously. This makes choice B a better answer choice than choice A. The transition state is not an isolatable molecule, as it exists in a period of transition between the product and the reactant. Choices C and D can be eliminated.

538. D is the best answer. A reaction coordinate plots the progress of a reaction (x-axis) by its energy level (y-axis). The initial low point of the reaction coordinate is the reactants. The initial increase in energy is due to old bonds breaking and new bonds beginning to form. The change in energy of the reactants to the peak of the energy hill represents the activation energy, or the energy required for the reaction to fully proceed. The peak of the energy hill (point A) represents the fleeting moment exactly in-between old bond breakage and new bond formation, called the transition state. Choices B and C can be eliminated. At point B, the first reaction has been completed, and an intermediate has been formed. This intermediate will also undergo bond breakage and formation, eventually forming the final product at point D. Point C represents the highest point of this second reaction's energy hill, corresponding to another transition state. Choice A can be eliminated. Choice D is the best answer.

539. C is the best answer. The peaks of the energy hills (points A and C) correspond to transition states. The first labeled trough (point B) corresponds to the intermediate. The second labeled trough (point D) corresponds to the final product. The transition state is the exact moment wherein the old bonds are breaking and the new bonds are forming. The transition state only exists for a fleeting moment of time and therefore cannot be isolated. Choices B and D can be eliminated, as they include transition states. The intermediate is an actual compound that exists for a longer duration and can be isolated by lowering the temperature after its formation or via introduction of additional reagents. Choice A can be eliminated. The product is an actual compound that can also be isolated. Choice C is the best answer.

540. D is the best answer. An intermediate is a molecule that is made from reactants but is not yet the final product. The molecule shown is a transition state which only exists for fractions of a second. Intermediates exist for much longer, so choice D is better than choice A.

541. B is the best answer. Enzymes lower the activation energy by stabilizing the transition state, thus decreasing the energy of the transition state. The transition state is the same, just stabilized, so choice A is not the best answer. Choice C is also a feature of enzymes, but it is unrelated to the lowering of activation energy. Choice D is the opposite of what an enzyme does, eliminating it as a possible answer.

542. B is the best answer. The transition state is the high energy molecule that exists transiently between the reactants and products. On this curve, it will be the highest energy point, so choice B is the best answer.

543. A is the best answer. The energy of activation is measured from the energy of the reactants to the energy of the activated complex so choice A is the best answer. E_2 is the overall change in Gibbs free energy for the reaction so choice B can be eliminated. $E_1 + E_2$ is the activation energy for the reverse reaction, so choice C can be eliminated. $E_2 - E_1$ is not an value that represents any specific energy change for the reaction, so choice D can be eliminated.

544. C is the best answer. The energy of activation is measured from the energy of the reactants to the energy of the activated complex, so choice A is the activation energy for the forward reaction. E_2 is the overall change in Gibbs free energy for the reaction, so choice B can be eliminated. $E_1 + E_2$ is the activation energy for the reverse reaction, so choice C is a strong answer. $E_2 - E_1$ is not a value that represents any specific energy change for the reaction, so choice D can be eliminated.

545. B is the best answer. The energy to begin the reaction is E_1, which is positive, so choices C and D can be eliminated. The energy of the overall reaction is E_2 which is negative, so choice B is the best answer.

546. D is the best answer. Use the following diagram to answer the question.

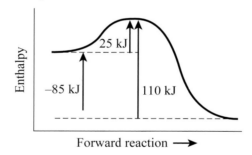

The energy values given in the problem are indicated in the appropriate places on the diagram. Examining the diagram, the activation energy of the reverse reaction is equal to the sum of the negative of the heat of reaction of the forward reaction and the activation energy of the forward reaction. So, 25 − (−85) = 110 kJ/mol, and choice D is the best answer.

Equilibrium

547. D is the best answer. All the coefficients of the reaction have been doubled. That means the powers in the equilibrium expression have been doubled, from 1 to 2. But that means all the concentrations have been squared, so the equilibrium constant must have been squared. $530^2 \approx 500^2 \approx 25{,}000 \approx 2.81 \times 10^5$, so choice D is the best answer.

548. B is the best answer. Compute the value of the equilibrium expression under these conditions is given by $[HI]^2/[H_2][I_2]$. This is $(5^2)/(0.2)(0.3)$ or about 350. Since the equilibrium constant is 50, at equilibrium there would be fewer products, and the hydrogen iodide concentration must therefore decrease to reach equilibrium, which eliminates choice A and makes choice B a strong answer. The system is not at equilibrium because the concentration of hydrogen iodide is presently too high but that does not mean there is an error in measuring the concentration, so choices C and D can be eliminated.

549. D is the best answer. Gases can be written either as concentrations or as partial pressures in equilibrium expressions, so choices A and B can be eliminated. Although both are appropriate, different values will result, so choice C can be eliminated, and choice D is the best answer.

550. A is the best answer. The formula relating the ΔG and the K_{eq} is $\Delta G = -RT\ln K_{eq}$. If the ΔG is negative, this means that all the values in the equation must be positive. Choices C and D can be eliminated. A reaction that has a negative ΔG is considered exergonic, meaning energy is released during a reaction. Most reactions favor the lowest thermodynamic energy state of the products, making choice A a better answer choice than choice B.

551. D is the best answer. The relationship between K_{eq} and ΔG is best described by the formula $\Delta G = -RT\ln K_{eq}$. A negative free energy change means a reaction is spontaneous and favors the products. In the lungs, CO_2 is released, so the more negative the ΔG, the more CO_2 would be released. As seen in the equation, the larger the K_{eq}, the more negative the ΔG becomes. Choice D is the best answer, as it has the largest K_{eq}. Remember that as the negative exponent becomes smaller, the closer the value is to zero and the larger the value.

552. C is the best answer. The equilibrium constant (K) is a value based on the concentrations of products and reactants at equilibrium. The concentrations listed in the table are at equilibrium because it is noted that the concentrations have stopped changing. $K = [NO]^4/[N_2O]_2[O_2] = (1 \times 10^5)^4/(2 \times 10^{-2})^{-2}(5 \times 10^1) = 5 \times 10^{21}$. Choice A can be eliminated. The reaction has reached equilibrium, as the concentrations of reactants and products have plateaued. Choice B can be eliminated. While K is an expression of the concentrations of reactants and products at equilibrium, Q is an expression of these concentrations at any given moment in time. Q is calculated the same way at K. When Q is less than K, it indicates that more product must be formed from reactants in order to reach equilibrium. $3.67 \times 10^{19}(Q)$ is less than $5 \times 10^{21}(K)$. N_2O (g) (a reactant) is expressed to decrease in concentration. Choice C is a strong answer. $2.13 \times 10^{22}(Q)$ is greater than $5 \times 10^{21}(K)$. When Q is greater than K, the concentration of products is expected to reduce as more reactants are made. $NO(g)$ is expected to decrease, not increase. Choice D is can be eliminated. Choice C is the best answer.

553. D is the best answer. Systemic errors are experimental errors that affect the accuracy of results. If the instrument reads 2.5×10^{-1} M when it should read zero, it is likely that every value has 2.5×10^{-1} M added to it. Although the results will remain somewhat questionable, the researchers would need to subtract 2.5×10^{-1} M from every value, and it is likely that the results will remain valid. Choice A is a weak answer. Although the researchers' only conducted the experiment once, the results will still remain valid as long as all errors were accounted for. Additional experiments would improve the validity. Choice B can be eliminated. Miscalculating the size of the reaction vessel represents another systemic error. After correcting for the size, molarity (mol L^{-1}) could be recalculated and concentration values can be fixed. Choice C can be eliminated. The equilibrium constant K is highly dependent on the temperature of the reaction. Without a known temperature, any ascertained values for K are meaningless. Choice A can be eliminated in favor of choice D. Choice D is the best answer.

554. C is the best answer. Choice A begins with a true statement, the reaction with a faster rate will deplete reactants faster however, if both reactions rely on the same reactant, this will slow both reactions. Reactions rates can vary depending on temperature, so choice B is a true statement but it is not clearly applicable to the scientists claim so there is probably a better answer. One major issue with the statement is that it ignores the role of reverse reactions. If the quick reaction also has a quick reverse reaction, the slower reaction may eventually dominate. Choice C is the best answer so far. Choice D can be eliminated because it is inaccurate—reactions are often in competition.

555. C is the best answer. As the concentration of reactants decreases, there are less collisions occurring but they still occur, so choice A can be eliminated. The dissociation of acetic acid does occur through an acid base reaction with ammonia; however, this will not stop the reaction, so choice B can be eliminated. Choice C defines an equilibrium state where forward and reverse reactions are occurring at the same rate, so this is a strong answer. Choice D can be eliminated because by definition, catalysts are not "used up" in reactions.

556. C is the best answer. The concentration of A and C are decreasing while B is increasing. So, A and C must be reactants and B must be the product. This eliminates choices A and B. The concentration of H_2 should be greater than that of N_2 because 3 moles of H_2 are needed for every mole of N_2. So, A should be H_2 and C should be N_2. This makes choice C the best answer.

557. C is the best answer. The reactants, A and C have not been used up because their concentration is not zero, so choice A can be eliminated. By definition, catalysts cannot be used up, so choice B can be eliminated. In the shaded area, the concentration of the reactants and products is no longer changing which is a feature of equilibrium, so choice C is a strong answer. The concentrations of the reactants and products have stopped changing, but no reactant has been used up, so the reaction has reached equilibrium, has no limiting reagent, and will not run to completion.

558. A is the best answer. Deal with each answer one by one. Choice A is a strong answer because it displays the reverse reaction where NH_3 forms H_2 and N_2. The H_2 is appropriately a higher concentration than the N_2. For choice B, the N_2 concentration is inappropriately higher than the H_2 concentration. Since 2 moles of NH_3 produce 1 mole of N_2 and 3 moles of H_2, the H_2 should be a higher concentration, so choice B can be eliminated. Choice C can be eliminated for a similar reason. Choice C depicts the forward reaction but incorrectly proportions the decline in concentration of H_2 and N_2. H_2 should fall at a faster rate since 3 are used for every 1 N_2, so choice C can be eliminated. Choice D is a non-real reaction that depicts NH_3 and H_2 as reactants and N_2 as the product. So, choice D can be eliminated, and choice A is the best answer.

559. A is the best answer. An equilibrium expression is products over reactants, so choice A is a strong answer. It is not appropriate to ignore either concentration, so choices B, C and D can be eliminated.

560. D is the best answer. Equilibrium expressions are products over reactants. However, solids are ignored. Choice A can be eliminated because it includes the solids Zn and ZnO. Choice B can be eliminated because it includes a solid, Zn. Choice C can be eliminated because it includes solids and is listed as reactants over products. Choice D is the best answer.

561. D is the best answer. Equilibrium expressions are products over reactants. However, pure liquids are ignored. Choices A, B and C can all be eliminated because they all include the concentration of H_2O. So, choice D is the best answer.

562. B is the best answer. A shortcut to answering this question would be to assume data are valid and laws are valid, so the conclusion must be invalid. First, recall that the law of mass action is the relationship between the equilibrium constant and the concentration of species. For this reaction above, it would be $K = [C]/[A][B]$. Using Beer's Law, which is $A = abc$ and assuming $b = 1$ cm, which it almost always does, the initial concentrations are 1 M, 1 M, and 0.1 M for A, B, and C, respectively. Calculating this is actually a waste of time and not helpful because the law of mass action only applies to reactions at equilibrium. At equilibrium, the concentrations are 0.1 M, 0.1 M, and 1 M. So $K = 1/(0.1 \times 0.1) = 100$ which is the same value listed in the table. So, the data are valid and the conclusion is not, making choice B is the best answer.

563. D is the best answer. Use Le Châtelier's principle to answer this question. Increasing the partial pressure of oxygen would drive the reaction to the right, so choice A can be eliminated. Decreasing the volume of the container favors the side of the reaction that has the fewest moles of gas. In this case, the reaction would be driven to the right, so choice B can be eliminated. There is no catalyst present, so choice C can be eliminated. By process of elimination, choice D must be correct but this can be rationalized with the following explanation. At lower temperatures, the $H_2O(g)$ will condense to $H_2O(l)$ which would drive the reaction to the right. Conversely, at high temperatures, the H_2O would remain in the gaseous state and the reaction would be driven to the left. So choice D is the best answer.

564. C is the best answer. Lowering the temperature of the surroundings would require the system (the reaction) to undergo a change to counteract this stress by releasing heat. The reverse reaction, which is exothermic, is preferred and the reaction is driven left. Choice A adds more of a left-hand reactant via a salt and would drive the equilibrium reaction further to the right. Choice B would decrease a product from the right-hand side and would also drive the reaction further to the right. Choice D is not the best answer because decreasing the pressure will generally drive the reaction toward the side with a greater number of moles, so also toward the right (3 moles of products versus 2 moles of reactants).

565. A is the best answer. Le Châtelier's Principle states that increasing the products will shift the reaction towards the reactants. The addition of heat increased the concentration of $SnO_2(g)$, a reactant. Heat can be thought of as a product, and reactions that generate heat are known as exothermic reactions. Choice A is a strong answer, and choice B can be eliminated. The addition of heat forms more reactants, decreasing the number of moles of gases. Gases have the greatest entropy of all phases, and as such, adding heat will decrease entropy. Choice C can be eliminated. According to Le Châtelier's Principle, increasing the temperature should increase $C(s)$, not lowering the temperature. Choice D can be eliminated. Choice A is the best answer.

566. B is the best answer. If the size of the vessel is reduced at constant temperature, total pressure increases. Following a pressure increase, Le Châtelier's Principle states that the reaction equilibrium will shift to the side with the least moles of gas. This will shift the given equation to the left. Because $CO(g)$ is a product, the addition of $CO(g)$ will shift the equilibrium to the left. Although this leftward shift will decrease the amount of $CO(g)$, it is unclear if the amount added is less than the amount lost due to the leftward shift. Choice A can be eliminated. There are 2 moles of solids in the reactants and 1 mole of solids in the products. A leftward shift will generate more moles of solids. Choice B is a strong answer. It is unclear how much $CO(g)$ has been added, so it is unclear what the final weight of the vessel is. Choice C can be eliminated. A leftward shift in the reaction equilibrium will decrease the mass of $Sn(s)$, not increase it. Choice D can be eliminated. Choice B is the best answer.

567. B is the best answer. Nearly all reaction rates increase with increased temperature, regardless of their enthalpy change. Choice A can be eliminated. If the reaction was exothermic, meaning that heat is a product, the equilibrium would shift to the left according to Le Châtelier's principle. This would reduce the yield of the reaction, likely making choice B the best answer. Pressure changes affect gas reactions but not reactions occurring in liquids. The mention of the aqueous catalyst gives the clue that the reaction is occurring in a liquid, eliminating choice C. There is no reason to believe high temperatures would break apart hydrogen, making choice D a weak answer choice.

568. A is the best answer. Both $NaOH(aq)$ and increased pressure drive the reaction to the left toward the magnesium hydroxide precipitate. Think of adding NaOH as simply delivering more OH^+ ions to the reaction, since NaOH is a strong base and Na^+ and OH^+ will easily dissociate in an aqueous environment. This increases the amount of right-hand product, so the reaction will be driven back to the left to try to mitigate the additional product. Adding pressure generally favors the side with less entropy, so it would favor the precipitation of the solid and drive the reaction to the left as well (think about pressure compacting loosely arranged molecules into highly ordered molecules). Choice B is not the best answer because while the first half is correct, the second half assumes added pressure will drive the reaction to the side with more entropy. Choice C is not the best answer because while some items are true, a decrease in precipitate mass and an increase in entropy and Mg^{2+} concentration would not be consistent with the reaction being driven left. Choice D is not the best answer because only one item, that Mg^{2+} will decrease under added NaOH, is consistent with a leftward driven reaction toward the precipitate.

Free Energy and Spontaneity

569. B is the best answer. The direction of a reaction under specific conditions can be predicted using the relationship between the equilibrium constant K and $\Delta G°$. Note that $\Delta G°$ is the change in Gibbs free energy under the specific case of standard conditions, namely at 1 bar, 298 K, and when all reactants and products are at 1 M. $\Delta G° = -RT\ln(K)$. The researchers noted that concentrations did not change when all compounds reached 1 M, indicating that equilibrium concentrations are 1 M. The equilibrium constant K must equal 1. $\ln(1) = 0$. $\Delta G°$ must equal zero. Choice B is the best answer.

570. A is the best answer. $\Delta G°$ is the change in Gibbs free energy under the specific case of standard conditions, namely at 1 bar, 298 K, and when all reactants and products are at 1 M. $\Delta G° = -RT\ln(K)$. It is noted that concentrations did not change after reaching 1 M, thus equilibrium is reached when all compounds are at 1 M. The equilibrium constant K must equal 1. $\ln(1) = 0$. $\Delta G°$ must equal zero. When concentrations are not 1 M, determining the ΔG under non-standard conditions will allow for determination of the direction of reaction progression. $\Delta G = \Delta G° + RT\ln(Q)$, where Q is equal to the reaction quotient. The reaction quotient is calculated the same way as K, except using concentrations that do not equal 1 M. $Q = 0.05^2/0.01 \times 0.05^5 = 1/0.01 = 100$. Without doing any calculations, note that R is greater than zero, the temperature is greater than zero, and $\ln(Q)$ is greater than zero. ΔG must be greater than zero, indicating that the reaction will proceed leftward. Choice A is the best answer.

571. A is the best answer. It is noted that $\Delta G° = -30$ kJ. $\Delta G°$, by definition, is the change in Gibbs free energy at standard conditions, namely at a defined temperature/pressure when the reactants and products are all at 1 M. $\Delta G°$ and K are related via the following equation: $\Delta G° = -RT\ln(K)$. Rearranging for $\ln(K)$, $\ln(K) = \Delta G°/-RT$. $2.3\log(x) \approx \ln(x)$. $2.3\log(K) = \Delta G°/-RT$, or $\log(K) = -\Delta G°/2.3RT$. Solving for K, $K = 10\Delta G°/2.3RT$. Filling in given values for $\Delta G°$ and T, $K = 10^{-30/2.3R(300)} = 10^{-30/690R}$. Choice A is the best answer.

572. B is the best answer. It is noted that $\Delta G° = -30$ kJ. $\Delta G°$ is defined as the change in Gibbs free energy at a given temperature/pressure when all reactants and products are 1 M. This reaction has a negative $\Delta G°$, indicating that, when $N_2(g)$, $H_2(g)$, and $NH_3(g)$ are all 1 M, the reaction will proceed towards product formation. Although $H_2(g)$ is expected to decrease, it is not the only gas expected to decrease. $N_2(g)$ is expected to decrease as well. Choice A can be eliminated. $NH_3(g)$ is expected to increase, as $NH_3(g)$ is a product. Choice B is a strong answer. $N_2(g)$ is a reactant and is expected to decrease, not increase. Choice C can be eliminated. The concentrations of gases will only remain the same when $\Delta G° = 0$. Choice D can be eliminated. Choice B is the best answer.

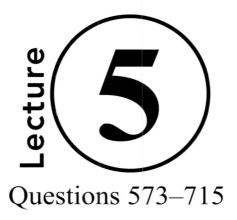

Lecture

5

Questions 573–715

Phases

ANSWERS & EXPLANATIONS

ANSWER KEY										
573. D	586. A	599. C	612. B	625. D	638. D	651. B	664. A	677. B	690. D	703. B
574. B	587. D	600. B	613. D	626. C	639. C	652. D	665. B	678. C	691. A	704. A
575. B	588. D	601. A	614. D	627. A	640. B	653. A	666. C	679. D	692. A	705. C
576. D	589. B	602. C	615. C	628. D	641. A	654. C	667. C	680. A	693. B	706. A
577. D	590. A	603. B	616. D	629. C	642. A	655. C	668. C	681. D	694. B	707. B
578. B	591. D	604. C	617. D	630. B	643. C	656. A	669. D	682. A	695. B	708. C
579. B	592. A	605. C	618. C	631. C	644. C	657. C	670. A	683. C	696. B	709. D
580. A	593. C	606. B	619. C	632. D	645. A	658. C	671. C	684. D	697. B	710. A
581. B	594. A	607. A	620. C	633. B	646. A	659. D	672. B	685. A	698. C	711. D
582. B	595. D	608. C	621. D	634. C	647. B	660. B	673. A	686. D	699. B	712. D
583. A	596. B	609. D	622. B	635. C	648. A	661. A	674. C	687. D	700. B	713. A
584. D	597. A	610. D	623. D	636. A	649. A	662. B	675. D	688. A	701. C	714. C
585. C	598. D	611. B	624. B	637. B	650. A	663. B	676. B	689. D	702. A	715. D

Behavior of Gases

573. D is the best answer. This question tests qualities of ideal gases. Ideal gases undergo elastic conditions, so choice A is not the best answer. Choice B can be ruled out because atoms lacking volume is one of the assumptions that define behavior of ideal gases. The ideal gas law is $PV = nRT$, and ideal gases do obey this. Choice C can be ruled out. Choice D is the best answer because the ideal gas law focuses on the lack of intermolecular forces, not intramolecular forces.

574. B is the best answer. The kinetic molecular theory defines an ideal gas and has four principles: 1) gas molecules have no molecular volume; 2) gas molecules do not exert attractive or repulsive forces on one another; 3) gas molecules have completely elastic collisions; 4) the average kinetic energy of a gas molecule is directly proportional to the temperature of the gas. An ester functional group is oxygen bonded to a carbonyl, which does not exist in isoflurane, eliminating choice A. The fluorine atoms could contribute to hydrogen bonding, which occurs between hydrogen and N, F, and O atoms. This would create attractive forces between molecules, which would make it less likely that isoflurane would behave as an ideal gas. Hydrogen bonds are a particular intermolecular force, so choice B is a strong answer. sp^2 hybridized bonds are generally found in atoms with double bonds, and no double bonds exist in isoflurane, making choice C unlikely. Single bonds contain s orbitals, but any molecule that contains single bonds also contains s orbitals. The presence of s orbitals alone does not mean that the molecule would violate any of the principles of the kinetic molecular theory, eliminating choice D. Choice B is the best answer.

575. B is the best answer. The question stem indicates that heat is released when two molecules of oxygen gas collide. One of the properties of an idea gas is that the collisions are completely elastic, meaning no energy is lost during a collision. Oxygen does not behave as an ideal gas, making choice A unlikely. When a gas is not an ideal gas, it is considered to be a real gas, which makes choice B a strong answer. Noble gases are found in column eighteen of the periodic table, while oxygen is found in column sixteen, which eliminates choice C. Halogens are found in column seventeen of the periodic table, while oxygen is found in column sixteen, eliminating choice D and making choice B the best answer.

576. D is the best answer. Remember both gases and liquids are fluids, and this gas behaves as an ideal fluid. Irrotational flow occurs when one portion of the fluid experiences drag forces that reduce its velocity relative to other portions of the fluid. This creates eddies and turbulence in the flow. Option I should be a component of the best answer. Acceleration is a change in velocity. An ideal fluid should not experience a change in velocity, as it should not have interactions with molecules that are attractive or repulsive, which would accelerate or decelerate the fluid, respectfully. Option II should be part of the best answer. Turbulence is similar to irrotational flow in that it is not streamlined laminar flow and flows in non-parallel lines. An ideal fluid displays laminar flow, not irrotational flow or turbulence, making choice D the best answer.

577. D is the best answer. One of the main properties of an idea gas is that the kinetic energy is directly proportional to the temperature. The formula for kinetic energy is $KE = \frac{3}{2}kT$, where T is in units of Kelvin. Thus, if the temperature in K doubles, as is noted in the question stem, then the kinetic energy should double. 60 J is double the 30 J of kinetic energy that Kr had at 300 K. Choice A mistakenly halves the kinetic energy. Choice B is the original kinetic energy and can be ruled out. Choice C increases the kinetic energy, but not by enough. Choice D is the best answer since it matches the doubling and calculations shown earlier in this explanation.

578. B is the best answer. The kinetic molecular theory defines an ideal gas and has four principles: 1) gas molecules have no molecular volume; 2) gas molecules do not exert attractive or repulsive forces on one another; 3) gas molecules have completely elastic collisions; 4) the average kinetic energy of a gas molecule is directly proportional to the temperature of the gas. If scientists found that they were unable to store more than a certain number of molecules in a container that cannot expand in volume, the molecular volume of the molecules may play the most prominent role, as the other forces could likely be overcome with continual increases in pressure. With increased pressure, repulsive forces could be overcome, eliminating choice A. If gases had a molecular volume, there would be a point at which the continued increase in pressure could not force molecules to be more compact, likely making choice B the best answer. This point would be when all gas molecules reach their minimum molecular volumes. Undergoing elastic collisions does not relate to volume of molecules. Choice C is unlikely. Choice D is also unlikely as having a velocity that is proportional to temperature do not necessarily relate to storing more molecules in a certain volume. Choice B is the best answer.

579. B is the best answer. At a temperature extreme like 0 K, a gas would most likely no longer be in gaseous phase, and would not obey the ideal gas law. Ideal gases lack intermolecular forces. Lack of a dipole would increase the likelihood of none of these forces being present, so choice B is a strong answer. Ideal gases are assumed to lack volume, so a large atomic radius would not promote ideal behavior, and choice C can be eliminated. Ionized gases would have extensive intermolecular interactions due to strong charge, so choice D is not the best answer. Choice B is the best answer.

580. A is the best answer. An ideal gas will exist as a straight line at 1 because $PV = nRT$ so $PV/nRT = 1$. The curve that deviates most from the ideal behavior will be the one with the greatest molecular volume and largest intermolecular forces. The order of the gases in increasing molecular volume would be: $H_2 \rightarrow N_2 \rightarrow O_2 \rightarrow CO_2$. It makes sense that the lines should be in order of molecular volume, ruling out choices B and C. Choice A is a stronger answer than choice D because the greatest molecular volume and highest degree of intermolecular forces would lead to the greatest deviation, meaning CO_2 is likely to be curve IV.

581. B is the best answer. For an ideal gas, internal energy is a function of temperature only. Changing pressure does not influence internal energy, ruling out option I, and choices A and C. Since there are no intermolecular forces in an ideal gas, changing the distance between the molecules while holding temperature constant does not affect the internal energy of an ideal gas. This rules out option III, and choices C and D. The kinetic energy of the molecules are a function of temperature from $K.E. = \frac{3}{2}RT$. Molecular rotational and vibrational energies are also a function of temperature. Choice B is the best answer as only option II is in the best answer.

582. B is the best answer. The question stem is asking about real liquids and gases, not ideal liquids and gases. Real gases experience intermolecular attractive and repulsive forces. Choice A can be eliminated. Real gases do, however, have fewer intermolecular attractive forces than liquids. This property allows gas molecules to be far more spread out than liquid molecules. For comparison, molecules in a liquid account for about 70% of the total volume occupied by a liquid at STP, whereas gas molecules account for about 0.1% of the total volume occupied by the gas. Choice B is a strong answer. Crystal lattice structures are atoms arranged in a network such that the intermolecular bonds form a lattice-like shape. Due to its rigidity, crystal lattices are typically only formed by solids. Choice C can be eliminated, as liquids and gases generally do not form these structures. Although real gases do sort themselves by density, so do liquids. Choice D can be eliminated. Choice B is the best answer.

583. A is the best answer. The table shows that gaseous reactants tend to react faster than liquid reactants. Validation of the research results requires a statement that explains why gases tend to react faster than liquids. A reaction can only take place if the reactants collide with each other with sufficient speeds (to overcome the activation energy) and correct spatial orientations. Compared to liquids, gas molecules move at much greater speeds, allowing for a greater reactant collision frequency, which could facilitate the speed of the reaction. Choice A is a strong answer. Although gases and liquids possess varying properties, these properties are independent of the quantity of molecules. There is also no indication from the research results that greater quantities of gases were used. Choice B can be eliminated. Although the research results indicate that gases form products faster than liquids, this does not explain the findings, but rather restates them. Choice C can be eliminated. Ideal gases exhibit no intermolecular attractive/repulsive forces, and while it is true that this property allows gases to travel at fast speeds that could allow for greater collision frequency, choice A is more direct in its reasoning. Choice D can be eliminated in favor of choice A, and choice A is the best answer.

584. D is the best answer. The question is more-or-less asking for an explanation as to why it is valid to assume that gas molecules have no intermolecular attraction. Although CO_2 molecules are nonpolar, recall that nonpolar molecules can still exhibit Van der Waals' interactions, which can be attractive. Choice A can be eliminated. Although the partial pressure of O_2 is likely to be greater than the partial pressure of CO_2, the partial pressure of CO_2 is not so low as to completely disregard it. This does not explain why the attractions between CO_2 molecules can be considered insignificant. Choice B can be eliminated. While gas movement at the capillary-alveolus interface is due to pressure gradients, this fact does not explain why intermolecular interactions are insignificant. Choice C can be eliminated. Coulomb's Law ($F = kq_1q_2/r^2$) can predict the force between two gas molecules with minor charges. Note that as the radius between the molecules increases, the force between the molecules decreases. Gases are distinct from other phases in that their molecules are extremely spread apart. This large intermolecular distance makes the force between molecules insignificant. Choice D is the best answer.

585. C is the best answer. The table displays the dipole moments of the four gases to be mixed. Note that a greater dipole moment indicates polarity, whereas a dipole moment of zero indicates that a molecular is nonpolar. Although H_2O and CH_3Cl are polar, and CCl_4 and CO_2 are nonpolar, ideal gases are assumed to have no intermolecular attractive/repulsive forces. Thus, polarity differences should not affect gaseous mixing. Choices A and B can be eliminated. A mixture of compounds in the gas phase will be homogeneous regardless of polarity differences, unlike liquids. This is because the molecules are so far apart that they exert negligible attractive/repulsive forces on each other. Choice C is a strong answer. Since it is true that the gas molecules are expected to mix together irrespective of chemical composition, choice D can be ruled out. Choice C is the best answer.

586. A is the best answer. A reaction can only take place if the reactants collide with each other with sufficient speeds that overcome activation energy and correct orientation to facilitate reaction. Compared to liquids, gas molecules move at much greater speeds, allowing for a greater reactant collision frequency. The mean free path is the distance travelled by a molecule between collisions. Because gases have a greater collision frequency, they also have a smaller mean free path. Choice A is a strong answer. Although real gases do exhibit non-negligible intermolecular interactions, so do liquids. This statement does not differentiate liquids from gases, and as a result, choice B is unlikely. Although it is true that a mixture of compounds in the gas phase tends to be homogenous, this does not explain the reaction rate phenomenon. Choice C can be eliminated. Gases tend to spread to fill their respective vessel, whereas liquids do not. This spreading, however, is a result of the increased kinetic energy (or increased speed) of the gas molecules. It is the increased kinetic energy that fundamentally increases the reaction rate, leading to a decreased mean free path. Choice D can be eliminated. Choice A is the best answer.

587. D is the best answer. There is no difference between He and Ne behavior when both are considered ideal gases. As a result, the estimate would be correct, ruling out choices A and B. The estimate would be correct regardless of how many atoms are in the molecule, as each molecule would behave the same. Choice C can be eliminated. Choice D is the best answer because it gives the correct reason that the estimate is correct. Under ideal conditions, all gas molecules can be considered the 'same' in many situations, including the one above.

588. D is the best answer. The ideal gas law is $PV = nRT$. P is pressure, V is volume, n is the number of moles, R is the gas constant, and T is temperature. V has nothing to do with speed or velocity, ruling out choices A and B. Choice C can also be ruled out as V more specifically means the total volume or the volume of the container. Choice D is the best answer.

589. B is the best answer. Pressure and temperature are directly proportional, based on the equation $PV = nRT$. Choice A can be ruled out as it shows an inverse proportion. The equation shows a linear, direct proportion, which fits with the graph for choice B. Choices C and D can be ruled out since those graphs are not linear. Choice B is the best answer.

590. A is the best answer. One strategy to solve this problem is the use of the ideal gas law. However, it is much quicker to realize that the conditions described are fairly close to STP. Under these conditions, one mole of gas should occupy about 22 L, and thus half of a liter should comprise about 1/40 of a mole. This is the closest to choice A, as $1/40 = 0.025$. Choice B is about 10 times the best answer and can be ruled out. Choices C and D are also factors of 10 higher. The heavy estimation and rounding done in this question is acceptable based on the large differences between the answer choices.

591. D is the best answer. According to the ideal gas law, the new temperature should be triple the value of the original. But, be careful! Temperatures must be expressed in Kelvins when using the ideal gas law. $25°C + 273 = 298$ K, which, when tripled, is almost 900 K. This is $900 - 273 = 627$ K, or about 600°C. Choice A can be ruled out as it is a third of the temperature in K. Choices B and C can be ruled out because they are based on forgetting to convert to Kelvin, which is necessary to use the ideal gas law and other laws derived from this one. Choice D is the closest answer, and exact discrepancies can be explained by rounding.

592. A is the best answer. Use the ideal gas law: $PV = nRT$. If the volume is cut in half, then the number of moles will be cut in half. In addition, the pressure is dropped to 90% of what it was, so the number of moles should drop by this factor as well. 90% of 50% is 45%, so the new number of moles is 0.45 times the old number of moles. Mass is proportional to number of moles, so $20 \times 0.45 = 9$ g. Choice A is the best answer. Choice B does not consider the change in pressure, and only halves the mass. Choice C shows the change in mass rather than the new mass. Choice D can be ruled out since this explanation shows how the answer was determined.

593. C is the best answer. There are 4 variables in the ideal gas law: $PV = nRT$. These are pressure, volume, moles, and temperature. Identical containers imply equivalent volume. The question stem also states that the temperatures and pressures are equivalent. 3 variables cannot be identical without the 4th, volume, being the same as well. Choices A and B can be ruled out. Choice C is a strong answer as the number of moles is determined and must be the same in both containers. Moles and temperature are actually inversely proportion, so choice D can be eliminated. Choice C is the best answer.

594. A is the best answer. Fifty grams of oxygen is a considerably smaller number of moles than fifty grams of hydrogen, because the molecular weight of oxygen is so much larger. For ideal gases, when determining pressure, it is the number of molecules that matters rather than the total weight. Thus, choice A is a strong answer as pressure is directly proportional to the number of moles. Choice B is unlikely since the pressure will be different due to the different number of molecules. Choice C describes the opposite of the true relationship. Choice D can be eliminated as the pressure relationship can be determined. Choice A is the best answer.

595. D is the best answer. Consider the ideal gas law, $PV = nRT$. P, R, and T are known, but V and n are not. If the volume was given, the number of moles and total mass could be found. However, with two unknowns, the volume and number of moles, which would be used to calculate mass, and only one equation, the equation cannot be solved. Choices A, B, and C can be ruled out, while choice D is the best answer.

596. B is the best answer. The ideal gas law works with partial pressures as well as total pressure. At 1 atmosphere and 0°C, 22.4 L would contain one mole of an ideal gas. Compared to the STP values, the volume and pressure are both cut in half, and the temperature is slightly higher, so the number of moles should be *about* $\frac{1}{2} \times \frac{1}{2} = 1/4$. The change in temperature, from 273 to 298 K, is not significant enough to warrant calculation. This is confirmed by the significant differences between answer choices, with each subsequent answer choice being double the numerical value of the previous choice. One-fourth of a mole of nitrogen gas (N_2) is about 7 g. Choice A is unlikely because it shows the mass of $\frac{1}{8}$ mole of nitrogen gas. Choice B is the best answer, as it matches the calculation. Choice C gives the mass of one nitrogen atom, while choice D gives the mass of one nitrogen molecule. Both can be ruled out.

597. A is the best answer. The ideal gas law, $PV = nRT$, shows that pressure is directly proportional to moles assuming all else is held constant. If volume is constant, then the change in moles per unit volume will be proportional to the change in moles. Since concentration is all about moles per unit volume, choices C and D are less likely. Pressure is not the same as concentration, and though choice D could be true, it does not explain why pressure can be used. Choice A is a better answer than choice B because it more accurately describes the relationship between pressure and moles.

598. D is the best answer. At a glance, this question seems like it can be solved based on the ideal gas equation, $PV = nRT$. Since pressure and volume are inversely proportional, choice A is a tempting answer. Choice B is simply the original pressure, and is unlikely to be the best answer since the volume is changing. Choice C is double the original pressure and changes in the wrong direction. The best answer is actually choice D since temperature is also in the ideal gas law, and there is no information on how temperature is affected in the scenario.

599. C is the best answer. As a balloon rises, external pressure decreases because the total weight of air above the balloon and number of gas molecules present decreases. Choice A is not the best answer because volume and temperature should be directly proportional according to Charles' law. Although choice B makes sense on the basis of Boyle's law, it is not consistent with the decreasing pressure at higher altitudes. Choice C is consistent with Boyle's law and the observation of decreasing pressure as the balloon rises. Choice D is not the best answer because even though the balloon is impermeable to gases, changes in external pressure can cause changes in volume since a balloon is a container that can change size. Choice C is the best answer.

600. B is the best answer. The volume at standard pressure of 1 atm or 760 mmHg can be found using Boyle's law. The volume at standard pressure is equal to (570 mmHg/760 mmHg) × 2 L = 1.5 L. This problem can be solved quickly by realizing that the answer must be between 1 L and 2 L. Choice B is the best answer. Choice A can be ruled out since 570 mmHg is much more than half of 760 mmHg. The volume should change in response to the pressure increase, so choice C can be eliminated. Pressure and volume are inversely related, so if all other variable are held constant and the pressure increases, the volume should decrease. Choice D can be eliminated.

601. A is the best answer. The initial pressure can be calculated from Boyle's law and is 4 atm × ($\frac{1}{2}$) = 2 atm. The answer to this problem can also be reasoned by understanding that pressure and volume are inversely proportional, so a decrease in volume would cause an increase in pressure. This means that the initial pressure would be lower than the final pressure, which only corresponds to choice A. With that change in volume, the pressure should change, ruling out choice B. Choices C and D represent higher initial pressures, and are weaker answers based on how volume is affected by an increase in pressure. Choice A is the best answer.

602. C is the best answer. By rearranging Boyle's law, the ratio of final pressure to initial pressure can be found to be $\frac{5}{4}$, or 1.25. The change in pressure should be the reciprocal of the change in volume ($\frac{4}{5} \rightarrow \frac{5}{4}$) given the number of moles and temperature remain constant. This makes sense because compression, or a decrease in volume, would cause an increase in pressure according to Boyle's law. This would create a ratio that is larger than 1, eliminating choices A and B. The ratio of pressures is the reciprocal of the ratio of volumes, due to inverse proportionality, so choice C is the best answer. Choice D does show an increase but by the wrong factor.

603. B is the best answer. The relationship between pressure and volume in the lungs is best explained by Boyle's law. Choice A is not the best answer because Charles' law states that volume and temperature are directly proportional. Choice B is the best answer because Boyle's law states that pressure and volume are inversely proportional. Choice C is not the best answer because Avogadro's law states that number of moles of gas and volume are directly proportional. Choice D is not the best answer because Dalton's law states that total pressure in a mixture of gases is equal to the sum of the individual pressures of the gases. Choice B is the best answer since the law describes the two variables discussed in the question stem.

604. C is the best answer. Based on Boyle's Law, which states that pressure and volume are inversely proportional, the pressure must be tripled to 3×850 torr = 2550 torr. This is because the volume is reduced to ⅓ of its original value. That means the additional pressure needed is $2550 - 850 = 1700$ torr. Choice A gives ⅓ of the original pressure of 850 torr. Choice B can be ruled out since this is just the original pressure. Choice C is the best answer since it gives the change in pressure required. Choice D is a tempting, but unlikely answer since it actually gives the pressure needed, rather than the amount of additional pressure required.

605. C is the best answer. According to Charles' law, an increase in temperature at constant pressure causes an increase in volume. Choice A is not consistent with any gas laws, nor is choice B. Choice C is consistent with Charles' law, and choice D is the opposite of choice C. Choice C is the best answer.

606. B is the best answer. Choice A can be ruled out since all oxygen molecules have the same molecular weight since they consist of two oxygen atoms. Choice B is a strong answer since the question does not specify the temperature of the samples, and this difference could certainly lead to the pressure difference. Choice C can be ruled out since volume and moles are only two of the four unknowns in the ideal gas law. When using proportional reasoning, be careful to make sure that all other factors are constant. Although choice D is a true statement, it's technically only true when temperature and number of moles are both constant. Choice B is the best answer.

607. A is the best answer. This figure shows 6 points, but the only ones relevant to the question stem are A and F. The A → F change represents an increase in volume with constant pressure. If volume increases and pressure and moles remain constant, then from $PV = nRT$, the temperature must increase. Choice A is a strong answer, and choice B is the opposite and can be eliminated. The temperature is unlikely to stay constant if volume changes as it must change in response based on the ideal gas law. Choice C can be ruled out. Choice D cannot be determined to be true based on the information in the question stem. Choice A is the best answer.

608. C is the best answer. The temperature can be found using $PV = nRT$. However, since P and V increase, so must T. Choice C is the only positive answer. Choices A and B describe decreases in temperature, so these two choices can be ruled out. Choice D is unlikely because if P and V both increase, and n stays constant, T must increase.

609. D is the best answer. This question involves Charles' law, which states that temperature and volume of a gas are directly proportional. The first step is to convert the temperatures to Kelvin by adding 273. 27°C equals 300 K, and 77°C equals 350 K. The ratio of the final volume to the initial volume is equal to the ratio of the final temperature to the initial temperature, or 350/300. This ratio comes out to be 7:6. Choices A and B are based on using Celsius to calculate the volume change. Kelvin must be used in these calculations. Choice C is the inverse of the calculated ratio, and choice D is the best answer.

610. D is the best answer. The final temperature of the gas can be found using Charles' law. 25°C is equal to 298 K. Doubling 298 K leads to 596 K, which is equal to 323°C. Choice is A is a trick answer because it involves doubling temperature before converting to units of Kelvin. Choice B is another distractor that simply gives the difference between Kelvin and Celsius units. Choice C is a close answer, but not as exact as 323°C. Choice D is the best answer as it matches the earlier calculation.

611. B is the best answer. Charles' law is best explained by the greater kinetic energy of gas molecules at higher temperatures, which leads to a proportional increase in volume. Choice A is not the best answer because it restates Avogadro's law rather than Charles' law. Choice B is the best answer because it explains Charles' law using the change in average speed of gas molecules due to a change in temperature. Choice C is not the best answer because it restates Henry's law rather than Charles' law. Choice D is not true because pressure should actually decrease as volume increases, according to Boyle's law. Choice B is the best answer.

612. B is the best answer. This question can be solved using Charles' law. The height of a cylindrical piston is proportional to the volume of the piston, assuming constant cross-sectional area. Therefore, height can be used as a substitute for volume in Charles' law. The initial temperature of the gas is equal to (5 cm/10 cm) × 300 K = 150 K. Choice A can be ruled out since this actually represents ¼ of the final temperature. Choice B is the best answer since it is half of the final temperature. Choices C and D represent increases in temperature, and temperature should not increase based on the situation described in the question. Choice B is the best answer.

613. D is the best answer. This question tests the principle of Avogadro's law which states that any two gases at constant temperature and pressure will occupy a volume proportionate to the number of moles in the gases, regardless of the chemical composition of the gases. A balloon will allow that gas to remain at the room's pressure and temperature, so the Avogadro's law may be applied as follows:

$$14 \text{ L}/0.3 \text{ mol} = \text{Final volume in L}/0.4 \text{ mol}$$

$$14 \text{ L} \times 0.4 \text{ mol}/0.3 \text{ mol} = \text{Final volume in L}$$

$$\text{Final volume in L} = 18.7 \text{ L}$$

Choice A is half of the calculated answer. The volume should change by 25% based on the number of moles added, so choices B and C can be ruled out. The difference between these values and 14 L is not large enough. Choice D is the best answer.

614. D is the best answer. It is helpful to remember that 1 mole of an ideal gas at STP occupies 22.4 L of volume. Using Avogadro's law, it is then possible to determine how much volume 3 moles of gas occupies at STP. This can be shown through the calculation $(3 \text{ mol}/1 \text{ mol}) \times 22.4 \text{ L} = 67.2 \text{ L}$. Choice A provides the numerical value of the number of moles, and can be ruled out. Choice B is the volume that would be taken up by $\frac{1}{3}$ mole of gas at STP, rather than 3 moles. Choice C is the volume of one mole of gas at STP. Choice D is the best answer since it matches the final answer from the calculation above.

615. C is the best answer. This question tests the principle of Avogadro's law which states that any two gases at constant temperature and pressure will occupy a volume proportionate to the number of moles in the gases, regardless of the chemical composition of the gases. If pressure, volume, and temperature are equal as in this case, the composition of the gases is irrelevant, and the moles will not change. Choices A and B are based on estimations that increase the original value by a ratio of $^{32}/_{21}$. These can be ruled out. Choice C is a strong answer since the number of moles should not change. Choice D represents a decrease in moles by a ratio of $^{21}/_{32}$, ruling out choice D. Choice C is the best answer.

616. D is the best answer. Avogadro's law is used to find the balloon's final volume. Initially, the balloon contains 0.5 moles of He, and after adding more He, the balloon contains 2.5 moles. The final volume is equal to $(2.5 \text{ mol}/0.5 \text{ mol}) \times 5 \text{ L} = 25 \text{ L}$. Choice A gives the number of moles after the addition of the 2 moles of helium, but does not factor in how this affects the volume. It can be ruled out. Choice B gives the numerical factor that the original volume should be multiplied based on the change in moles. Choice C can be ruled out since it comes from multiplication of the volume and pressure together, which is not applicable here. Choice D is the best answer.

617. D is the best answer. Because Avogadro's law establishes that volume and moles of gas are directly proportional, the percent change in volume should be equal to the percent change in moles of gas. This percent change can be calculated as (30,000 molecules/50,000 molecules) × 100 = 60%. Choice A comes from an error in division by powers of 10. Choice B is half of the calculated answer. Choice C comes from an arithmetic error, and is actually 20,000/50,000. Choice D is the best answer.

618. C is the best answer. The first step to this question is to balance the reaction. After balancing both sides, the coefficient for $SO_2(g)$ is 2, the coefficient for $O_2(g)$ is 1, and the coefficient for SO_3 is 2. Three moles of gaseous reactants form two moles of gaseous product. Choice A comes from mistakenly calculating that the number of moles will reduce to $\frac{1}{3}$ of the original value. Choice B comes from mistakenly assuming that two reactants becoming one product means that the volume can just be halved. Using Avogadro's law, the final volume is calculated to be $(2 \text{ mol}/3 \text{ mol}) \times 6 \text{ L} = 4 \text{ L}$. Choice C is the best answer. Choice D is a weaker answer as the volume will change based on the change in number of moles of gas.

619. C is the best answer. Avogadro's law can be used to find the moles of gas that escaped from the balloon. This is applicable here as pressure and temperature are constant. The number of moles remaining in the balloon after deflation is equal to $(0.45 \text{ L}/1.8 \text{ L}) \times 1 \text{ mol} = 0.25$ moles. Choice A is unlikely as this gives the amount remaining rather than the amount that escaped. Choice B is the result of a miscalculation when considering how moles and volume relate. The number of moles that escaped from the balloon is equal to 1 mol − 0.25 moles = 0.75 moles. Given this information, choice C is the best answer. Choice D can be ruled out, as it is impossible that the entire mole of gas escaped.

620. C is the best answer. Although the kinetic-molecular theory defines temperature in terms of the average speed of the molecules, it allows for variations in the speed of each individual molecule. This makes option I unlikely, and essentially rules out choices A, B, and D. Considering option II, gas molecules are assumed to have negligible volume. The last option, that no attractive forces are exerted on other molecules, is also true. Choice C is the best answer.

621. D is the best answer. In any gas, individual molecules have a wide range of speeds. In a gas at 300°C, the average kinetic energy of molecules will be greater than in a gas at 150°C, but the spread will be very wide in both cases. Certain molecules in each mixture will move faster and slower, so statements concerning every single molecule like in choices A and B can be ruled out. Temperature has no impact on the mass of molecules, so choice C can be ruled out. Choice D is the best answer since the other choices can be eliminated. The fact that temperature is actually proportional to kinetic energy and not speed further rules out choices A and B. The masses of gas molecules in each container are not given.

622. B is the best answer. This type of question can be solved by finding the unit that the final answer should have. Choice A gives g/mol × m⁶, which is not energy. Choice B gives mol × J/mol K × K. This simplifies to J, which is a unit for energy, making choice B a strong answer. Choices C and D give the units of force, so these answers can be eliminated. This kind of dimensional analysis can often help narrow down the answer choices on a formula-type question.

623. D is the best answer. The molar heat capacity of an isobaric polyatomic gas is $4R$ and because R is 8.13 J/mol K, the best answer is 33.24 J/mol K.

624. B is the best answer. Heat capacity is defined as the amount of energy (q) required to increase the temperature of a compound by 1 K. When energy is transferred into a system, not all of the energy goes into increasing the temperature of the compound. A compound can also absorb energy as atoms in a molecule increase motion and stretch intramolecular bonds. Intramolecular bonds are between valence electron shells, not atomic nuclei. Choice A can be eliminated. The more bonds a molecule has, the more energy it can divert into bond stretching rather than into raising temperature. Choice B is a strong answer. Choice C states the definition of heat capacity and does not explain the research findings. This can be tricky, because though it is true, it is not relevant to the question. Choice C can be eliminated. Although gravitational potential energy does increase with weight, this type of energy does not affect temperature. Choice D can be eliminated. Choice B is the best answer.

625. D is the best answer. The heat capacity of an isovolumetric diatomic gas is ½ nR, and because R is 8.13 J/mol K, the correct answer is 62.35 J/ K.

626. C is the best answer. Changes in the rotational axis of a molecule are best characterized by changes in internal energy. A constant volume calorimeter, rather than a constant pressure calorimeter, best measures the changes in internal energy. Choices A and B can be eliminated. One hint that neither of these answers is correct is that the two choices are incredibly similar. Gauge pressure is the recorded pressure minus the atmospheric pressure, which would be the pressure recorded in a constant volume calorimeter. Choice C is a better answer than choice D.

627. A is the best answer. Measuring the heat released from a reaction implies that the enthalpy of a reaction was measured, which is best recorded by a coffee cup calorimeter. As the reaction takes place, heat flow is represented by a change in the temperature of the fluid in the coffee cup. Choice A is the best answer. A bomb calorimeter measures changes in internal energy, which is alluded to by the question stem, eliminating choices B and C. As a coffee cup calorimeter would measure the enthalpy change and would be perfect for this goal, so choice D can be eliminated in favor of choice A.

628. D is the best answer. Rotational energy is one component of internal energy, along with translational energy in each of the three dimensions. This eliminates choices A and B since they discuss enthalpy rather than internal energy. A coffee cup calorimeter is a constant pressure calorimeter that measures changes in enthalpy, not internal energy. This eliminates choice C. A bomb calorimeter is a constant volume calorimeter and measures changes in internal energy, making choice D the best answer.

629. C is the best answer. The First Law of Thermodynamics for a system at rest states that $\Delta U = q + w$. The energy added to a system is q, whereas work done by the system is w. Note that a change in internal energy (ΔU) represents a change in temperature. Choice A restates the question but includes the definition of heat capacity. Choice A does not explain why the types of heat capacities are different, so this answer can be ruled out. At a constant pressure, the volume of the system is able to change. When the system expands, work is done on the surroundings, decreasing the internal energy of the system. When heated, a system at a constant pressure could lose internal energy due to work on the surroundings. At a constant volume, work cannot be done on the environment. When heated, a system at constant volume will not lose internal energy due to work on the surroundings. Thus, following a heat transfer, a constant volume system will exhibit a greater change in internal energy than a constant pressure system. Choice B can be eliminated. At a constant volume, work cannot be done on the surroundings, allowing for more energy to be diverted towards increasing the temperature. Choice C is a strong answer. At a constant pressure, the volume can change, and PV work can be done. Choice D can be eliminated. Choice C is the best answer.

630. B is the best answer. Protein structure denatures at particularly high temperatures and extremely low/high pH levels. When these proteins denature, their function decreases. Hemoglobin A is likely to reduce its oxygen-carrying capacity due to denaturation. 37°C is normal body temperature. Choice A can be eliminated. 67°C is well above normal body temperature, providing a risk for protein denaturation. Choice B is a strong answer. Converting 310 K to °C requires subtracting 273. Choice C is 37°C, which is normal body temperature. Choice C can be eliminated. $328 - 273 = 55$°C, which is less than choice B. Choice D poses less of a risk to protein denaturation than choice B and can be eliminated. Choice B is the best answer since it is the highest, most extreme temperature of the four choices.

631. C is the best answer. Reactions generally proceed fastest at higher temperatures due to the increased rate at which reactants are able to collide. With more temperature and kinetic energy, there are more collisions, and these collisions occur with more energy. All else equal, a reaction should proceed slowest in the coldest environment. 301 K is greater than 291 K. Choice B can be eliminated. K = °C + 273. 17°C + 273 = 290 K. Choice A can now be eliminated in favor of choice C. 23°C + 273 = 296 K, which is greater than choice C. Choice D can be eliminated, and choice C is the best answer.

632. D is the best answer. According to the ideal gas law, both pressure and volume are directly proportional to (absolute) temperature. Thus, plotting either pressure or volume against temperature would result in a line with the temperature axis intercept at absolute zero. Choices A and B are both methods for determining absolute zero, making choice D the best answer. Choice C can also be shown to be true, as the product of P and V is also proportional to temperature based on the ideal gas law, $PV = nRT$.

633. B is the best answer. 1 Pa is approximately $1/10^5$ atm. 1 torr = 1/760 atm. 1 mmHg = 1 torr = 1/760 atm. Based on these conversions, an atm is the largest, followed by mmHg and torr which are equivalent. The smallest is a Pa, so choice B is the best answer.

634. C is the best answer. All else being equal, a faster molecule exerts more force on the wall. Likewise, more collisions also mean more force and pressure on the wall. Options I and II are likely to both be in the final answer. Choices A and B can be ruled out. The volume of gas molecules is not related to average force or pressure. In fact, ideal gases are considered to have no molecular volume. Option III can be ruled out, so choice C is the best answer.

635. C is the best answer. The pressure at the bottom of the cylinder would be due to the weight of the air inside the cylinder. This pressure is 1 atm, so $P = F/A = mg/A = 1$ atm = 1.01×10^5 Pa. Force can be calculated by pressure since the area is known: 1.01×10^5 Pa/1 m^2 = 1.01×10^5 N of weight. $F = mg$, so $1.01 \times 10^5/10 = 1.01 \times 10^4$ kg. Choices A and B are the result of errors in dividing by powers of 10. Choice C is the best answer since it matches the calculation above. Choice D can be ruled out since it simply provides the number of Pa in one atm of pressure.

636. A is the best answer. By converting parameters like pressure and force to their basic units, this question can be solved. Plug each combination of parameters in to see if they describe F/A or pressure. For choice A: $\Delta mv = F_{avg}\Delta t$. $P = F/A$. $P = \Delta mv/A\Delta t$. Thus, choice A is a strong answer. Dividing kinetic energy instead would result in P(m/s) as the unit rather than just pressure. Choice B can be ruled out. Parameters in choices C and D including number of molecules and temperature of the fluid molecules has very little to do with pressure in this question. These choices can be ruled out.

637. B is the best answer. The mercury in the right side of the tube is lower than the mercury in the left. That means that atmospheric pressure is pushing harder than the pressure of the gas in the bulb. ρgh is a measure of how much lower the gas pressure is. Choice A can be ruled out since if this was the case, then the mercury levels on both sides would be equal. Choice B is the best answer. Choice C is the opposite of choice B, and if it were true, then the pattern of mercury height would be reversed. The pressure of the gas relative to atmospheric pressure can be determined, so choice D can be ruled out.

638. D is the best answer. The equation in the passage says that pressure change is proportional to temperature change. From $PV = nRT$, this is only true if volume stays constant. Also, the passage says that the mercury level on the left must be brought to zero. This requires the gas volume to be constant. Finally, the reservoir and the right side of the tube must remain at the same level because they are both exposed to atmospheric pressure. Since the reservoir is larger than the tube, when it is lowered, more mercury moves into the reservoir, lowering both sides of the mercury-filled tube. When it is raised, it holds less mercury, so the mercury in the right and left sides of the tube rises. By raising and lowering the reservoir, the mercury in the left side of the tube is adjusted to the zero mark. Choice A can be ruled out since the gas does not remain at atmospheric pressure except for at a specific temperature. Choices B and C can be ruled out because the gas changes temperature and pressure, and this is converted to a reading on the thermometer. Choice D is the best answer since the goal is to maintain volume.

639. **C is the best answer.** This question illustrates the importance of understanding restrictions imposed on equations. Boyle's law could lead to choices A or B, but Boyle's law only applies if temperature and number of moles are constant. T and n are not constant here based on the info in the question stem. Choice C is the best answer because weight on the piston does not change, so the force per area, or pressure, on the top of the piston is constant. Since this pressure must be matched by the gas pressure in order to support the piston, the pressure in the container must be the same for both recordings. Choice D can be ruled out.

640. **B is the best answer.** 60 L of gas at 0°C and 1 atm will contain 2.7 moles because the molar volume of any gas at STP is 22.4 L/mol. Using $PV = nRT$ will also work if 8.2×10^{-2} L atm K^{-1} mol^{-1} is used for R and 273 is used for T. However, this math takes a lot of time, so using the molar volume of a gas is preferred. Choice A results from dividing 22.4 L/mol by 60 L. Notice the units for the calculation would be mol^{-1}, which is why choice A is not the best answer. Choice C is a result of attempting to use $PV = nRT$ but using 760 Torr for P and 8.3 J K^{-1} mol^{-1} (alternative units would be L kPa K^{-1} mol^{-1}) for R. This R cannot be used with Torr, only kPa. Choice D results from forgetting that 60 L of gas are present and simply plugging in the standard volume of 1 mole at STP.

641. **A is the best answer.** The molar volume of gas, 22.4 L is defined at 0°C. Choice B is room temperature, which is sometimes used for STP, though not as accurate as choice A. Choice C is body temperature, which is used in experiments related to medicine. Choice D is the boiling point of water.

642. **A is the best answer.** In this graph, the only work done on the gas that could be isovolumetric is the hypotenuse. Because the hypotenuse passes through 1 atm at 273 K (STP), and contains 1 mole of gas, the volume must be 22.4 L. Choice B represents the volume of 2 moles of gas at STP, while choice C represents 0.5 moles of gas at STP. Choice D can be ruled out as it represents an answer close to the volume of 1 mole at STP but is not quite right.

643. **C is the best answer.** The equation in this question must be balanced to yield the following:

$$2HNO_3 + Na_2CO_3 \rightarrow 2NaNO_3 + CO_2 + H_2O$$

Because one mole of gas is produced per 2 moles of nitric acid, 0.5 moles of carbon dioxide will be produced at STP. Since the molar volume of any gas at STP is 22.4 L/mol, the volume of gas produced in this reaction will be 11.2 L. Choices A and B are the result of arithmetic errors when calculating number of moles and converting to volume. Choice D is a distractor that is close to molar volume at STP.

644. **C is the best answer.** At 0°C or 273 K, one mole of gas occupies 22.4 L. The best way to find the answer to this question is to use ratios, as shown below:

$$\frac{1 \text{ mol}}{22.4 \text{ L}} = \frac{x \text{ mole}}{38 \text{ L}}$$

By cross-multiplying and solving for x, there are around 1.7 moles of gas, making choice B the best answer. Choice A can be ruled out since 1 mole is 22.4 L, and 38 L is well over this value. Choice C can be ruled out since 2 moles at STP would occupy a volume of 22.4 × 2 = 44.8 L. This is much more than 38 L, so choice D can also be ruled out.

645. **A is the best answer.** 22.4 L is the volume of a gas at STP, but the temperature component of STP is very different from 100 K. Choices C and D can be eliminated because 1 mole of gas is 6.022×10^{23} molecules. Between choice A and choice B, choice A is the best answer because the researchers have made a systematic error. The error of the assumption will be applied to each trial equally, so there will not be a greater dispersion or error in reliability. The error will affect validity, making choice A the best answer.

646. **A is the best answer.** Note that water is formed in the liquid phase. Because the molar volume of any gas at STP is 22.4 L/mol, 60 liters of oxygen is equal to 60/22.4, or 2.68 moles. Because 2 moles of water are formed for every 1 mole of oxygen reacted, 5.36 moles of water will be formed. The molecular weight of water is 18 grams/mol. Therefore, 96.48 grams of water will be formed. Using the density of water (1 g/mL), the volume of water can be calculated to be 0.096 L. Choice A is the best answer. Choice B is the number of moles of oxygen that will be reacted, so choice B is not the best answer. Choice C is the number of moles of water that will be formed. Because the question asks the volume of water that will be formed, choice C is not the best answer. Choice D is the volume of water vapor that would be formed, if the reaction resulted in a vapor product. However, because the reaction creates liquid water, choice D is not the best answer.

647. **B is the best answer.** The total pressure is 760 torr at STP, so the partial pressure of the nitrogen must be 760 − 200 − 10 − 8 = 542 torr. Choice A is the non-nitrogen partial pressure. Choice B is the best answer as evidenced by the calculations shown above. Choice C is the total pressure at STP. Choice D mistakenly adds the components described in the question stem to the baseline pressure of 760 torr.

648. **A is the best answer.** At STP, the total pressure is 1 atmosphere, or 760 torr. The partial pressure is just the mole fraction multiplied by the total pressure, or 0.8 × 760 torr = 608 torr, choice A. Choice B is the pressure of STP. Choice C represents more pressure than the standard level, ruling it out. Choice D is unlikely as the pressure can be estimated as shown above in the explanation.

649. A is the best answer. At STP, a gas is at one atm of pressure. According to Dalton's law, there are $1 - 0.3 - 0.45 = 0.25$ atm of helium. The total number of moles of gas can be calculated by $10/22.4$, so approximately 0.4 moles. 0.25 atm $\times$ 0.4 moles/atm $= 0.1$ moles, choice A. Choice D gives the pressure of the helium rather than the number of moles.

650. A is the best answer. At STP, a gas is at one atmosphere of pressure. According to Dalton's law, there are 0.25 moles of helium, or 2.5 L of carbon monoxide. That's roughly $1/10$ of 22.4 L, the volume of one mole of any gas at STP, so choice A is the best answer.

651. B is the best answer. Use the formula:

$$P_a = \chi_a P_{total}$$

P_{total} is 1 atm, and the mole fraction (χ) is 0.21, so the best answer is choice B. Choice A is $1/10$ of the calculated answer. Choice C represents the combined pressure of non-oxygen gases. Choice D is the total atmospheric pressure at sea level.

652. D is the best answer. The question stem implies that the concentration of oxygen that enters a patient's lungs increases due to the administration of supplemental oxygen. The lungs have a fixed inspiratory volume, meaning supplemental oxygen administration would be likely to increase the concentration of oxygen entering the lungs. This would increase the mole fraction, the partial pressure of oxygen, and the mass of oxygen administered, as the inspiratory volume is fixed. This eliminates choices A, B, and C. Because the volume of inspiration of the lungs is fixed, the inspired volume of air would not be changed, just the concentration of oxygen in that fixed volume. Choice D is the best answer.

653. A is the best answer. The mole fraction is the ratio of the partial pressure to the total pressure. Since 5 atm $= 5 \times 760$ torr, a mole fraction can be calculated with: $35/(5 \times 760) = 0.009$. Choice A is the best answer. Choice B is the result of mistakenly considering the total pressure to be 1 atm rather than 5 atm. Choice C can be ruled out as this is $35 \times 5/760$, mixing up various parts of the calculation above. Choice D can be eliminated, as the mole fraction was determined above.

654. C is the best answer. A mole fraction of 1 would mean that helium is replacing all gas molecules present. Choice A is unlikely. Choice B can be ruled out since a mole fraction can not be greater than 1. If the total pressure of the gas doubles, then 50% of the gas composition has to be replaced by helium to maintain the partial pressure of the oxygen. Although it is tempting to use molar mass to calculate this, the moles of a gas are proportional to volume, so the helium should comprise half of the moles in the mixture, making choice C the best answer. Choice D is $1/10$ of the best answer.

655. C is the best answer. Answering this question without a calculator requires some rounding. Change 1.45 atm to 1.5 atm. Change 19% to 20%. The pressure of oxygen required for life on earth is 0.2×1 atm $= 0.2$ atm. The question says assume the same pressure (not mole fraction) is required for life on Titan. 0.2 atm on Titan would be 13.3% of the atmosphere ($0.2/1.5 = 0.133$). This means that other gases would have to decrease proportionally. Choice A results from simply calculating the mole fraction of oxygen on Titan and can be eliminated. Choice B results from assuming oxygen needs to be 20% of the atmosphere, so nitrogen and other gases comprise the other 75% and 5%, respectively. Choice D is the original percent of nitrogen, so it can be eliminated. This leaves choice C by process of elimination. The math is difficult to do without a calculator, but because nitrogen is 95% of the atmosphere originally, it must be reduced by 13.3×0.95, which is a number that rounds to $13.95 - 13 = 82$, so choice C is the best answer.

656. A is the best answer. First, rule out the answers that do not match the pressures described in the question stem. The partial pressure of carbon dioxide is lower in the alveoli while oxygen is lower in the blood. Choice D can be ruled out since carbon dioxide is higher in the blood. Choice A is a strong answer since carbon dioxide is lower in the alveoli, resulting in carbon dioxide moving down its gradient into the alveoli. Choice B can be ruled out as the movement of carbon dioxide would be in the opposite direction. Choice C can be ruled out since oxygen should move from the alveoli to the blood based on the partial pressures given.

657. C is the best answer. Dalton's law is best observed at low pressures. While gasses of low molecular weight might be reactive, they may also be inert. At higher pressures, reactivity increases, and Dalton's law is best observed with inert gases. Dalton's law can hold true in rigid containers, with gases with larger molecular weight, and when the ratios are lopsided. Choices A, B, and D can be ruled out. Choice C is the best answer.

658. C is the best answer. In this case, the identity and moles of the reactants are irrelevant because there is no evidence to show that the reaction has consumed all of the carbon in the reactants. Choices A and B can be eliminated. Dalton's law is required because the partial pressure of CO_2 equals the atmospheric pressure minus the vapor pressure, and the volume in the cylinder can be measured, followed by an application of the ideal gas law. Bernoulli's law does apply to gases, but is less relevant to this case where flow is not a major factor. Choice D can be ruled out.

659. **D is the best answer.** The partial pressure of a gas can be related to the composition of a gas, as the partial pressures of all the individual gases must sum to equal the overall pressure of a gas. The percentage of a gas in the atmosphere remains constant despite changes in elevation, as each component is affected equally by altitude changes. At various elevations, the total pressure can change, but the composition remains the same, eliminating choice A. While nitrogen does make up 78% of the atmosphere, this fact does not further support the scientist's conclusions regarding argon. Choice B can be eliminated. Similarly, although oxygen does make up 21% of the atmosphere, its composition does not directly determine the composition of argon, eliminating choice C. The pressure at sea level is 1 atm. If argon makes up 1% of the atmosphere, its partial pressure at that altitude would be (0.01)(1 atm) = 0.01 am. This finding would support the researcher's conclusion, making choice D the best answer.

660. **B is the best answer.** There are many ways to approach this problem. First of all, the mole fraction is 30/760 = 0.04. Imagine there were 100 moles of gas present. There would be 4 moles of carbon, with a mass of 4 × 44, or 176 grams. That represents 10% of the total mass, so the other species must have nine times that mass, or about 1600 grams. Since the other species would have 96 moles present, its molar mass would be 1600/96, or about 17 g/mol. Of the choices, only methane (CH^4) is close. Choice B is the best answer, while choices A, C, and D can be ruled out since those molecular weights are not close to 17.

661. **A is the best answer.** The partial pressure of a gas is related to the mole fraction of a gas by the following formula: $P_{Gas} = (\chi_{Gas})(P_{Total})$. As long as the total pressure and the volume of the gas are known, the partial pressure of a gas can be determined. Breathing out is called expiration, while breathing in is called inspiration. Choice A is likely a better answer choice than choice B. Oxygen and argon are the other two main components of atmospheric air, but other gases contribute minor fractions. Only measuring the partial pressures of oxygen and argon would not give the exact partial pressure of nitrogen, eliminating choices C and D.

662. **B is the best answer.** The composition of atmospheric air is approximately 20% oxygen, 80% nitrogen, and since oxygen and nitrogen are roughly similar in molar mass, it can be estimated that according to Dalton's Law, approximately 600 mmHg of standard air pressure is due to nitrogen. To quadruple the nitrogen partial pressure to 2400 mmHg, the pressure must quadruple. That is, an additional 3 atmospheres, or 90 feet of water pressure could cause nitrogen narcosis. Choice B is the best answer. Choices A, C, and D are miscalculations based on multiples of the 30 feet/1 atm that was used to determine the depth that a partial nitrogen pressure of 2400 mmHg would occur.

Real Gases

663. **B is the best answer.** Kinetic molecular theory describes certain ideal gas characteristics that are not shared by a real gas. Ideal gases have completely elastic collisions, meaning no energy is lost during collisions. Real gases therefore have incompletely elastic collisions. Choice A can be eliminated. The average kinetic energy of ideal gas molecules is directly proportional to the temperature of the gas. This is not always true of real gases. Choice B is a strong answer. Both ideal gases and real gases fill to the size of their containers. Choice C can be eliminated. The Van der Waals's equation is a modified ideal gas law that is used to account for real gas deviations from ideal behavior. Choice D can be eliminated, and choice B is the best answer.

664. **A is the best answer.** Gases deviate from ideal behavior when their molecules are close together, which occurs at high pressure and low temperatures. High pressures cause deviation from ideal behavior because gas molecules are pushed together. Also, molecules tend to settle together due to low temperature. Choices C and D can be ruled out. Choices A and B are the most likely answers at this point. Choice A is the best answer as it states the conditions that would bring molecules closest to one another.

665. **B is the best answer.** Gases deviate from ideal behavior when pressure is high and temperature is low. The experimental design indicates that balloon A would display behavior associated with real gases while balloon B would exhibit ideal gas behavior. Choice A is not the best answer as balloon A would not display ideal behavior. Choice B is a strong answer as the conditions in this container allow for more ideal behavior. Choice C is not the best answer as the different conditions in each balloon mean that they will not both behave ideally. Choice D can be eliminated as the best answer was determined above.

666. **C is the best answer.** An ideal gas has no molecular volume and has completely elastic collisions. Octane contains eight carbons, while methane contains one carbon. It is reasonable to assume that octane violates the ideal gas law more than methane due to the additional size. Octane would generate more heat during collisions due to its size and the opportunity for more atoms to collide, eliminating choice A. Even if choice A were true, it would not explain the more real behavior of octane. Octane is a larger molecule, meaning it takes up more molecular space, eliminating choice B. Octane would likely have less elastic collisions due to its size, making choice C most likely to be the best answer. Due to its larger size, octane would likely have more intermolecular interactions, eliminating choice D.

667. **C is the best answer.** Real gases deviate from ideal behavior when their molecules are close together, which occurs at high pressures and low temperatures. High pressures cause gas molecules to be compressed. This makes the distance between the molecules smaller and significant, increasing the magnitude of electrostatic interactions between adjacent gas molecules. Choice A can be eliminated. Increased pressure would increase *inter*molecular collision frequency, not *intra*molecular collision frequency. Choice B can be eliminated. Coulomb's law ($F = kqq/r^2$) would predict that this decreased intermolecular distance would increase the attractive force between gas molecules. Note that ideal gases are assumed to have no electrostatic interactions between molecules. Choice C is a strong answer. Choice D can be eliminated because it does not explain the deviation as directly and completely as choice C.

668. **C is the best answer.** Note that if the a and b variables of the Van der Waals' equation were zero, this equation would collapse to the ideal gas law: $PV = nRT$. This indicates that, as the a and b variables increase, the gas tends to deviate further away from ideal behavior. A characteristic of ideal gases is that gas molecules have no volume. Gases with greater molecular mass tend to deviate more from ideal behavior because these gases tend to have greater sizes. The volume difference is what is represented by this variable. Since SO_2 has the greatest size of the analyzed gases, choice C is the best answer. Choices A and B are both smaller gas molecules, while choice D can be eliminated since the answer can be reasoned out.

669. **D is the best answer.** Smaller a and b variables indicate that a gas molecule is less likely to deviate from ideal conditions. Note that ideal gases do not exert attractive or repulsive forces on one another. Anything that would increase the likelihood of intermolecular force generation would likely result in increased a and b variables. Greater electronegativity typically indicates greater polarity, which would generally increase attractive and repulsive forces, but the question stem indicates that CCl_4 has smaller a and b variables than SO_2. Choice A can be eliminated. As per Coulomb's law ($F = kqq/r^2$), greater packing could reduce the distance between molecules, increasing intermolecular force. However, the question stem indicates that CCl_4 has smaller a and b variables than SO_2. Choice B can be eliminated. Although decreased electrostatic interactions would allow CCl_4 to exhibit less non-ideal behavior that SO_2, this would not be due to the number of p orbitals. Choice C can be eliminated. CCl_4 has a tetrahedral geometry with no lone pairs, making it nonpolar and less likely to exhibit electrostatic interactions than SO_2, which is polar. Choice D is the best answer. These intermolecular attractive forces disrupt ideal behavior and increase real behavior of gases.

670. **A is the best answer.** The value of PV/RT for all gases shown at high pressures is greater than one. Real V is greater than ideal V due to molecular volume. Gases can be packed together by high pressure to a point where the molecular sizes become significant factors. Choice A is the best answer. Intermolecular attraction does increase when distance between molecules is decreased, but the classic factor with extreme high pressure is molecular volume. Choice B can be ruled out. Temperature and molecular shape are less important to this deviation at high pressure like molecular volume, ruling out choices C and D.

671. **C is the best answer.** Increased molecular mass and complexity tend to coincide with greater molecular volume and greater intermolecular forces. Choices A and B both seem to be strong answers, making choice C a great answer. Molecular characteristics certainly impact deviations from ideal behavior, as every type of gas molecule does not deviate identically. Choice D is unlikely.

672. **B is the best answer.** The value of PV/RT for CO at 100 atm is less than one. At a high pressure like 100 atm, the molecules will be closely packed, making molecular size a huge factor in deviation from ideal behavior. This happens regardless of the number of molecules, making choice B a better answer than choice A. Temperature is not the explanation for deviation in a high pressure scenario, ruling out choice C. The deviations observed are less due to exact shape than simply the bulk of having molecular volume while packed together. Choice D can be ruled out.

673. **A is the best answer.** The two most important assumptions of ideal gas behavior are that there are no intermolecular forces between particles, and that the particles themselves take up no volume. At low temperatures, gas molecules move slowly, and intermolecular forces have a greater chance of becoming significant. Therefore, at low temperatures, intermolecular forces cannot be considered negligible, and gases deviate from ideal behavior. Choices B and D are unlikely since they contain high temperature in the answer. At high pressures, the gas molecules are packed more tightly together, and collide more often. At this point, the volume becomes too significant to neglect. Because the excluded volume assumption can no longer be made, gases deviate from ideal behavior at high pressures. Choice A is the only answer that has both these conditions, and is the best answer. Choice C can be ruled out.

674. C is the best answer. The ideal gas law is as follows: $PV = nRT$. The researchers used the ideal gas law to calculate the pressure, but, in reality, gases can deviate from ideality. The question is more-or-less asking why a deviation from ideality would result in decreased pressure. Humans inspire all the gases in the atmosphere, not just $O_2(g)$. It just so happens that $O_2(g)$ has the greatest physiological impact, but all gases will contribute to pressure. Choice A can be eliminated. Real gases do account for the volume of gas molecules. It is ideal gases that assume gas molecules have no volume. Choice B can be eliminated. Real gases exhibit intermolecular attractive/repulsive forces. Since the predominant intermolecular forces are attractive, gas molecules are pulled inward toward the center and slow before colliding with container walls. This results in less force against the container walls. Recall that Pressure = Force/Area. Less force results in less pressure. Choice C is a strong answer, except for the fact that it only mentions $O_2(g)$ and not other atmospheric gases. Although it is true that ideal gas molecules have completely elastic collisions while real gases do not, this answer does not touch on the fundamental reason of why pressure is decreased: weaker wall collisions. Choice D can be eliminated. While choice C is not perfect, it is the best answer.

675. D is the best answer. The most likely reason for non-ideality would be strong intermolecular forces and large molecular size. Choices A, B, and C are all small nonpolar molecules, attracted only by London Dispersion forces. Choice D exhibits hydrogen bonding, which is a much stronger attraction than LDF. It is also the largest molecule in terms of number of atoms, making choice D the best choice. Choices A, B, and C are all nonpolar. Thus, they will behave more ideally.

676. B is the best answer. As the volume of the container is decreased, the molecules in the container approach each other more frequently, leading to an increase in the number and strength of intermolecular attractions among the molecules. This is based on Coulomb's law, where distance is in the denominator. This means that as distance decreases, strength of force increases. As these attractions increase in magnitude, the number and intensity of collisions between the molecules and the wall decrease, thus decreasing the pressure exerted by the gas. The pressure is lower rather than higher, ruling out choices C and D. This is due to intermolecular forces rather than molecular volume, making choice B a better answer than choice A.

677. B is the best answer. At lower temperatures, the potential energy due to the intermolecular forces is more noticeable compared to the kinetic energy. Molecules move more slowly and intermolecular interactions have more time to form and strengthen. Choice A can be ruled out because volume of gas molecules is not the main factor at low temperature; it becomes more of a cause for deviation at higher pressure. Choice B is a strong answer since it is these attractive forces that are a larger factor at low temperature. Choices C and D are unlikely since pressure does not deviate upward at low temperature.

678. C is the best answer. Real gas molecules have volume making real volume greater than ideal volume. Option I is likely to be in the right answer. Real gas molecules exert attractive forces on one another, decreasing their velocity and lowering the pressure. Option II is likely to be in the right answer. The rms velocity of ideal or real gas molecules is directly proportional to the temperature. Furthermore, temperature only gives information on the average kinetic energy and speed of all molecules, but it does not say that all molecules in the sample move at the same speed. Choice C is the best answer.

679. D is the best answer. An ideal gas has no volume, does not have intermolecular interactions with another gas, and has laminar flow. By the ideal gas law, $PV = nRT$, the volume should not change as long as the pressure and temperature do not change. Option I is a component of the best answer. Laminar flow is streamlined flow and should exist in an ideal gas. Option II is a component of the best answer. Similar to volume, the pressure of a gas should be fixed at a constant volume and temperature. Option III is a component of the best answer. Choice D is the best answer, as it contains options I, II, and III.

680. A is the best answer. Using less gas means fewer molecular interactions. Fewer molecular interactions results in behavior more like that of an ideal gas. The reduced number of interactions is the result of there being fewer molecules and fewer instances where molecules are close together. Choice A is a better answer than choice B. The question stem says the thermometer is most accurate when the gas behaves like an ideal gas, but does not mention characteristics of the fluid in the gauge. Choices C and D are unlikely to be the best answer.

681. D is the best answer. The ideal gas law is as follows: $PV = nRT$. Rearranging for n, the equation becomes $n = PV/RT$. Note that, for one mole of a given gas, PV/RT will always equal one. A positive deviation is when this number is greater than one, and a negative deviation is when this number is less than one. Although it is true that real gases exhibit intermolecular forces, this fact would likely lead to decreased pressure, which leads to a negative deviation. Choice A can be eliminated. While it is true that real gases will have less kinetic energy due to imperfectly elastic collisions, this would likely lead to gas molecules colliding with the vessel wall at decreased velocities, generating a lower force. Recall that Pressure = Force/Area. Less force results in less pressure, leading to a negative deviation. Choice B can be eliminated. It is true that gases deviate from ideality in high pressure, low temperature environments, but this broad statement does not describe why a positive deviation might occur. Choice C can be eliminated. Real gases have volume. Note that increasing the volume term in PV/RT would lead to a number greater than one. Choice D is the best answer.

682. A is the best answer. An ideal gas is defined by the formula $PV = nRT$. When $n = 1$ mole, $PV/RT = 1$ for an ideal gas. Deviations from ideal behavior are greatest at lower temperatures. T_1 shows the greatest deviation, so it is the lowest temperature, followed by T_2, then T_3. Choice A is the best answer. Choice B is the opposite of choice A, the best answer. The relationships only make sense when degree of deviation correlates with either lower or higher temperature, ruling out choices C and D.

683. C is the best answer. T_3 is the closest to a straight line at $PV/RT = 1$, which would be true if the gas was an ideal gas. Choice C is the best answer. Choices A and B have curves that extend further up the graph than the ideal line, and they are not similar in degree of ideality, ruling out choice D.

684. D is the best answer. Since $n = PV/RT$, doubling the number of moles, doubles the PV/RT. At 600 atm and 1 mole, T_1 has a PV/RT value of 2. Doubling the number of moles to two moles would give a value of 4. Choice A would be the value for a mole of ideal gas. Choice B would be the value at 600 atm and T_1 for 1 mole. Choice C is another distractor that is the result of arithmetic errors. Choice D is the best answer.

685. A is the best answer. If the ideal gas law is correct, one mole of gas will result in a value of one for PV/RT when R equals 0.08206 L atm K^{-1} mol^{-1}. According to the graph, this occurs at pressures of 0 atm and 500 atm for CO_2. With the graph above, this is where the curve intersects with $y = 1$. Choice B is not where ideal behavior occurs for any of the gases displayed in the graph, ruling out choice B. Choice C only gives one value where CO_2 behaves ideally. Choice D is well above where any of the gases intersect with $y = 1$.

686. D is the best answer. Using the ideal gas law, PV/RT equals 1. In the real methane, $PV/RT < 1$ at 200 atm, and $PV/RT > 1$ at 600 atm. The calculated V must be greater than the real V at 200 atm and less than real V at 600 atm. Choice D is the best answer, and all other choices include at least one wrong prediction of real volume.

687. D is the best answer. The graph does not give information about temperature because the samples are all at the same temperature. Choices A and B are unlikely since the information is not present in the graph. At high pressures, $PV/RT > 1$ for all samples. A greater than one value for PV/RT indicates a deviation due mainly to volume because real volume is greater than ideal volume. Choice D is a stronger answer than choice C. Choice C represents lower than expected pressure due to attractive forces.

688. A is the best answer. a reflects how strongly the molecules are attracted to each other. b is a measure of the actual volume occupied by just the molecules in a gas. Increasing molecular mass and structural complexity increases attractions and volume. Since both factors increase deviation, choice A is the best answer and all other choices can be ruled out.

689. D is the best answer. These are all noble gases, so they have comparable structural complexity. Thus, a and b values will tend to increase with molecular size. Choice D, the largest gas molecule/atom will be the least ideal gas. Choices A, B, and C are smaller and can be ruled out since they will behave more ideally.

The Liquid and Solid Phases

690. D is the best answer. All molecules exert LDFs, but they are not very strong. Choice A is a possibility. Hydrogen bonds may only occur when a hydrogen atom is bonded to fluorine, oxygen, or nitrogen. This is not the case in acetone, ruling out choice B. Because the question asks for the bonds between molecules, covalent bonds do not apply. Choice C can be ruled out. Acetone has polar bonds, so the primary interaction between the molecules is dipole-dipole. Choice D is a stronger answer than choice A.

691. A is the best answer. Liquids possess more intermolecular bonds than gases, indicating that, at STP, water possesses more intermolecular bonds than carbon dioxide. Recall that hydrogen bonding occurs between a hydrogen atom that is covalently bonded to a fluorine, oxygen, or nitrogen atom and a fluorine, oxygen, or nitrogen atom from another molecule. The difference in electronegativity between the hydrogen and other atoms generates a dipole moment, which allows for hydrogen bonding to occur. Note that water is able to hydrogen bond, whereas carbon dioxide cannot. Choice A is a strong answer. These stronger interactions reduce the likelihood of transitioning to gaseous phase. Although water has a bent molecular geometry, it is the dipole moment that allows for hydrogen bonding, not the geometry itself. Choice B can be eliminated. Although carbon dioxide has a greater molar mass than water, this does not affect intermolecular bonding. Choice C can be eliminated. Carbon dioxide possesses a greater number of orbitals and, intuitively, these orbitals would generate greater electron repulsion within an individual carbon dioxide molecule. However, this intramolecular repulsion does not explain intermolecular bonding capabilities and discrepancies in phase change. Choice D can be eliminated. Choice A is the best answer.

692. A is the best answer. Cyclohexane has no net dipole moment, so the only intermolecular interactions are London dispersion forces. Choice A is the best answer. Choices B and D can be ruled out since the lack of dipole moment makes hydrogen bonding and dipole-dipole interactions impossible. Because the question asks for the bonds between molecules, covalent bonds, choice C does not apply.

693. B is the best answer. There is no hydrogen bonding in hydrocarbons since they purely consist of carbon and hydrogen. Choice A is eliminated. Choice B involves saturated hydrocarbon flexibility and fitting closer, increasing intermolecular forces between chains and tails. Choice B is a strong answer. Saturated hydrocarbons do not form dimers, ruling out choice C. As for choice D, energy is not needed for the phase change from liquid to solid.

694. B is the best answer. The length of the chain affects the fluidity because longer chains are able to form stronger London dispersion forces. Hydrocarbons have primarily nonpolar bonds, so LDFs are the major intermolecular force. There are few dipole-dipole interactions and hydrogen bonding, ruling out choices A and C. Choice D is an intramolecular bond, not intermolecular. Choice B is the best answer.

695. B is the best answer. Molecules of a solid vibrate in place, even though this phase is the most closely packed of the three main phases. Choice A can be ruled out since the molecules are not motionless. Choice B is a strong answer. Choices C and D describe liquids and gases respectively, so both can be eliminated.

696. B is the best answer. Although water does contain covalent bonds, they do not break during melting. Intermolecular forces define phases and phase change, not intramolecular forces. This rules out options I and II, leaving only option III, choice B.

Calorimetry

697. B is the best answer. Choice A can be ruled out since the value is too small. The temperature in this problem is given in terms of change in temperature. Change in temperature is the same when measured in Kelvin or degrees centigrade. Thus, choice B is the best answer as the mass and temperature change magnitude are still the same. Choice C mistakenly adds 273, the conversion factor between Celsius and Kelvin, to the initial 35 cal. Choice D is too high of a value, and can be ruled out.

698. C is the best answer. From the equation $q = mc\Delta T$, the large pot requires more energy than the small pot. Choices A and B can be ruled out. Since the pot is losing heat to its surrounding environment throughout the heating process, the most efficient way to heat it is quickly. If heating is slow, more energy is lost to surroundings so more total heat is required. Choice C is the best answer, and choice D can be ruled out.

699. B is the best answer. Choice A is a possible answer, but the best answer here is choice B. "Specific" in thermodynamics indicates per unit mass. Specific heat is the energy necessary to change the temperature of 1 g of a substance by 1 K. Heat capacity is a more general term that can be used applied to various objects and masses. Choice C applies to a whole mole, and choice D applies to a specific volume, not mass. Choices C and D can be ruled out.

700. B is the best answer. Heat capacity could be considered a measure of how hard it is to change the temperature of a substance. Since block X changes temperature more easily, it must have lower specific heat and heat capacity. Choice A can be ruled out. Choice B is a strong answer. No conclusions can be drawn about the volumes and densities of the metals since the masses are identical. Choices C and D can be ruled out.

701. C is the best answer. A high heat capacity means that water gains or loses energy with smaller changes in temperature. This corresponds to options I and III, basically stating that the baseline temperature of the body is resistant to change. Since option II is not in the final answer, choice C is the best answer.

702. A is the best answer. Reactions in coffee cup calorimeters take place at constant pressure. At constant pressure, the energy transfer (q) is approximately equal to the enthalpy change. Choice A is the best answer. Coffee cup calorimeters do not measure entropy, Gibbs free energy, or total energy change, so choices B, C, and D can be ruled out.

703. B is the best answer. Convection through a single Styrofoam cup is already effectively zero: convection requires some fluid (liquid or gas) to pass through the surface. Choice A can be ruled out. Choice B is a strong answer since conduction is less likely to occur through two layers of insulation. Choice C can be ruled out since the calorimeter's heat capacity is irrelevant and the main concern is heat capacity of the solvent within the calorimeter. Choice D is a distractor and can be ruled out. Tipping over the cup is not a major concern, and the risk of doing so is unlikely to be affected by having two Styrofoam cups instead of one.

704. A is the best answer. The solution will heat up during an exothermic reaction making the solution hotter than the environment. If the experimenter leaves the lid off, energy escapes from the top and the temperature of the solution does not rise as much as it should, so ΔT is low. From $q = mc\Delta T$, the calculated q will be lower than if the lid was properly kept on. That means that the ΔH will be low. Choice A is a strong answer. Choice B is the opposite of the best answer. Choice C can be ruled out since some heat is lost to the environment. Choice D can be ruled out since the enthalpy change will always be underestimated in terms of magnitude.

705. C is the best answer. The internal energy of a system and the enthalpy of a system cannot be measured with a coffee cup calorimeter, ruling out options I and II. Change in enthalpy can be measured and calculated based on the change in temperature of the solvent present within the calorimeter. Option III only, choice C, is the best answer.

706. A is the best answer. The experimenter observes a temperature change and uses the temperature change to calculate the amount of heat released (or absorbed) in the reaction. If the heat capacity of part of the system is ignored, then the heat generated or absorbed will be underestimated. Thus, choice A is the best answer. Choice B is the opposite of the best answer. Choice C can be ruled out since the value will not be accurate if part of the system is ignored. The heat of solution will be underestimated every time, ruling out choice D.

Phase Changes

707. B is the best answer. Melting requires energy, making it an endothermic process. Choice A can be eliminated. Choice B is a strong answer since the temperature is likely to remain constant, as with phase change for most substances. Energy goes into changing intermolecular bonding, not changing temperature. Choice C can be ruled out because while additional kinetic energy is added, the molecules begin to move more freely. Nothing present in the question stem supports the statement in choice D, ruling it out.

708. C is the best answer. Ice, water, and water vapor are all present. The ice and water are at the interface temperature between liquid and solid, the freezing/melting point. There is water vapor present in the air of the room, making choice C the best answer.

709. D is the best answer. During each process, added energy goes into breaking bonds, not increasing temperature. Thus, temperature stays consistent throughout each of the processes listed in options I, II, and III. Choice D is the best answer.

710. A is the best answer. The heat of fusion is used when a solid changes to a liquid; vaporization is the conversion of liquid to vapor; and sublimation is the conversion of a solid to vapor. So sublimation should be the two processes together. No heat added for the purpose of temperature change is needed since this is a direct change. The sum will be just the two heats of phase change. Choice A is the best answer. Both processes of melting and boiling require heat, so subtraction does not make sense. Choice B can be ruled out. Choices C and D can be ruled out since heat transfer in processes like this would not be multiplied or divided. The heat of sublimation would be the sum of the two heats of simpler phase changes.

711. D is the best answer. One gram of H_2O would require 80 cal to melt it, 100 cal to raise the temperature to 100°C, and 540 cal to boil it. One hundred grams requires 100 times that much heat. Choice A can be ruled out since it only adds the heats of fusion and vaporization for 1 gram. Choice B can be ruled out since it does not consider heat added to increase temperature. Choice C only considers heat added to increase temperature and does it incorrectly by a factor of 10. Choice D is the best answer since it correctly multiplies the sum of heat of fusion, heat required for temperature change, and heat of vaporization, by 100 g.

712. D is the best answer. For 1 gram, 80 calories are required to heat the water from 20°C to 100°C, but 540 calories are required to convert it to steam. This is because $540/80 > 6$. Thus, more than six times the original time period is required to turn water to steam as to heat it up. Since this is true for one gram, it is true for any amount. Choices A, B, and C all represent times that are less than or equal to an hour, so these choices can be ruled out. It would actually take more than one hour to vaporize all of the water, making choice D the best answer.

713. A is the best answer. Solid phase is on the left part of the diagram, followed by liquid phase in the upper right, and gas phase on the lower right. This is an important detail to memorize for the exam. One way to memorize this is to consider the pressure extreme. At high pressure and low to normal temperature, the molecules will be packed into a solid. At low to normal pressure, and high temperature, the molecules will be spread out into gas phase. Liquid phase is in the middle. Choice A is the best answer. All other choices mistakenly assign regions to phases.

714. C is the best answer. Consider which temperatures allow for the transition between liquid and gas since this temperature is the boiling point of water. Only T goes through the equilibrium line between liquid and gas. Thus, choice C is the best answer. Water can undergo deposition at the temperatures represented by lines R and S, while U represents the temperature at the critical point of water. Choices A, B, and D can be ruled out.

715. D is the best answer. A phase diagram with pressure and temperature on it is required to answer this question. The impact of pressure on melting point varies between substances. For example, for most substances it will increase melting point. However, with substances like water, whose solid phase is less dense than liquid phase, a pressure increase will decrease melting point. Choices A, B, and C can be ruled out. Choice D is the best answer.

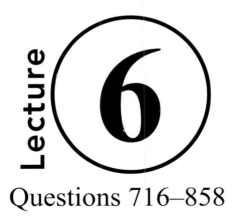

Lecture 6

Questions 716–858

Solutions and Electrochemistry

ANSWERS & EXPLANATIONS

ANSWER KEY										
716. C	729. A	742. D	755. B	768. B	781. A	794. C	807. A	820. B	833. B	846. B
717. C	730. A	743. C	756. B	769. A	782. C	795. A	808. A	821. C	834. A	847. D
718. A	731. D	744. D	757. D	770. B	783. D	796. C	809. D	822. C	835. D	848. B
719. C	732. A	745. C	758. C	771. A	784. C	797. B	810. C	823. B	836. D	849. B
720. C	733. D	746. A	759. C	772. B	785. D	798. A	811. A	824. A	837. A	850. B
721. C	734. B	747. D	760. D	773. A	786. D	799. C	812. A	825. B	838. A	851. C
722. C	735. B	748. C	761. D	774. B	787. B	800. C	813. C	826. C	839. A	852. C
723. A	736. C	749. A	762. A	775. C	788. C	801. D	814. A	827. D	840. B	853. A
724. D	737. C	750. B	763. A	776. B	789. A	802. D	815. B	828. D	841. C	854. A
725. D	738. D	751. B	764. C	777. C	790. C	803. A	816. B	829. B	842. D	855. C
726. A	739. A	752. C	765. C	778. B	791. A	804. B	817. C	830. A	843. B	856. D
727. D	740. B	753. C	766. B	779. B	792. B	805. D	818. A	831. B	844. C	857. C
728. B	741. A	754. A	767. C	780. B	793. A	806. B	819. C	832. D	845. C	858. D

Solution Chemistry

716. C is the best answer. The molarity of a solution is the number of moles of solute per liter of solution; since density changes with temperature, the volume of the solution can change when the temperature changes. So, option I does change with temperature, and choices A and D can be eliminated. The molality of a solution is the number moles of solute per kilogram of solvent; both of these variables are temperature-independent. So option II must be a component of the best answer, and choice B can be eliminated. The mole fraction of a solution is the number of moles of solute divided by the number of moles of solution. So option III is a component of the best answer, which confirms choice C is the best answer.

717. C is the best answer. Molarity is defined as moles per liter of *solution*, not per liter of solvent. In options I and II, the volume of water is added to the solute which would make the final volume the volume of solution. So, options I and II are components of the best answer, and choices A and B can be eliminated. The procedure described in option III would yield 500.0 mL of solvent rather than of solution. When the sodium chloride is added to the 500.0 mL of solution, the volume would increase slightly and the volume of solution would be slightly greater than 500.0 mL and the molarity would be slightly less than 2.000 M. So, option III is not a component of the best answer, and choice D can be eliminated. This leaves choice C as the best answer.

718. A is the best answer. Assume that 1.8 kg of water is 1.8 L since at room temperature, the density of water is very close to 1 g/mL. 18.0 grams of sucrose is 0.1 moles because (18.0 g)/(180 g/mol) = 0.1 mol. Molarity is moles per liter. So the molarity of the solution is 0.1 mol/1.8 L = 0.056 M, and choice A is the best answer.

719. C is the best answer. The molality of a solution is the number of moles of solute per kilogram of solvent. To find the moles of NaOH first determine the molecular weight, which is ~40 AMU. So the number of moles of NaOH is (30 g)/(40 g/mol) = 0.75 mol. The number of kilograms of solvent is (100 g)(1 kg/1000 g) = 0.1 kg. This gives a molality of 0.75 mol/0.1 kg = 7.5 m.

720. C is the best answer. Parts per million is equal to mg/liter. 0.1 moles of NaCl is 5.8 grams or 5800 milligrams because the molecular weight of NaCl is ~58 g/mol and (58 g/mol) × (0.1 mol) = 5.8 g. Round this to 6000 milligrams and divided by 60 liters. This gives 100 ppm. The closest answer is choice C.

721. C is the best answer. First of all, note the position of the elements on the periodic table: they are all in the same period. Density is a trend that is difficult to predict from periodic table trends. Mass increases from left to right but volume is variable depending on the electron shells. This variability results in the highest density elements being in the middle of a period and the lower density elements on the sides. So choices A and B can be eliminated. Between choices C and D, the lowest density element for any period is always the one in the first group, so choice C is the best answer.

722. C is the best answer. Diamond is solid so it will be the densest, and choice A can be eliminated. Choices B, C and D are all diatomic gases. Between choices B, C, and D, nitrogen is the least dense because it has the smallest mass and density is mass divided by volume. The volume can be thought of as the atomic radius. The elements further to the right on a period have a smaller atomic radius because they have a more positive nucleus that pulls in the electrons closer to the nucleus. With increased mass and decreased volume, element to the right of a period generally have the highest density. This trend is not perfect but it works on MCAT® questions.

723. A is the best answer. Density is mass divided by volume. The mass of an element increases from left to right down a period. The volume, which can be approximated by atomic radius, is more difficult to predict because it depends on the charge of the nucleus and which electron shells are present. Argon is naturally a monoatomic mass. Chlorine is a diatomic gas so it is has more mass and likely a higher density. So, choice A is better than choice B. Phosphorus occurs naturally as a solid, so choice A is still the best answer, and choice C can be eliminated. Sulfur is naturally a solid, so choice A is the best answer, and choice D can be eliminated.

724. D is the best answer. The volume of the block is $3 \times 5 \times 8$ cm $= 120$ cm$^3 = 1.2 \times 10^{-4}$ m^3. The density is 2 kg/1.2 $\times 10^{-4}$ m$^3 = 1.67 \times 10^4$ kg/m^3.

725. D is the best answer. Radioactive decay generally occurs through emission of a small particle like an alpha, beta, or positron particle. Argon is likely not a radioactive decay product of xenon because the atomic numbers are so far apart. Choice A can be eliminated. Choice B may be a factual statement but it does not answer the question. If argon is the most stable, it would probably be the most abundant in the universe. Choice B is not completely ruled out but there is likely a better answer. Greenhouse gases are made by the combustion of hydrocarbons and include CO_2, CH_4 and O_3. Argon is not made in the process so choice C can be eliminated. Choice D is factual and logical. The density of argon is similar to that of nitrogen whereas helium has a very low density. Helium rises up to the top of the atmosphere and escapes completely, making it less abundant. Since argon has a similar density to the atmosphere, it remains mixed in the atmosphere unable to escape, so choice D is the best answer.

726. A is the best answer. It is a general trend that the solubility of salts increases with temperature. So, choice A is a strong answer, and choice B can be eliminated. Adding more NaCl to a solution will increase the concentration of the solution by not the maximum concentration that can dissolve, so choice C can be eliminated. Adding water will increase the amount of NaCl that will dissolve, but it will not increase the concentration, so choice D can be eliminated.

727. D is the best answer. Solubility increases with increasing temperature, so choice A is not the best answer. The solvent is the liquid that is dissolving the solute. Typically, the solvent is water but if the solvent was ethanol, the K_{sp} would certainly change so choice B is the best answer. For K_{sp} the reactants are solid and thus ignored in the calculation, so choice C is not the best answer. Solubility is a relative concept. Typically, compounds with solubility less than 0.01 mol/L are considered insoluble, so choice D is not true and thus is the best answer.

728. B is the best answer. Recall that the hydroxide of Ba is considered soluble while the carbonates are insoluble except for alkali metal and ammonium compounds. The sulfides are insoluble except for alkali metal, ammonium ion, and Ba^{2+}, Ca^{2+}, and Sr^{2+} compounds. Barium hydroxide dissociates into three particles, so the equation will be $K_{sp} = [Ba^{2+}][OH^-]^2 = (x)(2x)^2$. For barium hydroxide x is greater than 0.01. $NiCO_3$ and FeS each dissociate into two particles, so their solubility is given by $K_{sp} = x^2$. x for these compounds is less than 0.01.

729. A is the best answer. Ion pairing removes ions from the equilibrium expression shifting the equilibrium to the right. So, choice A is a strong answer. Although K_{sp} does change with changes in temperature, the final equilibrium will not change if the solution becomes warm. Eventually, heat generated from the exothermic reaction would dissipate and at equilibrium the K_{sp} would again be the one in the table. So, choice B is the best answer. Choice C is not the best answer because this fact is already considered in the formula for K_{sp}. Choice D is already taken into account by the equilibrium expression and a basic solution would shift the equilibrium to the left.

730. A is the best answer. Silver nitrate is soluble. The silver ions dramatically decrease the solubility of the silver carbonate due to the common ion effect, so choice C can be eliminated. The remaining compounds all dissociate into the same number of particles and none are affected by the common ion effect. So, the compound with the highest K_{sp} will be the best answer.

731. D is the best answer. An unsaturated solution is not in equilibrium like a saturated solution. In a saturated solution there is an equal amount of solvent leaving and entering the aqueous state at all time which describes equilibrium. There is no clear applicability of this term to an unsaturated solution, so choice A is not the best answer. Choice B describes a supersaturated solution but does not apply to an unsaturated solution, so choice B is not the best answer. Choice C describes a saturated solution in the same way choice A does, so choice C is not the best answer. A decrease in temperature decreases solubility so an unsaturated solution may become saturated, and choice D is the best answer.

732. A is the best answer. Both sodium and nitrate ions form highly soluble salts, so choices B and D can be eliminated. The dissolution of $PbCl_2$ is given by the following reaction: $PbCl_2(s) \rightarrow Pb^{2+}(aq) + 2Cl^-(aq)$, giving $K_{sp} = [Pb^{2+}][Cl^-]^2$. The final volume of the mixture is 1000 mL, so there will be some dilution.

$[Pb^{2+}] = (0.01 \text{ M}) \times (900 \text{ mL}/1000 \text{ mL}) = 0.009 \text{ M}$, while $[Cl^-] = (0.2 \text{ M}) \times (100 \text{ mL}/1000 \text{ mL}) = 0.02 \text{ M}$.

So Q is less than $(0.009 \text{ M}) \times (0.02 \text{ M})^2 = 3.6 \times 10^{-6}$), which is less than K_{sp}. Therefore, the solution is unsaturated and lead(II) chloride will not precipitate making choice A the best answer.

733. D is the best answer. Fill in the units for each number to find the correct answer. 1.8×10^{-10} is the K_{sp} which has units of $(\text{mol/L})^2$ because $K_{sp} = [Ag^+][NO^{3-}]$. 6.0 is M or mol/L. 20.0 is mL. 58.4 is the g/mol of NaCl. 1000 is mL/L. The only way the units cancel out to give grams (g) is if the 6.0 is in the denominator and the 20.0 is in the numerator, so choice D is the best answer.

734. B is the best answer. Choice A is not the best answer because temperature is proportional to the square of the velocity: $KE = 3/2kT$. A greater proportion of heat energy is absorbed by the vibration of the hydrogen-oxygen bonds of water than by the bonds of most molecules, so choice B is the best answer. Choice C is not the best answer because bond breakage would lead to a phase change; it is not a significant factor in determining the heat capacity of a phase. Choice D is not the best answer because bond formation releases energy.

735. B is the best answer. The fluid is probably somewhat polar in order to mix with water, so choice A can be eliminated. Since it is not completely miscible with water at room temperature, choice C can be eliminated. It is hard to know if Fluid X is more or less polar than water however the hint is in the paragraph included before the figure. The paragraph states Fluid X is organic meaning it is composed of C, H and O. Hydrocarbons, even those that are oxygenated are less polar than water, so choice B is the best answer.

736. C is the best answer. Gases almost always exist in one phase unless there is a large difference in density. There is not in the case of water and ether, so choice A is not the best answer. The ether and water will separate into two liquid phases due to the polarity difference, so choice B can be eliminated. Choice D can be eliminated because liquids have a vapor pressure, which is a force that allows molecules to enter the gas phase. This leave choice C as the best answer.

737. C is the best answer. Solvent layers are visibly distinct layers stacked on top of each other inside a fluid-filled beaker. Two solvent layers are formed when aqueous compounds do not have favorable interactions with each other and instead remain in a "layer" with other molecules that they do have favorable interactions with. Methanol (CH_3OH) has a permanent dipole moment, indicating that it is a polar molecule. Other polar molecules would have favorable interactions with methanol and not form a second solvent layer. Toluene (choice A) is nonpolar and would not have favorable interactions with methanol. Choice A can be eliminated. Although the alcohol group of choice B does have a permanent dipole, the remainder of the molecular is a nonpolar hydrocarbon. Choice B can be eliminated. Acetone (choice C) has a strong permanent dipole across the carbonyl double bond. This is likely to result in favorable dipole-dipole interactions with methanol, resulting in a single solvent layer. Choice C is a strong answer. Phenylalanine (choice D) possesses a bulky, non-polar side group that will not bond favorably with methanol. Choice D can be eliminated. Choice C is the best answer.

738. D is the best answer. Water is being poured into a beaker of diethyl ether: water is a solute, and diethyl ether is the solvent. Water is a polar molecule capable of hydrogen bonding with itself. Diethyl ether is nonpolar, does not exhibit a dipole moment, and cannot hydrogen bond. Nonpolar molecules are held together by weak intermolecular bonds between instantaneous dipoles. These weak bonds cannot break the much stronger hydrogen bonds of the solute. Choice A can be eliminated. The solvent is nonpolar. Choice B can be eliminated. Although the nonpolar solvent does exhibit weaker intermolecular interactions, this does not accurately describe what happens when water is poured into diethyl ether. Choice C can be eliminated. Water's permanent dipole moment is what allows it to hydrogen bond with itself and what makes its intermolecular interactions much stronger than that of diethyl ether. Choice D is the best answer.

739. A is the best answer. Note that all alkanes are nonpolar molecules. Nonpolar molecules can exhibit intermolecular interactions, called London dispersion forces or Van der Waals' forces, due to instantaneous dipole formation. Instantaneous dipoles occur because electrons move about, and at any given moment they may not be distributed exactly between two bonding atoms even when the atoms have equivalent electronegativity. More electrons allows for more instantaneous dipoles, allowing for greater intermolecular interactions and higher boiling points. Choice A is a strong answer. Although molecular weight does increase with boiling point, this increase is due to increased Van der Waals', not the molecular weight itself. Choice B can be eliminated in favor of choice A. Increased *inter*molecular interactions generate greater boiling points, not *intra*molecular interactions. Choice C can be eliminated. Although London dispersion forces do increase the boiling point, this is independent of hydrogen ion concentration. Choice D can be eliminated. Choice A is the best answer.

Vapor Pressure

740. B is the best answer. Gases become less soluble in water as the water temperature increases; at higher temperatures, the increased entropy of the gas is more of a factor, so choice B is the best answer, and choices A, C, and D can be eliminated.

741. A is the best answer. Fractional distillation distills based on differential boiling points of two liquids in a solution. For water and ethanol, there exists a point where the distillation cannot proceed. This occurs at the trough in the diagram above. Essentially, at this point, the mole fraction of ethanol in the vapor is equal to that of ethanol in solution, so boiling no longer selectively removes water. At the trough, the solution is 95% ethanol and has a boiling point of 79.2°C, so choice A is the best answer. Choice B is the boiling point of pure ethanol, which cannot be obtained by this method. Of note, this is why alcohol that is bought for consumption almost never exceeds 190 proof, which is 95% ethanol. Chemists can purchase pure ethanol, but it is not obtained via fractional distillation. Choice C is a made up number that has no significance in the figure. Choice D is the boiling point of pure water.

742. D is the best answer. Volatile liquids have very high vapor pressures, meaning many molecules exist in the gas phase just above the liquid. So, the mole fraction (χ) of molecule A should be greater than molecule B, and choices A and C can be eliminated. Choice B is too extreme, molecule B is weakly volatile so some will be present above the solution. Choice D is the best answer.

743. C is the best answer. Remember from vapor pressure that solids and liquids can be in equilibrium with their vapor pressures. So, choices A and B can be eliminated, and choice C is a strong answer. Choice D is not the best answer because the triple point is the point on a phase diagram where all phases are in equilibrium.

744. D is the best answer. Density does not always predict a change in boiling point, so choice A is not the best answer. A lower boiling point is associated with greater kinetic energy of molecules, so choice B is not the best answer. Cooling a liquid would not change the boiling point, which is independent of the present temperature of a solution, so choice C is the best answer. The solute molecules occupy some of the positions at the surface of the liquid and block liquid molecules from escaping the liquid. This lowers vapor pressure. Boiling occurs when vapor pressure equals atmospheric pressure, so a lower vapor pressure results in a higher boiling point, and choice D is the best answer.

745. C is the best answer. Skip the long Raoult's law calculation: the vapor pressure of an ideal solution must be intermediate between the vapor pressure of its components, and only one answer satisfies this requirement. Choices A, B and D can be eliminated, and choice C is the best answer.

746. A is the best answer. High altitudes have lower atmospheric pressure. Water boils when its vapor pressure equals its atmospheric pressure, so water boils at a lower temperature and at high altitudes. So, boiling water is actually hotter at low altitude. It is not the boiling that cooks the egg, it's the temperature. So, an egg will cook more quickly at low altitudes, and choice A is the best answer. Choice B is the opposite of what occurs, water takes longer to boil because it must get hotter at low altitudes. Choice C is also an opposite, water is hotter a lower altitudes. Choice D is also an opposite; water has a lower vapor pressure when boiling at high altitudes.

747. D is the best answer. Choices A, B and C can be eliminated because they are too absolute. Remember: there are always exceptions to "always" statements. Choice C is a weaker answer than choice D because there can be deviations to Raoult's law causing a lower of vapor pressure even when adding a substance with a higher vapor pressure.

748. C is the best answer. The rate of evaporation is dictated by the temperature, so it remains constant, so choices A, B and D can be eliminate. As molecules fill the space above the liquid, the rate of condensation (molecules reentering the solution) increases until the rates are equal making choice C the best answer.

749. A is the best answer. At higher temperatures, vapor pressures are higher, so choice A is better than choices B and D. Nonvolatile solutes (such as salts) lower vapor pressure, so choices C can be eliminated, and choice A is the best answer.

Solubility

750. B is the best answer. Choice A would not increase mass, so it can be eliminated. Both choices B and C give a mechanism for adding mass to the solution, but in case choice C this will not be detected. This is because the mass of a solution is always calculated by taking the total mass of the solution and container and subtracting the mass of the container. If some of the container dissolves, it does not matter—its mass (the tare) will still be subtracted from the total. Choice D would result in a decreased, not increased mass, so choice D can be eliminated, and choice B is the best answer.

751. B is the best answer. The names of polyatomic anions containing oxygen include the suffixes –ite and –ate. –ate is used for the most common oxyanion. –ite is used for the anion with the same charge but one less oxygen. Hypo- means low, indicating the species with one less oxygen than the –ite species. The prefix per- is added to the beginning of the name for the species with one more oxygen than the -ate species. So, choice A is hypochlorite. Choice B is chlorite. Choice C is chlorate. Choice D is perchlorate. Choice B is the best answer.

752. C is the best answer. The bicarbonate ion is the conjugate base of carbonic acid: H_2CO_3 which is HCO_3^-, so choice C is the best answer. The other ions are not formed by dissociation of H_2CO_3.

753. C is the best answer. Alkali metals, nitrates, ammonium salts, and sulfates (with noted exceptions) are soluble in water. So, choice A is not the best answer. Choice B is not the best answer because the sulfate salts it names as exceptions are the ones that are insoluble. Choice C is the best answer because carbonate ions are usually insoluble. Choice D is not the best answer because ammonium salts are soluble.

754. A is the best answer. Halogen compounds are soluble except for salts of silver, mercury, and lead which are choices B, C and D, respectively.

755. B is the best answer. Hydroxides are insoluble except for calcium, barium, strontium, and the alkali metals, so choices A, C and D can be eliminated, and choice B is the best answer.

756. B is the best answer. Sulfur compounds are insoluble except for calcium barium, strontium, alkali metals, and ammonium salts. So choices A, C, and D can be eliminated, and choice B is the best answer.

757. D is the best answer. Choice A describes part of a hydration reaction but is incomplete. Choice B describes a part of hydration where intramolecular solute bonds are broken, but choice B is incomplete. Likewise, choice C describes park of hydration where water-solute bonds are formed, but choice C is still incomplete. Choice D is the best answer because it describes two of the three things that occur in a hydration reaction. Water-water bonds are broken, solute-solute bonds are broken, and solute-water bonds are formed. Choice D is the most complete and is thus the best answer.

758. C is the best answer. Hydrochloric acid, or HCl, acts as the acid in this reaction. Choice A is not the best answer. The base in this reaction must then be H_2O, so choice B is also not the best answer. It is important to note that the common convention is to call reactants the "acids" and "bases", while calling the products "conjugate acids" and "conjugate bases". If H_2O is the base in this reaction, then the conjugate acid should be H_2O with an added hydrogen ion. This new molecule would be H_3O^+, so choice C is the best answer. HCl is the "acid" in this reaction, then the conjugate base should be the same molecule with a hydrogen ion removed. Cl^- is the conjugate base, so choice D is not the best answer.

759. C is the best answer. Salts that are dissolved in water dissociate into their respective ions. Each ion is surrounded by water molecules of opposite charge in order to neutralize the charge of the ion. The water molecules point their partially positive hydrogen atoms towards the anions and their partially negative oxygen atoms towards the cations. This process is called hydration, and the number of water molecules that surround a given ion is called the hydration number. The number of water molecules that must surround an ion for hydration to occur increases with increasing size and charge of the ion. SO_4^{2-} has the same absolute value of charge than Ca^{2+} but has a greater size. SO_4^{2-} likely has a greater hydration number. Choice A can be eliminated. HCO_3^- is larger than Na^+ and likely has a greater hydration number. Choice B can be eliminated. Cl^- has a smaller charge and size than Ca^{2+}, so Ca^{2+} likely has a greater hydration number. SO_4^{2-} has the same absolute value of charge than Ca^{2+} but has a larger size. SO_4^{2-} likely has a greater hydration number than Ca^{2+}. Choice C is a strong answer. Choice D would be correct, except for the fact that it incorrectly lists a positive charge above what should be HCO_3^-. Choice D can be eliminated. Choice C is the best answer.

760. D is the best answer. Choice A describes the solubility of an ion, which is not related to the hydration number, so choice A is not the best answer. Choice B describes the exact opposite of the hydration number, so choice B is not the best answer. Choice C is describing a concept related to the solubility of an ion, so choice C is not the best answer. When an ion is hydrated, it is surrounded and bonded by water molecules. The average number of water molecules bonding to an ion is that ions hydration number. The hydration number varies but is often 4 or 6. This is described in choice D, so choice D is the best answer.

761. D is the best answer. The heat of hydration is the enthalpy change when a gaseous solute is dissolved in water. It involves the breaking of water-water bonds, which is endothermic, and the forming of solute-water bonds, which is exothermic. (Since the solute is gaseous, there are no solute-solute bonds.) The net result can be either endo- or exothermic, so choice D is the best answer. "Always" statements are often not the best answers on the MCAT®.

762. A is the best answer. Acidic solutions have fewer hydroxide ions and increase solubility of calcium hydroxide based on the common ion effect, so choice A is the best answer. In neutral and basic solutions, there are more hydroxide anions which push the solubility reaction towards formation of solid, so choices B, C and D can be eliminated.

763. A is the best answer. Le Châtelier's principle, also known as the common-ion effect, can be used with the following equation:

$$NaCl(s) \rightarrow Na^+(aq) + Cl^-(aq)$$

Because hydrochloric acid will add chloride to the solution, it will drive the reaction to the left and reduce the solubility of sodium chloride. So choice A is the best answer, and choices B, C and D can be eliminated.

764. C is the best answer. Adding protons pushes the reaction toward formation of HF which allows more CaF_2 to dissolve, so choices A and B can be eliminated. The chloride ions are spectator ions and have no effect on the reaction, so choice D can be eliminated, and choice C is the best answer.

765. C is the best answer. Adding protons pushes the reaction toward formation of HF which allows more CaF_2 to dissolve. The question says a very small amount of calcium was then added, this implies the amount of calcium is much less than the amount of HCl. So, there is unlikely to be a precipitate and choices A and B can be eliminated. Supersaturated solutions are usually made by changing the temperature, so choice D is not the best answer, and choice C should be selected.

766. B is the best answer. Due to the parietal cell production of HCl, the stomach is a highly acidic environment (pH < 7). Magnesium hydroxide (Mg_2OH) dissociates into $Mg^{2+}(aq)$ and $2OH^-$. The presence of H^+ in the stomach leads to the following reaction: $H^+ + OH^- \rightarrow H_2O(l)$. This decreases the concentration of OH^-. Further note that OH^- is a product in the solvation of Mg_2OH. Decreasing the concentration of OH^- thus increases the solubility of Mg_2OH. This will result in equilibrium with more Mg^{2+}, but there is no indication that this equilibrium will be reached any faster. Choice A can be eliminated, and choice B is a strong answer. The H^+ ions increase the solubility of Mg_2OH due to the OH^- neutralization reaction with H^+. Choice C can be eliminated. This reaction only generates aqueous ions, no gases. Choice D can be eliminated. Choice B is the best answer.

767. C is the best answer. Iodine is I_2, iodide is I^-. The reaction of iodine with iodide continually removes iodine from solution. This reaction is $I_2 + I^- \rightarrow I_3^-$. By Le Châtelier's principle, the equilibrium for the reaction $I_2(s) \leftrightarrow I_2(aq)$ shifts to the right. For choice A, there are two problems: first, iodine and iodide are different species; second, the common ion effect suppresses solubility, rather than enhancing it. Choice A can be eliminated. Choice B sounds plausible, except that iodide is a reducing agent so choice B can be eliminated. Choice D confuses iodine and iodide and can be eliminated.

768. B is the best answer. The question stem describes the formation of a complex ion in solution, which is comprised of one or more ligands attached to a central metal cation. In this case, there are 6 water molecules bound to the iron ion. The reaction rarely goes to completion. Instead the reaction will form products until a steady state is reached, and the concentrations of the reactants and products are constant. This makes choices B and D more likely than choices A and C to be the best answer. The hydroxide ion would likely have a stronger association to the iron atom, given its negative charge. In order to form the hydrated complex, the hydroxide ion would not be included in the reaction, as it would compete with water, making choice B a better answer than choice D.

769. A is the best answer. This question is testing the concept of complex ion formation which increases the solubility of an ionic compound in water. In this case, the least soluble compound would be most affected by the mystery aqueous solution if the solution contained a complex ion. NaCl, Lysine, and $AgClO_3$ are already readily soluble in water while AgCl is a classic example of a slightly soluble compound that becomes readily soluble in the presence of a complex ion in aqueous solution

770. B is the best answer. When answering this question, try using the process of elimination. From the solubility rules, one can expect $AgNO_3$ to be a soluble solid. Adding more silver ions would actually decrease the solubility of AgCl, due to the common-ion effect. Choice A is not the best answer. Ag^+ and NH_3 react to form the complex ion $Ag(NH_3)_2^+$. This information is not readily given to the reader, and is not expected knowledge. However, further answer elimination can be performed. Decreasing the temperature actually decreases the solubility, so choice C is not the best answer. Increasing the amount of AgCl in the solution does not affect the solubility of the solid. Solubility is an intensive property, and is not affected by the amount of material in question. Adding more AgCl might result in a higher concentration of Ag^+ and Cl^- ions, but the solubility itself will stay the same. Choice D is not the best answer. By process of elimination, choice B must be the best answer. By reacting with Ag^+ to form the complex ion, $Ag(NH_3)_2^+$, the ammonia removes with Ag^+ from the solution. By Le Châtelier's Principle, more AgCl will dissolve. This effect is known as the complex-ion effect.

771. A is the best answer. $AgI(s)$ dissociates into $Ag^+(aq)$ and $I^-(aq)$. It is noted that $Ag^+(aq)$ can further react with $CN^-(aq)$ to form a complex ion. A complex ion is, by definition, a metal ion bound to one or more ions in an aqueous solution. According to Le Châtelier's Principle, increased HCN levels would likely facilitate the formation of more $Ag(CN)_2^-(aq)$. This would decrease the concentration of $Ag^+(aq)$. According to Le Châtelier's Principle, this would result in the formation of more $Ag^+(aq)$ and $I^-(aq)$ from $AgI(s)$. Thus, individuals with increased HCN would have less circulating $AgI(s)$. Choice A is a strong answer. Although the increased dissociation of $AgI(s)$ would lead to elevated concentrations of $Ag^+(aq)$, this $Ag^+(aq)$ would then feed into the complex ion formation. It is not clear if $Ag^+(aq)$ would be elevated. Choice B can be eliminated. HCN is an acid. Its dissolution would result in more H^+ ions, lowering the pH. Choice C can be eliminated. It is only noted that a bluish-grey skin discoloration occurs. It is not noted that there are varying degrees of this skin discoloration. Choice D can be eliminated. Choice A is the best answer.

772. B is the best answer. $AgI(s)$ dissociates into $Ag^+(aq)$ and $I^-(aq)$. It is noted that $Ag^+(aq)$ can further react with CN^- to form a complex ion. A complex ion is, by definition, a metal ion bound to one or more ions in an aqueous solution. Consumption of the iodized salt will result in increased concentrations of $Na^+(aq)$ and $I^-(aq)$. According to Le Châtelier's Principle, increased $I^-(aq)$ will decrease the solubility of $AgI(s)$, leading to greater circulating quantities of solid silver iodide. Choice A can be eliminated Decreasing the solubility of $Ag(s)$ will result in less circulating $Ag^+(aq)$, leading to less $Ag(CN)_2^-(aq)$ formation. Choice B can be eliminated, and choice C is a strong answer. The iodized salt will have an effect on blood chemistry, as the increased $I^-(aq)$ concentrations will affect $AgI(s)$ dissolution and the complex ion formation.

773. A is the best answer. A complex ion is a metal ion bound to one or more ions in an aqueous solution. The formation constant K_f is the equilibrium constant representing the $[\text{products}]^x/[\text{reactants}]^y$, where x and y represent the coefficient in the chemical equation. The complex ion formed is $Ag(CN)_2^-$. The reactants are Ag^+ and $2CN^-$. The K_f is therefore $[Ag(CN)_2^-]/[CN^-]^2[Ag^+]$. Choice A is the best answer. Note that choice B reverses the numerator and denominator. Choice C represents the equilibrium constant for the solvation of solid silver iodide. Note that this answer choice does not include $AgI(s)$, as solids are not included in equilibrium constants. Choice D also represents the equilibrium constant for the solvation of solid silver iodide, but it incorrectly lists the solid in the denominator.

774. B is the best answer. Poor stomach acidity is often solved by administering Vitamin C, but in a healthy patient administering a drug with more acid is unlikely to help dissolve the drug any more than the standard HCl concentration is the stomach could. Likewise, de-acidifying the stomach acid is also going to be impractical unless more is known about the pK_a of the drug. Administering the drug with a lipid is not going to help a metal ion dissolve, as ions are hydrophilic. A large ligand with a lone electron pair results in complex ion formation, significantly improving the solubility of a compound. Choice B is the best answer.

775. C is the best answer. This is an example of complex ion formation assisting to dissolve a relatively insoluble compound. In this reaction, when silver and chloride dissociate, the ammonia ions give lone pairs to empty hybridized orbitals. Lone electrons cannot accept orbital pairs from ammonia, so choice A is unlikely. Choices B and D do not reflect complex ion formation, which is a key consideration when dealing with an electron pair donor and transition metal salt.

776. B is the best answer. For a given reaction, K_{sp} depends *only* on temperature, so choices A and C can be eliminated. Solubility, on the other hand, is affected by the common ion effect, so choice D can be eliminated, and choice B is the best answer.

777. C is the best answer. This question relates to the common ion effect and Le Châtelier's Principle. When sodium bicarbonate ($NaHCO_3$) is added to this solution, it dissociates into Na^+ and HCO_3^-. HCO_3^- is a common ion. The equilibrium shifts left in an attempt to restore the disruption in the equilibrium caused by the addition of HCO_3^-. This shift to the left causes a decrease in H^+ in the blood, causing blood to become less acidic, meaning the pH increases. Choice C is the best answer.

778. B is the best answer. Increasing the amount of gas in the surrounding atmosphere pushes more of it into water, thus increasing its solubility, so choice B is the best answer, and choices A, C and D can be eliminated.

Chemical Potential and Redox Reactions

779. B is the best answer. "Agents" are always reactants, so the correct answer must be choice A or B. The reducing agent is the compound that contains the element being oxidized, which in this case is iron because Fe loses electrons to become Fe^{2+}. Remember the mnemonic OIL RIG; Oxidation Is Losing, Reduction Is Gaining. So, choice B is the best answer.

780. B is the best answer. The reducing agent is the molecule that is oxidized. Oxidation occurs when a species gains an oxygen because this is associated with a loss of electrons. The chlorine in $NaClO_3$ loses an oxygen and its oxidation state changes from +5 to +4, so option I is not a component of the best answer. SO_2 gains two oxygens to become SO_4^{2-}. In this process, the oxidation state of sulfur changes from +4 to +6. So option II is a component of the best answer. The H_2SO_4 in the reaction only acts as an acid catalyst and is not reduced or oxidized, so option III is not a component of the best answer. This makes choice B the best answer.

781. A is the best answer. In sodium hydride, hydrogen has an oxidation state of -1. In water, it has an oxidation state of +1, in sodium hydroxide it has an oxidation state of +1, and in H_2 it has an oxidation state of 0. In the reaction, the H^- and H^+ undergo oxidation and reduction respectively to become H_2. The H^+ from water is reduced, so water is the oxidizing agent, and choice A is the best answer.

782. C is the best answer. Nitrogen has an oxidation number of +4 in NO_2. That increases to +5 in HNO_3 but decreases to +2 in NO. So it is both oxidized and reduced, and choice C is the best answer. This kind of reaction, where the same compound is both the oxidizing and reducing agent, is called a disproportionation reaction.

783. D is the best answer. In nitrogen gas, the nitrogen has an oxidation state of 0. In ammonia gas, the oxidation state is −3, so nitrogen must be reduced by a reducing agent, and choice D is the best answer. Some bases are reducing agents and some acids are oxidizing agents, but choice A is not as accurate as choice D.

784. C is the best answer. Choice A does not make sense because oxidizing agents are reduced. Rusting is a form of oxidation, so the magnesium must be oxidized preferentially. So choice B can be eliminated, and choice C is likely the best answer. Choice D has the same problem as choice A, reducing agents are oxidized, so choice D can be eliminated, and choice C is the best answer.

785. D is the best answer. Redox reactions do not necessarily represent actual transfers of electrons. For instance, the charge on an atom does not necessarily change. So choices A and B can be eliminated. Oxidation states represent a model to help understanding of redox reactions. When oxidized, an atoms oxidation state becomes more positive. So choice C can be eliminated, and choice D is the best answer.

786. D is the best answer. Assume the sulfurs are S^{2-} because this is sulfurs most common oxidation state, especially when it is not bound to oxygen. Since the salt is neutral, and the sulfurs are contributing at total of −6 charge, the irons must be contributing +6 charge, or +3 each. This makes choice D the best answer.

787. B is the best answer. Assume that K is K^+ and O is O^{2-} because this is the most common oxidation states of these atoms. If the K is contributing +4 charge and the O is contributing −12 charge, the Xe must be contributing +8 charge to keep the molecule neutral and choice B is the best answer. Be wary of statements like the one in choice D. This type of answer is rarely correct on the MCAT®.

788. C is the best answer. This is a salt called potassium bisulfate. The oxidation state of potassium is +1 as is the oxidation state of H. Choices A and B cannot both be correct, so they both must be wrong. Oxygen's oxidation state is −2, so choice D is not the best answer either. For potassium bisulfate to be neutral, the sulfur must be in the +6 oxidation state, so choice C is the best answer.

789. A is the best answer. The question states the strongest base with have the lowest oxidation state. In CrO, chromium has an oxidation state of +2. In CrO_2, chromium has an oxidation state of +4. So choice A is better than choice B. In CrO_3 chromium has an oxidation state of +6, so choice A is better than choice C. In Cr_2O_3 chromium has an oxidation state of +3, so choice A is better than choice D.

790. C is the best answer. Oxidation and reduction always occur together. Half reactions can never occur by themselves. This rules out choices A, B and D and makes choice C the best answer.

791. A is the best answer. At equilibrium, by definition, $Q = K$, so option I is a component of the best answer, and choices B and C can be eliminated. At equilibrium, E and ΔG will be zero whereas $E°$ and $\Delta G°$ will depend upon the half reactions. It is unlikely that $E = E°$ or $\Delta G° = \Delta G$, so choice D can be eliminated, and choice A is the best answer.

792. B is the best answer. The applicable formula is $\Delta G = -nFE$, so choices A and C can be eliminated. The formula $\Delta G° = -nFE°$ applies only at standard state which is 1 M for all concentrations. Since the question states the reactants are at 1.4 M, then choice D can be eliminated, and choice B is the best answer.

793. A is the best answer. At standard conditions, the concentration of all reactants and products is 1 M. Only one species contributes to the pH of the solution, H^+. The pH is $-\log[H^+] = -\log(1) = 0$. If the pH is changed to 7, there is significantly less H^+ around. If there is less reactant, the reaction will have less potential driving it forward and the voltage will decrease. Choice A is the best answer, and choices B and C can be eliminated. Choice D is overly specific, even if the voltage at pH 7 is 1 V, there is no reason that the change would be asymptotic. So, choice D can be eliminated, and choice A is the best answer.

794. C is the best answer. When $K > 1$, a reaction favors products which would produce a positive standard potential, so option I is a component of the best answer, and choices A and B can be eliminated. A positive potential also means that a reaction is spontaneous, which is why option III is a component of the best answer. There is no particular entropy requirement for a cell to be spontaneous, so option II is not necessary. So, option II is not part of the best answer, which leaves choice C.

795. A is the best answer. When $K > 1$, a reaction is favoring products. Favoring products is associated with a positive cell potential so option I is not a component of the best answer, and choices C and D can be eliminated. For a reaction to proceed in the forward direction, Q must be less than K, and option II must be a component of the best answer, and choice A can be selected. Do not be confused between this statement the one about option I. Some product can be made spontaneously so $Q < K$, but there is still more product than reactant so $K < 1$.

796. C is the best answer. Positive potentials correspond to spontaneous reactions, and thus negative free energies. So, choices A and B can be eliminated. The "standard" in standard potential refers to the conditions. Choice D can be eliminated because, at equilibrium, the free energy change of any reaction is 0.

797. B is the best answer. The oxidant is at the cathode in a galvanic cell, so choice A is not the best answer, and choice B is a possible answer. Changing the internal resistance will not change the emf, so choice C is not the best answer. Raising the temperature will not necessarily increase the emf, so choice D is not the best answer.

798. A is the best answer. Oxidizing agents are reduced. F^- and I^- cannot be reduced any further, so choices B and C can be eliminated. The strongest oxidizing agent "wants" to be reduced the most. The reduction potential of Cd^{2+} is -0.40 and Na^+ is -2.71. This means Cd^{2+} requires the least amount of energy to be reduced, so choice A is the best answer, and choice D can be eliminated.

799. C is the best answer. Reducing agents are oxidized. Na^+ and Cd^{2+} cannot be oxidized any further, so choices A and D can be eliminated. The strongest reducing agent "wants" to be oxidized the most. The oxidation potential of F^- is -2.87 and I^- is -0.54. This means I^- requires the least amount of energy to be oxidized, so choice C is the best answer, and choice B can be eliminated.

800. C is the best answer. In the table, sodium is shown being reduced and iodide is shown being oxidized. Combine them into an oxidation-reduction reaction with a cell potential of $-0.54 + (-2.71) = -3.25$ V. But galvanic cells utilize spontaneous reactions, and spontaneous reactions have positive voltages, so the actual reaction must be the reverse reaction, with a voltage of 3.25 V.

801. D is the best answer. The question stem states the reactions are listed from highest to lowest potential. So, the lowest metal will have the lowest potential and is least likely to be spontaneous. Copper is below hydrogen, while the other choices are above hydrogen. So, choice D is the best answer.

802. D is the best answer. Oxidizing agents are reduced so choices A and C can be eliminated because these species are already reduced. The reactions are listed from highest to lowest oxidation potential. The reverse reaction would be the reduction potential and the reduction potentials are lowest to highest. So, choice D is the best answer and choice B can be eliminated.

803. A is the best answer. Reducing agents are oxidized, so choices B and D can be eliminated because these species are already oxidized. The reactions are listed from highest to lowest oxidation potential, so choice A is the best answer, and choice C can be eliminated.

804. B is the best answer. Choice A is a reduction in acidic solution, but it is not balanced with respect to oxygen. Choice B is a reduction in an acidic solution that is balanced so it is a strong answer. Choice C is a reduction but is not in acidic solution, so it can be eliminated. Choice D is a reduction in an acidic solution, but it is not balanced, so choice D can be eliminated.

805. D is the best answer. Choice A is not balanced with respect to oxygen so it can be eliminated. Choice B is not balanced with respect to oxygen so it can be eliminated. Choice C is not balanced with respect to hydrogen, so it can be eliminated. Choice D is balanced, so it is the best answer.

806. B is the best answer. In iodometry, iodine is gaining electrons while $S_2O_3^{2-}$ loses electrons. A good way to determine this is to calculate the oxidation numbers of both the products and the reactants; the oxidation number of the iodine atom goes from $-\frac{1}{3}$ to -1, while the oxidation number of the sulfur atom changes from $+2$ to $+2.5$. Therefore, I_3^- is the oxidizing agent, while $S_2O_3^{2-}$ is the reducing agent. Because a standard solution of $S_2O_3^{2-}$ is added to an unknown solution of I_3^-, it makes sense this titration is used to find the molarity of I_3^-. Choice A is not the best answer, because the goal of this titration is not to find the molarity of $S_2O_3^{2-}$. Choice B is the best answer, because the goal is to find the molarity of the triiodide ion, which is the oxidizing agent. Choice C is not supported in the question stem; there is no information about the voltage of this reaction, so this choice is not the best answer. While this reaction does result in tetrathionate as a product, it is unlikely that this is the goal of a titration reaction. Choice D is not the best answer.

807. A is the best answer. The equivalence point of a redox titration is not when the voltage of the solution is 0; in fact, because there is a spontaneous reduction and oxidation taking place, the voltage is most likely above 0. Choice A is the best answer. The equivalence point can be defined as when all the moles of the reducing agent are converted to their most oxidized form. Because of this, choice B is not the best answer. In common titration terminology, the solution of unknown concentration is known as the analyte, with the titrant being the solution of known concentration. Choice C is not the best answer. The equivalence point can be determined by using an indicator that changes color. However, one can also use a voltmeter to get a more accurate measurement of the voltage at the equivalence point, which can be calculated using standard reduction potentials. Choice D is not the best answer.

808. A is the best answer. The equivalence point occurs when all of the moles of the reducing agent in the solution have been completely oxidized. The reducing agent donates electrons. Fe^{2+} is the reducing agent, and it is donating electrons to Ce^{4+}. The equivalence point will occur when the number of moles of Fe^{2+} exactly equals the number of moles of Ce^{4+}. First calculate the number of moles of Fe^{2+}. $(5 \times 10^{-2}$ L$)(2 \times 10^{-1}$ M$) = 10 \times 10^{-2}$ moles $= 1 \times 10^{-2}$ moles Fe^{2+}. Note that Fe^{2+} reacts with Ce^{4+} in a 1:1 ratio, meaning that, for every 1 mole of Fe^{2+} consumed, 1 mole of Ce^{4+} will also be consumed. Therefore, 1×10^{-2} moles of Ce^{4+} will be consumed. Now, calculate the volume of Ce^{4+} added to reach this number of moles. $(1 \times 10^{-2}$ moles$)(4 \times 10^{-1}$ M$) = 0.25 \times 10^{-1}$ L $= 0.25$ L $= 25$ mL. Choice A is the best answer.

Electrochemical Cells

809. D is the best answer. It is easiest to work this problem out using electrons. Three moles of zinc, according to the first half-reaction, produce 6 moles of electrons. And 6 moles of electrons, according to the second half-reaction, can reduce 6 moles of MnO, so choice D is the best answer.

810. C is the best answer. Metal plating can be achieved through electrolytic cells so choice A is not the best answer. Solid purification can be achieved through a variety of methods including electrolytic cells, so choice B is not the best answer. Galvanic cells allow the chemical energy of redox reactions to be utilized as electrical energy, so choice C is a strong answer. Galvanic cells do not allow oxidation without reduction—that would require creation of electrons (which occurs during some radioactive decay). Choice D can be eliminated, and choice C is the best answer.

811. A is the best answer. Electrons flow from higher on the redox table to lower on the redox table, so the metal composing electrode B should be higher up on the table. In this case, only choice A fits this rule.

812. A is the best answer. ΔG is a measure of work so choices A and B are strong answers. $\Delta G°$ is the Gibb's energy for standard conditions only, so it does not cover all cells. This makes choice A more accurate than choice B. E and $E°$ are not measures of work, so choices C and D can be eliminated.

813. C is the best answer. An electrochemical cell is a battery, so option I is a component of the best answer, and choices A and B can be eliminated. A pH meter is a type of electrochemical cell but memorizing that is not required to answer this question. Option III is a non-spontaneous process, because gold is very stable. Thus, choice C is the best answer, and choice D can be eliminated.

814. A is the best answer. The cathode can be remembered as the cA+hode, because it Attracts +. If it attracts, positive, the cathode must be negative, so choices C and D can be eliminated. Also recall the Red Cat, which is a mnemonic for reduction taking place at the cathode. So, choice A is the best answer.

815. B is the best answer. In a Galvanic cell, the oxidation half reaction takes place at the anode while the reduction half reaction takes place at the cathode. A good mnemonic to use is RED CAT; AN OX. Choice B is the best answer as it incorrectly describes where the half reactions take place within a galvanic cell.

816. B is the best answer. In an electrolytic cell, the anode is positive and the cathode is negative. Choices A and D are not the best answers, as a positively charged cathode and a negatively charged anode are seen in galvanic cells. Negatively charged molecules should be attracted to the anode, as it is positive. Because of this, choice B is the best answer. The negatively charged nucleic acids are unlikely to travel to a negatively charged cathode; therefore, choice C is not the best answer.

817. C is the best answer. An electric voltage is applied to a gel that contains DNA samples that have been uniformly coated in order to separate them based on length. Sodium dodecyl sulfate (SDS) is used when running macromolecules on a gel. SDS is one of many agents that can be used to denature samples. If the student forgot to use a denaturing agent, the sample should not migrate at all, eliminating choice A. The concentration of polyacrylamide would make the band run slower or faster, with higher and lower concentrations of polyacrylamide, respectively. It would not change the direction the band migrates, eliminating choice B. The electric field drives the migration of the DNA through the gel. If the polarity of the electric field were reversed, this would drive the DNA in the opposite direction, likely making choice C the best answer. An electric field, not a magnetic field, is applied to the gel. This eliminates choice D.

818. A is the best answer. The zinc is not present at the anode. So, choice A is a stronger answer than choice B. Zinc ions are present, but are completely oxidized, so choice D is not the best answer. That leaves only the silver electrode and the water. To determine which is oxidized, consult the table. The oxidation potential of silver is -0.80 V; that of water is -1.23 V. Therefore, the silver is preferentially oxidized, and choice A is the best answer.

819. C is the best answer. The zinc electrode cannot be reduced any further, so choice A is not the best answer. To decide among the other choices, consult the table: the reduction potential of water is -0.83 V, the reduction potential of silver ions is $+0.80$ V, and the reduction potential of zinc ions is -0.76 V. Since the silver ions have the greatest reduction potential, the silver ions must be reduced, and choice C is the best answer.

820. B is the best answer. Sodium is much easier to oxidize than zinc, so the anode reaction would involve sodium over zinc or water, and choices C and D can be eliminated. Zinc ions are easier to reduce than either sodium ions or water, so the zinc would be reduced at the cathode, which makes choice B the best answer.

821. C is the best answer. Water will be oxidized at the anode and reduced at the cathode. Choices A and B are just an acid base reactions, not redox reactions, so they can be eliminated. Choice D is not the best answer because water is capable of being both oxidized and reduced.

822. C is the best answer. Corrosion occurs via oxidation so choices B and D can be automatically eliminated. Between choices A and C, zinc has a more spontaneous oxidation than iron whereas tin is less spontaneous, so choice C is the best answer.

823. B is the best answer. Strong electrolytes dissociate completely (or almost completely) in water. Option I is a component of each answer choice, so it must be true. Most salts are in fact strong electrolytes. Strong bases are strong electrolytes because they dissociate completely, so option II is part of the best answer, and choices A and C can be eliminated. Weak acids are not strong electrolytes because they do not dissociate well, so option III is eliminated, and choice B is the best answer.

824. A is the best answer. Choice A does not create ions in solution, so it is a non-electrolyte. Choice B, although molecular, is a weak base, and thus a weak electrolyte. Choices C and D are both salts and thus strong electrolytes.

825. B is the best answer. Hydrochloric acid contains two nonmetals, so it must be a molecule. Molecules are covalently bonded, so choices A and B are possible, and choice C and D are eliminated. Hydrochloric acid is also a strong acid, which means, when placed in water, it will break up into in ions. This makes it a strong electrolyte, so choice B is the best answer.

826. C is the best answer. The strength of an electrolyte is independent of its solubility. For example, acetic acid is a weak electrolyte that is very soluble in water. So choices A, B, and D can be eliminated, and choice C is the best answer.

827. D is the best answer. Potassium oxide contains a metal and nonmetal, which makes it a salt. Salts contain ionic bonds so choices A and B can be eliminated. Potassium salts dissolve well in water so potassium oxide is a strong electrolyte, and choice D is the best answer.

828. D is the best answer. The ANode Attracts Negative, meaning the anions. So choices B and C can be eliminated. The cathode is the site of reduction (recall the mnemonic "red cat") so the electrons must be migrating there. So, choice D is the best answer.

829. B is the best answer. From the mnemonic An Ox, Red Cat, reduction occurs at the cathode so electrons flow toward the cathode, so choices A and D can be eliminated. The highest potential energy will occur when the electron is farthest from the cathode, so choice B is the best answer.

830. A is the best answer. In an electrolytic cell, the electrons flow UP the redox chart, from gold to silver. Metal ions also flow in that direction, causing the silver to be plated. The redox potential difference is sufficiently high to cause this plating with an external power source, which is part of an electrolytic cell. The voltage of the battery changes the speed of plating, but not direction. Choice A is the best answer.

831. B is the best answer. Electrons flow from the anode to the cathode, so choices A and C can be eliminated. The zinc solid dissolved and Cu^{2+} formed copper solid in the first experiment, so zinc must lose electrons and copper must gain electrons, and choice B is the best answer.

832. D is the best answer. The EMF of the cell can be calculated using a version of the Nernst equation,

$$E_{cell} = E°_{cell} - \frac{0.059}{n} \times \log \frac{[Oxidized\ Ion]}{[Reduced\ Ion]}$$

where n is the number of electrons that are transferred, which is two in this example. The species with the most positive $E°$ is reduced, which is silver in this example. This means that zinc is oxidized. The zinc reduction potential is turned around to be positive, as it is oxidized, meaning the $E°$ of the cell is 1.56 V. The.

$$E_{cell} = 1.56\ V - \frac{0.059}{2} \times \log \frac{[0.1\ M]}{[1\ M]} = 1.59\ V.$$

Choice D is the best answer.

833. B is the best answer. Both half-reactions are written as reductions, so one must be reversed. Reverse the one that will lead to a positive total when combined, which in this case is the lithium half-reaction. So the total voltage is $-(-3.05\ V) + (-0.76\ V) = 2.29\ V$, so choice B is the best answer. Do not double the first reaction to balance the overall reaction; potentials do not change when a reaction is multiplied by a constant.

834. A is the best answer. A spontaneous reaction has a negative ΔG and a negative ΔG corresponds to a positive emf because $\Delta G = -nFE$. So choice A is the best answer and choice B can be eliminated. Choices C and D can be eliminated because ΔG depends on enthalpy and entropy. A negative ΔG can occurs with positive or negative enthalpy.

835. D is the best answer. Temperature changes the rate of reactions which would change the emf, so choice A is not the best answer. Choices B and C can be ruled out because the emf of a cell is fully dependent on the reactions and the concentrations of reactants. The emf is an intensive property, thus volume of solution does not affect it, so choice D is the best answer.

836. D is the best answer. Temperature changes the rate of reactions which would change the emf, so choice A is not the best answer. Choices B and C can be ruled out because the emf of a cell is fully dependent on the reactions and the concentrations of reactants. The length of the wire doesn't affect the emf of a galvanic cell, so choice D is the best answer.

837. A is the best answer. The standard reduction and oxidation potentials will cancel exactly so $E°$ will be 0, and choice A is the best answer. Choice B is from the $E°$ for the reaction in the question stem but that is not appropriate to use here because the oxidation and reduction are occurring simultaneously. So choice B can be eliminated. Choices C and D are completely made up numbers and can be eliminated.

838. A is the best answer. The cathode can be remembered as the cA+hode, because it Attracts +. So the silver ion concentration must be higher at the cathode than the anode, which makes choice A the best answer. Choice D might be appealing but do not be tricked by answers like this on the MCAT®. Choice D does not even answer the question.

839. A is the best answer. The cathode can be remembered as the cA+hode, because it Attracts +. So the zinc ion concentration must be higher at the cathode than the anode, which makes choice A the best answer. Choice D might be appealing but do not be tricked by answers like this on the MCAT®. Choice D does not even answer the question.

840. B is the best answer. Remember An Ox Red Cat. So, at the cathode, silver ions are being reduced to solid silver and at the anode solid silver is being oxidized to silver ions. Q is always products/reactants, and solids are not included in the formula. The products are the silver ions at the anode, and the reactants are the silver ions at the cathode, so choice B is the best answer.

841. C is the best answer. If electrons are flowing to the sample then current must be flowing to the reference. Current flows from the cathode so the sample and probe are the cathode and the reference is the anode. So choices A and B can be eliminated. If current is flowing to the reference then the sample is at higher H^+ concentration and lower pH than the reference. So choice C is the best answer.

842. D is the best answer. Choices A and B do not explain the production of hydrogen gas, so they can be eliminated. Reduction occurs at the cathode, so choices A and C can be eliminated. This leaves choice D as the best answer.

843. B is the best answer. It's easiest to work with electrons: (3 mol Cu^+)(1 mol e^-/1 mol Cu^+)(1 mol Mg/2 mol e^-) = ³⁄₂ mol Mg, so choice B is the best answer.

844. C is the best answer. Electrolytic cells use reactions that are forced to proceed by an external power source. They are not effective power sources themselves. Choice A is a common commercial use of electrolytic cells. Choice B is tricky because electrolytic cells are usually not a power/recharging source. But if the electrolytic cell is the "electrochemical cell" that is being recharged; during the recharging process it is an electrolytic cell. Choice B is a better answer than choice A but probably not the best answer. Electrolytic cells are not power sources, so choice C is a strong answer. Choice D is a common commercial use of electrolytic cells and thus not the best answer.

845. C is the best answer. Thermodynamics are physical laws so they cannot be broken, and choice A can be eliminated. Entropy is a part of a free energy calculation, so choice B is not the best answer. Electrolytic cells are always driven by an external power source; this external source gains its power from a spontaneous reaction, so choice C is a strong answer. The flow of free energy is independent of the charge of the species, so choice D can be eliminated.

846. B is the best answer. Electrolytic cells can be used to drive non-spontaneous processes by converting electrical energy to chemical energy. These processes often require an external battery. They cannot be used as a voltage source, so option I is not a component of the best answer, and choice C and D can be eliminated. Therefore, either options II or III must be true. The dissolution of a gold bar is a non-spontaneous process, because gold is very stable, so option III is most likely true. Therefore, choice B is the best answer.

847. D is the best answer. If the anode is silver, and oxidation occurs at the anode, the anode is oxidized to Ag^+. (Note that the zinc cathode cannot be further reduced so this is the only option initially). The oxidation of silver is associated with a production of -0.8 V. The electrons released have two options—they can reduce silver or zinc. Reduction of silver is more favored because of the positive reduction potential. So, silver ions are reduced at the cathode and solid silver plates the zinc cathode. This make a no net chemical reaction and is known as metal plating. Choice D is the best answer.

848. B is the best answer. An electrolytic cell requires a non-negative voltage to run, so choice B is the best answer. Since no chemical reaction takes place, and everything is under standard conditions, no voltage is necessary. In reality, internal resistance and the like necessitate some voltage, but the problem says to ignore these considerations.

849. B is the best answer. If the silver electrode is the anode, that electrode is oxidizing solid silver to silver ions, so choice A can be eliminated. The electrons travel across the salt bridge and will reduce either water or zinc. The reduction of zinc has a less negative reduction potential, so choice B is the best answer.

850. B is the best answer. The presence of a salt bridge is irrelevant. The direction of electron flow is determined by an external power supply; thus, it must be an electrolytic cell, and choice B is the best answer. The other types of cells produce power instead of consuming it, so choices A, C and D can be eliminated.

851. C is the best answer. To answer this question quickly, compare the answer choices. Choice A has the 3 on top, while the others have it on the bottom. 3 is the current. With more current, should it take more or less time to reduce a fixed amount of copper? Since it should take less time, the time and current should be inversely proportional, and the 3 should be in the denominator. So choice A can be eliminated. The only other difference is the 2: does it belong on top, on the bottom, or nowhere? The two must be the number of electrons each copper atom is gaining. As an example, would reducing Fe^{3+} to Fe take more or less time than it would take to reduce Fe^{2+} to Fe? Since the answer is *more* time, the time must be proportional to the change in oxidation number. Thus the 2 belongs in the numerator, and choice C is the best answer.

852. C is the best answer. The molar mass of Zn(s) is 65.38 g. Round to 65 g. 130 g Zn(s)/65 g per mole = 2 moles Zn(s). The current must be sustained long enough to generate 2 moles of solid zinc. Note that $ZnSO_4(aq)$ will dissociate into the following ions: $Zn^{2+}(aq)$ and $SO_4^{2-}(aq)$. For every mole of Zn^{2+} in solution, 2 moles of electrons must react to form Zn(s). (2 mol Zn^{2+})(2 mole electrons per mole Zn^{2+}) = 4 mole electrons. Note that Faraday's constant (F) = 96,485 C/mole e^-. Round up to 100,000 C/mole e^-, or 1×10^5 C/mole electron. (4 mole electron)(1×10^5 C per mole electron) = 4×10^5 C. Note that 10 A is equal to 10 C per second. (4×10^5 C)/(1×10^1 C per second) = 4×10^4 seconds = 40,000 seconds. Note that the answer must be slightly below 40,000 seconds because Faraday's constant (which was put in the denominator of a division problem) was rounded up. Choice C is the best answer.

853. A is the best answer. Use the following calculation:

(0.108 g Ag)(1 mol Ag/108 g Al)(1 mol e^-/mol Ag) (96,485 C/mol e^-)(1 sec/2 C) = 48 seconds; choice A is the best answer.

854. A is the best answer. Use units to solve this one. g = (197 g/mol Au × 2 c/s × 30 s)/(96,500 c/mol e^- × 3 mol e^-/mol Au) so 2 c/s must be in the numerator of the equation and 3 mol e^-/mol Au must be in the denominator, and choice A is the best answer.

855. C is the best answer. Handle this question be process of elimination. Choice A can be eliminated because the emf does not control the speed of a reaction. Choice D can also be eliminated because the fact that gold requires more electrons to make solid gold means that it would take longer to plate. Choices B and C are both true statements, copper will plate faster because it requires 2/3 the number of electrons as gold. But, gold has an atomic mass of ~197 g/mol and copper has a mass of ~64 g/mol. So, gold weighs 197/64 ≈ 200/64 ≈ 25/8 ≈ 3. Since 3 > 2/3, the weight of gold means that the gold spoon will be plated with 1 g of gold more quickly, and choice C is the best answer.

856. D is the best answer. When a vehicle is moving, the battery powering the motor is being discharged. While discharging, the battery is behaving like a Galvanic cell. To recharge a battery, the half reactions taking place must be reversed. When being charged, the battery is acting as an electrolytic cell as a large voltage must be used to push the reverse reaction to completion. Choice D is the best answer as it accurately describes this phenomenon.

857. C is the best answer. A salt bridge is usually required to keep one half-cell from accumulating a surplus of charge. But the battery described does not have separate half-cells, so the question becomes: How can the automobile battery function without separate half-cells? Choice A does not answer this question, so it can be eliminated. Choice B also does not answer this question and can be eliminated. Choice C is a reasonable explanation, so choice C is probably the best answer. Choice D is a true statement, but it does not answer the questions, so choice D is not the best answer.

858. D is the best answer. These batteries are rechargeable, so option I is correct. In order to be rechargeable, they must both discharge energy and be able to store energy. In other words, they must be able to act as both a galvanic and an electrolytic cell. Choices A, B, and C are all good answers, as they describe some of the properties of nickel-cadmium batteries, but they are not the best answer. Choice D is the only answer that describes all the properties of these batteries and is the best answer.

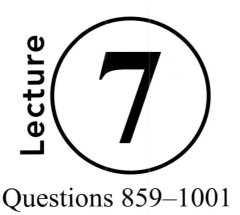

Lecture

7

Questions 859–1001

Acids and Bases

ANSWERS & EXPLANATIONS

ANSWER KEY

859. B	872. D	885. A	898. B	911. D	924. A	937. A	950. B	963. C	976. B	989. B
860. A	873. C	886. A	899. B	912. D	925. C	938. A	951. C	964. B	977. C	990. C
861. A	874. D	887. B	900. D	913. D	926. A	939. D	952. B	965. B	978. D	991. A
862. C	875. A	888. D	901. D	914. C	927. C	940. D	953. C	966. A	979. B	992. A
863. A	876. D	889. A	902. C	915. D	928. C	941. B	954. C	967. B	980. B	993. D
864. B	877. D	890. B	903. A	916. C	929. B	942. B	955. D	968. D	981. B	994. B
865. B	878. C	891. A	904. C	917. D	930. A	943. B	956. C	969. C	982. A	995. A
866. B	879. D	892. C	905. B	918. B	931. B	944. B	957. A	970. C	983. C	996. B
867. A	880. D	893. D	906. D	919. B	932. B	945. C	958. D	971. C	984. C	997. A
868. D	881. B	894. C	907. C	920. A	933. D	946. B	959. A	972. C	985. C	998. C
869. B	882. B	895. B	908. D	921. A	934. C	947. C	960. D	973. D	986. A	999. D
870. A	883. D	896. B	909. C	922. D	935. C	948. C	961. C	974. C	987. C	1000. D
871. A	884. C	897. B	910. B	923. B	936. A	949. A	962. D	975. D	988. B	1001. C

Acids and Bases

859. B is the best answer. Acids increase [H^+], so choice A is not the best answer. Acids decrease the pH of a solution, so choice B is a possible answer. Acids increased the pOH of a solution, so choice C is not the best answer. Acids decrease the [OH^-] of a solution, so choice D is not the best answer.

860. A is the best answer. Arrhenius acids must produce hydronium ions in water by releasing protons. HCl dissociates to H^+ and Cl^-, so option I is a component of the best answer. Neither CH_3CH_2OH nor BF_3 produce H^+ directly, so options II and III can be eliminated, and choice A is the best answer.

861. A is the best answer. The Brønsted-Lowry and Lewis definitions are in terms of a particular reaction; a substance can act as a Lewis acid in one reaction and as a Lewis base in another. Therefore, since the sign seems to be talking about substances that are always either acids or bases, it cannot be using the Lewis or Brønsted-Lowry definitions. The definition the sign writer has in mind is probably the Arrhenius one, so choice A is the best answer, and choices B, C, and D can be eliminated.

862. C is the best answer. Brønsted-Lowry acids are capable of donating protons. Option I certainly can donate a proton, so choice B can be eliminated. Although ethanol is not an Arrhenius acid, since it will not donate its proton to water, it can be deprotonated by sufficiently strong bases so in some instances it is a Brønsted-Lowry acid, and option II is a component of the best answer. Choice III has no protons to donate, so it cannot be a Brønsted-Lowry acid. So, choice D is eliminated, and choice C is the best answer.

863. A is the best answer. A Brønsted-Lowry acid is a proton donor. In this reaction, NH_3 donates a proton to H^-. So, choice A is the best answer. H^- is the Brønsted-Lowry base, so choice B is not the best answer. NH_4^+ is not even part of the reaction, so choice C is not the best answer. NH_2 is the conjugate acid of NH_3 and H_2 is the conjugate base of H, so choice D is not the best answer.

864. B is the best answer. A Brønsted-Lowry acid is one that donates protons whereas a Lewis acid accepts electrons. The act of donating a proton requires accepting electrons so all Brønsted-Lowry acids are also Lewis acids but the reverse is not true. This makes choice B a stronger answer than choice A. Molecules can act as Lewis acids or bases or Brønsted-Lowry acid or bases depending on the solution they exist in, so choices C and D are not the best answers.

865. B is the best answer. CH_4 is not a Lewis acid or base except under very extreme conditions, so choice A is probably not the best answer. NH_3 is the only answer with a lone pair of electrons, so choice B is a strong answer. Choices C and D are both well-known Lewis acids. They have empty orbitals to receive electrons, so these are not the best answers.

866. B is the best answer. Choice A, C, and D all have lone pairs of electrons. Choice B is an ammonium ion so the lone pair of electrons found on ammonia is now used to form the bond with the fourth hydrogen. This makes choice B the best answer.

867. A is the best answer. When doing this type of question, it's helpful to check for the quicker possibilities first. The reaction is clearly not a combustion because it does not involved O_2, so choice D can be eliminated. It is also not Brønsted-Lowry acid/base, since what is transferred is an H^-, not an H^+, so choice B can be eliminated. This leaves redox or Lewis acid/base. Of the two, redox is easier to check; Lewis acid/base requires sketching several Lewis structures. The oxidation numbers are given below:

$$Ca(+2)H(-1)_2 + 2B(+3)H(-1)_3 \rightarrow 2B(+3)H(-1)_4^- + Ca(2+)$$

The oxidation numbers do not change, so choice C can be eliminated, and choice A is the best answer.

868. D is the best answer. The Lewis definition is the most general definition of an acid. *All* Brønsted-Lowry acids are Lewis acids. In addition, anything capable of accepting an additional bond is a Lewis acid. A compound may be able to accept an additional bond because the compound has a leaving group, a double or triple bond, or an incomplete octet. HCl has a leaving group (Cl^-), so option I is a component of the best answer. CH_3CH_2OH is able to accept an electron from H to give $CH_3CH_2O^-$ and H^+, so option II is a component of the best answer. BF_3 has an empty orbital for accepting electrons, so it is a common Lewis acid, and option III must be a part of the best answer making choice D the best answer.

869. B is the best answer. No oxidation numbers change, which eliminates choices C and D. The iron has empty orbitals that the lone pairs on the oxygen attach to, which makes it a Lewis base, so choice A can be eliminated, and choice B is the best answer.

870. A is the best answer. There is no change in oxidation number, so choices C and D can be eliminated. The ion needs to be protonated so an acid is necessary, and choice A is the best answer.

871. A is the best answer. This question can be solved by writing out the reaction in question: $HA + H_2O \rightarrow A^- + H_3O^+$. In the forward reaction HA transfers a proton to H_2O; in the reverse reaction, H_3O^+ transfers a proton to A^-. If HA is a strong acid, the equilibrium favors the forward reaction, and choice A is the best answer. Choice B is the opposite of the forward reaction so it can be eliminated. Choices C and D confuse the reactants and the products and are not the best answers.

872. D is the best answer. The acidity of the hydrogen halides increases moving down the periodic table, so choice A is the weakest acid, and choice D is the strongest.

873. C is the best answer. Choice A describes a hydrated metal, not a hydride, so choice A is not the best answer. Choice B describes a dehydration reaction, so choice B is not the best answer. A hydride contains hydrogen and one other element, so choice C is a strong answer. A compound containing hydrogen is too vague of a statement because organic molecules contain hydrogen but are not hydrides, so choice D can be eliminated, and choice C is the best answer.

874. D is the best answer. The strength of an oxyacid increases as the number of oxygen increases, so choice A is the weakest acid, and choice D is the strongest.

875. A is the best answer. On an oxyacid, when the central atom is different and each central atom has the same number of oxygens, the central atom with the greatest electronegativity produces the strongest oxyacid. The species with the greatest electronegativity is Cl, followed by Br, the I, so choice A is the best answer.

876. D is the best answer. If adding oxygen atoms improved an oxyacid's ability to "take on" protons, then adding oxygens would increase basicity of oxyacids, which is not the case, so choice A is not the best answer. Choice B is a true, in that oxygens are electron withdrawing, but if this stabilized hydroxide ions, oxyacids would be strong bases, not acids, so choice B is not the best answer. If the bond between oxygen and the acidic hydrogen were strengthened, then the oxyacid would be weaker, so choice C is not the best answer. The oxygens are electron withdrawing, which tends to polarize the bond on the acidic hydrogen increasing its likelihood of dissociating in water, so choice D is the best answer.

877. D is the best answer. Metal hydrides like NaH are basic or neutral, so choices A and C are not the best answers. Nonmetal hydrides like H_2O and HCl are acidic or neutral, so choice B is not the best answer, and choice D is the best answer. Ammonia, NH_3, is an important exception to this rule.

878. C is the best answer. The ionic hydrides are bases. Choices A, B and D are all hydrides and all strong bases, so choice C is the best answer.

879. D is the best answer. The hydride ion is a stronger base than the hydroxide ion so any base that produces hydride is stronger than the respective hydroxide base. This makes options I and II a component of the best answer. $HClO$ is a weak acid especially relative to HCl, so option III is also a component of the best answer. Select choice D.

880. D is the best answer. Choices A, B and C are three common strong acids on the MCAT®. Choice D is a weak acid. These acids are all worth memorizing.

881. B is the best answer. K_a and K_b are inversely proportional, so in general, strong acids must have weak conjugate bases, and choice A can be eliminated. However, because K_w is small, it is possible for K_a and K_b to be small and for a weak acid to have a weak conjugate base, so choice B is a possible answer. Choice C is not the best answer for the same reason as choice A. Choice D is not the best answer because the trend that as an acid becomes weaker, the conjugate base becomes stronger is true. This is in contrast to choice B which is too absolute in saying weak acids must have strong conjugate bases.

882. B is the best answer. $HClO_4$, HBr, and HNO_3 are all strong acids because they are prone to donate a proton to water to make H_3O^+. This makes H_3O^+ the weakest acid, and choice B is the best answer.

883. D is the best answer. Choices A, B, and C are very strong bases because they produce OH^- when reacting with water. So, by definition, choice D is the weakest base.

884. C is the best answer. KOH is a strong base, so choice A is not the best answer. $Ca(OH)_2$ is also a strong base, so choice B is not the best answer. $Mg(OH)_2$ is insoluble and thus not a strong base, so choice C is a strong answer. Compared to choice D, choice C is a weaker base because it does not dissolve in water to produce any OH^-, so choice C is the best answer.

885. A is the best answer. It is easiest to compare the conjugate acids here: $HClO$, H_3O^+, and HCl. HCl is a strong acid, and $HClO$ is a weak acid. By definition, a strong acid is a stronger acid than H_3O^+, and a weak acid is weaker than H_3O^+. So the acid strength is $HCl > H_3O^+ > HClO$. The strength of their conjugate bases will be in reverse order, so choice A is the best answer.

886. A is the best answer. Choice A is an ionic oxide because it is made of a metal and a nonmetal. Ionic oxides form bases in water, this is worth memorizing.

887. B is the best answer. Choices A and C can be eliminated because the conjugate ion of a weak acid must be a base. When deciding between choices B and D, consider the mathematics. If HF has a pK_a of 3.1, its conjugate, then has a pK_b of 11. Even though the acid is weak, the conjugate base is also weak. The accepted definition of a strong acid is one with $pK_a < 0$, and a strong base is one with $pK_b < 0$, so HF is a weak acid, and F^- is a weak base, and choice B is the best answer.

888. D is the best answer. Choices A and C can be eliminated because the conjugate ion of a weak acid must be a base. When deciding between choices B and D, consider the mathematics. If benzoic acid has a pK_a of 4.19, its conjugate, then has a pK_b of 9.81. Even though the acid is weak, the conjugate base is also weak. The accepted definition of a strong acid is one with $pK_a < 0$, and a strong base is one with $pK_b < 0$, so benzoic acid is a weak acid, and benzoate is a weak base, and choice D is the best answer.

889. A is the best answer. To form the conjugate base, remove a proton (H^+), which leave NH_2^-, so choice A is the best answer. Choice B is ammonia, so it can be eliminated. Choice C is the conjugate acid of ammonia, ammonium, so it can be eliminated. Choice D is hydroxide, which is made when ammonia is protonated to make ammonium, so choice D can be eliminated.

890. B is the best answer. To form the conjugate base, remove a proton (H^+), which leaves CO_3^{2-}, so choice B is the best answer. H_2CO_3 is the conjugate acid, so choice A can be eliminated. Choice C is water, so it can be eliminated. Choice D is hydroxide, which is made when HCO_3^- is protonated to make H_2CO_3, so choice D can be eliminated.

891. A is the best answer. To form the conjugate base, remove a proton (H^+), which leaves H_2O, so choice A is the best answer. H_3O^+ is the acid mentioned in the question, so choice B can be eliminated. Choice C is hydroxide, which is the conjugate base of choice A, so it can be eliminated. Choice D is hydrogen peroxide, which is not related to hydronium, water, or hydroxide, so choice D can be eliminated.

892. C is the best answer. To form the conjugate acid, add a proton (H^+), which results in $H_4PO_4^+$, so choice C is the best answer. $H_2PO_4^+$ is the conjugate base, so choice A can be eliminated. Choice B is phosphoric acid, which is mentioned in the question, so it can be eliminated. Choice D is hydronium, which is the conjugate acid of water, made when phosphoric acid dissociates into H^+, and it's the conjugate base. So, choice D can be eliminated.

893. D is the best answer. By definition, every acid has a conjugate base, so choice A is not the best answer. Furthermore, choice B defines this conjugate base, although it is only true of a Brønsted-Lowry acid because these produce protons in water. An example where choice C is true is the conjugate base of sulfuric acid which is HSO_4^- which has a pK_a of 2. So choice C is not the best answer. The conjugate base of the hydronium ion is water, H_2O and the conjugate base of water is hydroxide, so choice D is the best answer.

894. C is the best answer. K_a is an acid's equilibrium constant in water. Larger K_a is indicative of greater acid strength. Each acid has an associated conjugate base, which is formed upon removal of H^+. Each conjugate base as its own equilibrium constant, K_b. Larger K_b values indicate a stronger base. For an acid/conjugate base pair, K_a and K_b are related via K_w in the following equation: $K_w = K_aK_b$, where K_w is a constant. Thus, a larger K_a (of the acid) corresponds to a smaller K_b (of the conjugate base). Stronger acids have weaker conjugate bases. Of the conjugate bases listed in the answer choices, $C_6H_5COO^-$ is associated with the acid with the smallest K_a, meaning $C_6H_5COO^-$ has the largest K_b and is the strongest base. Choices A and B can be eliminated in favor of choice C. Note that CH_3COOH is not a conjugate base of any acids listed in the table, and because it does not have a negative charge, it is unlikely to be a stronger base than the other answer choices. Choice D can be eliminated. Choice C is the best answer.

895. B is the best answer. For an acid/conjugate base pair, K_a and K_b are related via K_w in the following equation: $K_w = K_aK_b$, where K_w is 1×10^{-14} at 25°C. K_b and K_w are known. Solve for K_a of the unknown compound via the following equation:

$$K_a = (1 \times 10^{-14})/(2.5 \times 10^{-11}).$$

At this point, treat the mantissa and the exponent separately:

$$1/2.5 = 0.4; \quad 10^{-14}/10^{-11} = 10^{-3}.$$

Now combine them together:

$$0.4 \times 10^{-3} = 4.0 \times 10^{-4}.$$

This is the listed K_a of nitrous acid. Choice B is the best answer.

896. B is the best answer. There are three major factors affecting acid strength: H–X bond strength, bond polarity and the stability of the conjugate base. A polar bond is weaker, so it is associated with a stronger acid and, choice A is not the best answer. A strong H–X bond will be more difficult to break making H–X less likely to dissociate and hence a weaker acid, so choice B is a possible answer. A stable conjugate base is associated with strong acids, so choice C is not the best answer. Temperature may increase pH but it does not change the intrinsic strength of an acid, so choice D can be eliminated.

897. B is the best answer. This is the definition of pH is pH $= -\log[H^+]$. This is worth memorizing. Choice B is the best answer.

898. B is the best answer. pH $= 7$ in a neutral solution only at 25°C, so choice A is a possible answer but there is probably a better answer. Choice B is a better definition because it applies to multiple temperatures. Choice C would be a very basic solution, so choice C is not the best answer. Choice D describes an unrealistic solution—there is always an equilibrium between donating and accepting protons.

899. B is the best answer. 3.0×10^{-4} is between 1.0×10^{-4} and $10 \times 10^{-4} = 1.0 \times 10^{-3}$, so the pH is between 3 and 4, and choice B is the best answer. It is not necessary to be more precise than this for the MCAT®, do not waste time doing formal calculations.

900. D is the best answer. With each pH, the hydrogen ion concentration increases by a factor of ten. So changing from 5 to 4 is a $10\times$ change in $[H^+]$. Changing from 5 to 3 is a $100\times$ change in $[H^+]$, and choice D is the best answer.

901. D is the best answer. KOH is a salt, and thus dissociates completely, giving an OH^- concentration of 0.01 M and a pOH of 2 because $pOH = -\log[OH^-]$. Since $pH + pOH = 14$, the pH is 12. Or, skip the calculations and realize that choice D is the only basic pH.

902. C is the best answer. KOH is a salt, and thus dissociates completely, giving an OH^- concentration of 0.01 M and a pOH of 2 because $pOH = -\log[OH^-]$.

903. A is the best answer. Since the pH is between 11 and 12, $[H^+]$ is between 1.0×10^{-12} and 1.0×10^{-11}. It is not necessary to be more precise than this for the MCAT®. Choices C and D can be immediately eliminated, but choices A and B should be considered carefully. Choice A is 5.5×10^{-12}, which is equal to 0.55×10^{-11}, which is between 1.0×10^{-12} (0.1×10^{-11}) and 1.0×10^{-11}, so choice A is the best answer. Choice B is larger than 1.0×10^{-11}, so it can be eliminated.

904. C is the best answer. Dilution by a factor of 10 increases the pH by 1 unit. Dilution by a factor of 100 increases the pH two factors of 10, and therefore the pH increases by 2, so choice C is the best answer. Dilution will not make the solution more acidic, so choice A can be eliminated. Dilution will change the $[H^+]$ and thus the pH, so choice B can be eliminated. Having a pH of 230 in water is not impossible but exceedingly unlikely. On the MCAT®, the pH of a solution usually falls between 0 and 14 so answers outside that range should be avoided. Choice D can be eliminated.

905. B is the best answer. Acetic acid is an acid, so choices C and D can be eliminated. Acetic acid is a weak acid, so choice B is probably the best answer but this can be checked with the following calculation.

$$pK_a = -\log[H^+][A^-]/[HA]$$

Since $[H^+] << [HA]$, assume that $[HA] = 0.1$ M.

Also assume $[H^+] = [A^-]$.

$$4.74 = -\log[H^+]^2/0.1$$
$$4.74 = -\log[H^+]^2 + \log 0.1$$
$$4.74 = -\log[H^+]^2 - 1$$
$$5.74 = -\log[H^+]^2$$
$$5.74 = -2\log[H^+]$$
$$2.87 = -\log[H^+] = pH$$

This answer is closest to choice B, so choice B is the best answer.

906. D is the best answer. An amphiprotic molecule is one that has acidic and basic side groups, such as an amino acid. Since substance X is amphiprotic, the pK_a and pK_b must be known to determine the pH. The pK_b is determined experimentally and cannot be calculated from the pK_a, so choice D is the best answer.

907. C is the best answer. The strongest base has the smallest pK_b. Since $pK_a + pK_b = 14$ for a pair of conjugates, SCN^- has a pK_b of 15.8, BF_4^- has a pK_b of 13.5, and IO^- has a pK_b of 3.5. So out of this group, IO^- is the strongest base, and choice C is the best answer.

908. D is the best answer. $pK_a = -\log[H^+][A^-]/[HA]$. A weak acid will be one where $[H^+] << [HA]$. So for a weak acid, the pK_a is the negative log of a small number, which is a number greater than 1. So, option I can be eliminated, and options II and III are the best answers—select choice D.

909. C is the best answer. For conjugates, $pK_a + pK_b = 14$. So, $14 - 4.74 = 9.26$, and choice C is the best answer.

910. B is the best answer. For conjugates, $pK_a + pK_b = 14$. So, $14 - 9.31 = 4.69$, and choice B is the best answer.

911. D is the best answer. The equation $pK_a + pK_b = 14$ applies to conjugates only. The pK_b of the carbonate ion, which is conjugate to the hydrogen carbonate ion, is indeed 3.75, but that is not what this question asks for, so choice B can be eliminated, and choice D is the best answer.

912. D is the best answer. As temperature increases, ionization tends to increase as well, so option I should be included, and choices A and C can be eliminated. The identity of an acid determines its pK_a, so option II should be included. The concentration of another acid can determine the percent ionization by Le Châtelier's principle. If another acid is present in solution, the ionization of a weak acid may decrease. So, choice D is the best answer.

913. D is the best answer. As concentration increases, percent dissociation tends to decrease, this is true of salts and acids, so choice A can be eliminated. Stronger acids dissociate to a greater extent, but even strong acids cannot dissociate completely in very concentrated solutions, so choice B can be eliminated. Increasing temperature usually increases the percent dissociation, so choice C can be eliminated. By definition, strong acids create more H^+ so they dissociate more, and choice D is the best answer.

914. C is the best answer. Consider the formula for pK_a:

$$pK_a = -\log[H^+][A^-]/[HA].$$

Option I will permit calculating the [H$^+$] of an acid. This problem is, as more base is added, a weak acid will continue to dissociate so the [H$^+$] will be equivalent to [HA] initially added to the solution. There is no way by this method to determine the [H$^+$] relative to the [HA] because the acid will continue to dissociate. Titration curves can be used to determine pK_a, and option I may sound similar to a titration. However, there is no description of graphing the pH, so option I cannot be used to calculate the pK_a of a weak acid, and choices A, B and D can be eliminated. To be certain, options II and II should be considered. Measuring the pH of a solution of known concentration of acid would give [H$^+$] and [HA] so the pK_a could be calculated, and option II is part of the best answer. For option III, finding the pK_b of a conjugate base would allow calculation of pK_a via the formula $14 = pK_a + pK_b$. So, choice C is the best answer.

915. D is the best answer. Both HI and HCl are readily soluble in water, so choice A can be eliminated. Both acids are strong acids, so choice B can be eliminated. Between choice C and D, the distinguishing feature is if the acids are stronger acids than water or hydronium. They are stronger than both, but the relevant statement is that they are stronger than hydronium. When each acid is added to water, the following reaction occurs, HX + H$_2$O → H$_3$O$^+$ + X$^-$ where X is either Cl or I. If hydronium (H$_3$O$^+$) was the stronger acid, the reaction would favor the reverse direction, so choice D is the best answer.

916. C is the best answer. Choice A is a true statement, but it does not answer the question because it does in explain why hydroiodic acid is more acidic than hydrochloric acid in an acetic acid solution only. Choice A can be eliminated. If the conjugate base of hydrochloric acid (Cl$^-$) was a stronger base than water, then HCl would be a weak acid, which it is not. So, choice B can be eliminated. Between choices C and D, choice D can be eliminated because acetic acid is an acid, thus it is a poor base. Choice C is the best answer by process of elimination, but consider what this answer is saying. When HI dissociates in water, the reaction is HI + H$_2$O $\rightleftharpoons$ H$_3$O$^+$ + I$^-$. In this reaction, water is acting as a base. When in acetic acid, the reaction is HI + CH$_3$COOH → CH$_3$COOH$_2^+$ + I$^-$. Since acetic acid is a weaker base, the later reaction is less likely to proceed to completion for any given acid. This allows the ability to distinguish the strength of acids that are otherwise indistinguishable when dissolved in water.

917. D is the best answer. Choice A states that the most acidic proton in a diprotic acid is the most acidic. This is true, so choice A can be eliminated. For each proton, there is an equivalence point as stated in choice B, so this answer can also be eliminated. In very concentrated solutions, the pH is very low so the dissociation of the second proton is negligible, and choice C can be eliminated. K_a is a measure of the acidity of a proton with a high K_a corresponding to very acidic protons. As stated previously, the most acidic proton is the first one, so choice D contradicts choice A and can be eliminated.

918. B is the best answer. If K_a is 1.2×10^{-2} then p$K_a \approx 2$. From the Henderson-Hasselbach equation, pH = pK_a + log[A$^-$]/[HA] so $2 \approx 2 + \log[A^-]/[HA]$. This means log[A$^-$]/[HA] must be very close to zero meaning [A$^-$] = [HA]. This is called the half equivalence point. In this problem HA is HSO$_4^-$, and A$^-$ is SO$_4^{2-}$, so choice B is the best answer.

919. B is the best answer. Alcohols are more water-soluble than alkanes, so choice A is possible. However it implies that propanol would have a lower pH, so choice A is probably not the best answer. Choice B is a reasonable explanation, if both propanol and ethane are such weak acids that essentially the only H$^+$ made is from the autoionization of water, then the pH of both solutions would be very close to 7. Choices C and D can be eliminated because propanol and ethane are exceedingly weak acids compared to water and hydronium.

Water and Acid-Base Chemistry

920. A is the best answer. Pure water reacts with itself to form hydronium and hydroxide ions in a reaction called the autoionization of water, as shown below. In this reaction, one water molecule (acting as an acid) donates a proton to another water molecule (acting as a base). The autoionization is only possible because water can act as both an acid and a base. Note that an amphoteric species is, by definition, a compound that can act as both an acid and a base. Water is therefore an amphoteric species. Choice A is a strong answer. Although water does have a large heat capacity, this does not contribute to its ability to autoionize. Choice B can be eliminated. Water's two lone pairs of electrons contribute to its ability to act as a base, but this does not specify its amphoteric nature. Choice C can be eliminated. Water is able to hydrogen bond to itself due to its polarity and the fact that it contains oxygen and hydrogen bound to each other, but this fact alone does not indicate that water can act as both an acid and base. Choice D can be eliminated. Choice A is the best answer.

$$H_2O + H_2O \rightleftharpoons H_3O^+ + OH^-$$

921. A is the best answer. pH is defined by $[H^+]$ where pH $= -\log[H^+]$. Since autoionization of water is endothermic, meaning it requires heat, increasing the temperature will increase the reaction. So, the $[H^+]$ will increase and the pH will decrease, and choice A is the best answer. Choice D is a common misconception—the pH depends only on the $[H^+]$. It does not matter that there is more $[OH^-]$ present as well.

922. D is the best answer. Water is an amphoteric species, meaning it can act as a base and acid. It will act as a base upon the addition of a weak acid, HA. Water would accept H^+, generating H_3O^+ (conjugate acid) and A^- (conjugate base). Option I is correct. Water will also act as an acid, allowing it to donate H^+ to the conjugate base of the weak acid, A^-. This will result in HA and OH^- (conjugate base). Option II is correct, and choice C can be eliminated. Pure water reacts with itself to form H_3O^+ and OH^-, a process called the autoionization of water. This occurs even without the presence of the weak acid. Option III is correct, and choices A and B can be eliminated. Choice D is the best answer.

923. B is the best answer. The equilibrium constant is 10^{-14}. This means hardly any of the products are formed and $[H_2O] \gg [H_3O^+]$. So the equilibrium lies far to the left, and choice B is the best answer.

924. A is the best answer. Pure water reacts with itself to form hydronium and hydroxide ions in a reaction called the autoionization of water, as shown below. The table indicates that addition of heat lowers the pH, which corresponds to increased hydronium ion concentrations. Addition of heat shifts the autoionization of water equilibrium to the right (favoring hydronium ions and hydroxide ions). The concentrations of hydronium ions and hydroxide ions will increase concurrently, and water will remain neutral, as $[H_3O^+]$ will always equal $[OH^-]$. Choice A is a strong answer. Because no acids are added to the pure water, water at a higher temperature will not be more acidic than water at a lower temperature. Note that comparing pH to determine acidity is only valid at a given temperature, not across varying temperature ranges. Choice B can be eliminated. $[H_3O^+]$ will always equal $[OH^-]$; choices C and D can be eliminated. Choice A is the best answer.

$$H_2O + H_2O \rightleftharpoons H_3O^+ + OH^-$$

925. C is the best answer. The pH decreases with increasing temperature because the equilibrium of the autoionization of water is shifted to the right (see below). Increasing $[H_3O^+]$ results in a lower pH (pH $= -\log([H_3O^+])$). Note that $[OH^-]$ is expected to increase concurrently with $[H_3O^+]$. Thus, increasing temperature would also lower pOH (pOH $= -\log([OH^-])$). Also note that, although pH and pOH are changing, water is still expected to remain neutral because, at all levels, pH is expected to equal pOH. Choice C is the best answer.

$$H_2O + H_2O \rightleftharpoons H_3O^+ + OH^-$$

926. A is the best answer. Endothermic reactions require heat from the environment. Place heat on the reactants (left) side of the autoionization reaction. According to Le Châtelier's Principle, increasing the temperature (adding more heat) should shift the reaction equilibrium towards the products (to the right). The K_w of water is equal to $[H_3O^+] \cdot [OH^-]$. Given that $[H_3O^+]$ and $[OH^-]$ are expected to increase with temperature, the K_w is also likely to increase. Choice A is the best answer.

927. C is the best answer. As a strong acid, 0.001 M HCl will completely dissociate into 0.001 M H^+ and 0.001 M Cl^-. The new pH of the solution is calculated based on this new H^+ concentration as follows: pH $= -\log(10^{-3}) = 3$. pH + pOH $= pK_w$, and pK_w is always equal to 14 at 25°C. pOH $= 14 - 3 = 11$. Choice C is the best answer.

928. C is the best answer. At 25°C, $K_w = 10^{-14}$. Note that $K_w = K_a K_b$. Round 1.76×10^{-5} to 2×10^{-5}. Rearranging the equation with the rounded value, $K_b = 10^{-14}/(2 \times 10^{-5}) = 5 \times 10^{-10}$. Because the number in the denominator was rounded up, the actual answer must be greater than 5×10^{-10}. Choice C is the best answer.

929. B is the best answer. The K_a is K_w divided by 55 which is the concentration of water (55 mol/L), so choice B is the best answer because it is the only answer smaller than K_w.

930. A is the best answer. The equilibrium constant for the autoionization of water is 10^{-14} meaning there is much more H_2O than H^+. In fact, since $K_w = K_a K_b$ the $[H^+]$ is 10^{-7} that of $[H_2O]$. 10^7 is 10,000,000 so for every H^+ there are 10,000,000 H_2O molecules, and choice A is a strong answer. Choices B and C are saying the same thing, so they can be eliminated. Choice D is the opposite of choice A and can be eliminated.

931. B is the best answer. $K_w = K_a K_b = [H^+][OH^-]$. For pure water, $[H^+] = [OH^-]$. Defining $[H^+]$ as x, the following equation can be formed: $K_w = 2.916 \times 10^{-14} = x^2$. Round 2.916 to 3, and recall that

$$\sqrt{3} = 1.7.$$
$$\sqrt{(3 \times 10^{-14})} = 1.7 \times 10^{-7} = x = [H^+].$$

Find the pH via the following formula:

$$pH = -\log([H^+]). \quad pH = -\log(1.7 \times 10^{-7}),$$

which equals something just below 7. Choice B is the best answer.

932. B is the best answer. The K_a and K_b of an acid/base conjugate pair in aqueous solution at 25°C are related by K_w via the following equation: $K_w = K_a K_b$. K_w at 25°C is 1×10^{-14}. Benzoate is the conjugate base of benzoic acid. Round 1.55×10^{-10} down to 1.5×10^{-10}. Solving for K_a of benzoic acid: $K_a = (1 \times 10^{-14})/(1.5 \times 10^{-10}) = 6.67 \times 10^{-5}$. $pK_a = -\log(K_a) = -\log(6.67 \times 10^{-5}) = 4.18$, which is closest to choice B. Note that the exponent in the pK_a calculation (-5) indicates that the answer choice must be between 4 and 5, and choice B is the only answer choice in this range. Note that choices A, B, and D could be chosen due to common mistakes. K_b and K_w have negative exponents. Using positive exponents instead will yield a pK_a of -3.82. 25°C is about room temperature, and if one incorrectly assumes that a fluid at room temperature should be roughly pH neutral, choice C would be chosen because it is closest to 7. If one incorrectly uses K_b to calculate pK_a, the pK_a calculation would resemble: $-\log(1.55 \times 10^{-10}.)$. This would equal a number between 9 and 10, leading a test-taker to incorrectly choose choice D.

933. D is the best answer. Due to its amphoteric nature, water reacts with itself to form hydronium ion and hydroxide ion in a process known as autoionization. $K_w = K_a K_b = [H^+][OH^-]$. The table indicates that K_w increases with temperature, further indicating that $[H^+]$ and $[OH^-]$ must increase with temperature. Because the autoionization of water results in an equal number of $[H^+]$ and $[OH^-]$, water is expected to remain neutral as temperature increases. Although choice A indicates this, this statement does not directly support the findings, which make a claim about the K_w of water, not its neutrality. Choice A can be eliminated. Water autoionizes more readily with increasing temperature, not decreasing temperature. Choice B can be eliminated. The K_w is changing with temperature, and as such, the autoionization equilibrium must be changing as well. Choice C can be eliminated. $K_w = [H^+][OH^-]$. K_w is increasing with temperature, and as such, hydronium and hydroxide ion concentrations must be increasing as well. Choice D is the best answer.

Titration

934. C is the best answer. In titration, an acid or base is added to a base or acid, respectively. In this process, the acidic or basic pH is neutralized, so choice C is a strong answer. Choices A, B and D may be occurring depending on the specific titration, but choice C is the best answer because it is true in all situations.

935. C is the best answer. Dilution of an acid or base could be done by slowly adding base or acid, respectively. It would not require precise measurement as is done in a titration. So choice A can be eliminated. The same is true for choice B. Choice C describes the purpose of a titration, to determine the concentration of an unknown acidic or basic solution, so choice C is a strong answer. Choice D, discovering the endpoint of an indicator, could be a rare use for titrations, but choice C is the best answer because it is the most common use for titrations.

936. A is the best answer. Using $M_1 V_1 = M_2 V_2$, $M_1(30) = (7.0)(21)$, $M_1 = 147/30 \approx 150/30 \approx 5$. But since the numerator is < 150, the actual number must be < 5, so choice A is the best answer. Note that there is no need to convert out of milliliters in this formula, since the conversion factor would affect both sides of the equation equally.

937. A is the best answer. Using $M_1 V_1 = M_2 V_2$, $(5.0)(25) = M_2 (50)$, $125/50 = M_2 = 2.5$ M, so choice A is the best answer. Note that there is no need to convert out of milliliters in this formula, since the conversion factor would affect both sides of the equation equally.

938. A is the best answer. Using $M_1 V_1 = M_2 V_2$, $M_1(100) = (7)(30)$, $M_1 = 210/100 = 21/10 = 2.1$, and choice A is the best answer. Note that there is no need to convert out of milliliters in this formula, since the conversion factor would affect both sides of the equation equally.

939. D is the best answer. 30 mL of 3 M acetic acid is $30 \times 3 = 90$ millimoles. 50 mL of 2 M sodium hydroxide is $50 \times 2 = 100$ millimoles of base. So there is more base than acid, and some of the base will be left over. Therefore, the final pH will be greater than 7, so choice D is the best answer.

940. D is the best answer. 30 mL of 3 M acetic acid is $30 \times 3 = 90$ millimoles. 45 mL of 2 M sodium hydroxide is $45 \times 2 = 90$ millimoles of base. Since there are equal amounts of base and acid, both reactants will be gone. The products of this reaction are water and (sodium) acetate. Since acetate is the conjugate of a weak acid, it is a weak base. Thus, the solution will be basic, and the pH will be greater than 7, so choice D is the best answer.

941. B is the best answer. 30 mL of 3 M acetic acid is $30 \times 3 = 90$ millimoles. 40 mL of 2 M sodium hydroxide is $40 \times 2 = 80$ millimoles of base. Since there is more acid than base, the acid will be left over. This time it is only a weak acid, however, and one of the products will be its conjugate base. Thus, a buffer has been formed. The pH of a buffer is generally fairly close to its pK_a (it might be off by one or two pH points), so the pH should be somewhere between 3 and 6, and choice B is the best answer.

942. **B is the best answer.** Here is the reaction: $HCl + NH_3 \rightarrow Cl^- + NH_4^+$. It is correct to say that the reaction goes nearly to completion because HCl is a strong acid which pushes the reaction to the right. Since ammonium is the conjugate of a strong base, it is a weak acid that dissociates to release a proton. Thus, the resulting solution is acidic. Choice A references a neutral solution, so it can be eliminated. Choice B references an acidic solution, so it is likely the best answer. Choices C and D can be eliminated because the reaction goes to completion and should not be represented as an equilibrium.

943. **B is the best answer.** Using $M_1V_1 = M_2V_2$ at the equivalence point, one can calculate the initial concentration of the acid, so option I is a component of the best answer, and choice C can be eliminated. Since the acid is weak, there will be a buffer region before the equivalence point, and in the middle of the buffer region, $pH = pK_a$ so option II is a component of the best answer, and choice A can be eliminated. From the titration curve alone, however, there is no way to determine the acid's molecular weight, so option III is not a component of the best answer, and choice D can be eliminated. Choice B is the best answer.

944. **B is the best answer.** The equivalence point is 50 mL for all six titrations. At the equivalence point the number of base molecules equals the number of acid molecules. 50 $mL_{NaOH} \times 0.1$ mol/L = 50 $mL_{acid} \times$ [acid S]. So, [acid S] is 0.1, and choice B is the best answer.

945. **C is the best answer.** To find the K_a, look at the half equivalence point, which occurs halfway to the equivalence point, in this case at 25 mL. At the half equivalence point, the pH equals the pK_a, so the pK_a is 4 for acid T. $pK_a = -\log(K_a)$ so K_a is 1×10^{-4}, and choice C is the best answer.

946. **B is the best answer.** After 45 mL of base have been added, the pH is 3. $pH = -\log[H^+]$ so $[H^+] = 10^{-3} = 0.001$, so choice B is the best answer.

947. **C is the best answer.** The pH of the conjugate of acid S can be found by looking at the equivalence point. At the equivalence, only the conjugate base of acid S is left. However, this solution has been diluted by 2 by the titrant, so the equivalence point reflects the pH of a 0.05 M solution of the conjugate base. The equivalence point is near 9 on the graph, so choice C is the best answer.

948. **C is the best answer.** The endpoint range should cover the equivalence point, which occurs for acid R at 50 mL where the pH is 10. Only choice C includes a pH of 10, so choice C is the best answer.

949. **A is the best answer.** At the beginning of the titration, the pH is about 4, so the concentration of H^+ is about 10^{-4}. This is the concentration of dissociated acid. The concentration of undissociated acid is the original concentration minus the amount dissociated, $0.1 - 0.0001$ which is essentially 0.1. So the percent dissociated is $0.0001/0.1 = 0.001 = 0.1\%$, which makes choice A is the best answer.

950. **B is the best answer.** Acid V has a starting pH of 1, so it is a strong acid. The titrant is a strong base, so the pH of the equivalence point must be 7, and choice B is the best answer.

951. **C is the best answer.** Choice A can be eliminated because it depicts an acid (low pH) being titrated by a base. Between choices B, C, and D, it is necessary to determine where the half equivalence point should be. Acid V is a strong acid because its starting pH is 1. The conjugate of acid S is a weak base. When a base is titrated with acid, the half equivalence point is when the concentration of the conjugate acid equals the concentration of the base: $[HA] = [A^-]$. When an acid is titrated by a base, the half equivalence point is when the concentration of conjugate base equals the concentration of acid: $[A^-] = [HA]$. These are the same positions regardless of which direction they are approached from. The half equivalence point for acid S is below 7, so choice C is the best answer.

952. **B is the best answer.** Water is a weak acid with a pK_a of 14 so if water was one of the acids, the half equivalence point would be around 14. It is hard to tell where acid Q's half equivalence point is, but it is probably not at 14, so choice A can be eliminated. Acid Q is in fact a weak acid because the pH prior to addition of base is 5.5, so choice B is a strong answer. Choices C and D can be eliminated because if acid Q was a base, the initial pH would be > 7.

953. **C is the best answer.** An acid buffers best at its half equivalence point, and the acid with a half equivalence point around pH 5 is acid T, so choice C is the best answer.

954. **C is the best answer.** Think about $M_1V_1 = M_2V_2$; there is no room for acid strength to play a role in the volume calculations, so choices A and B can be eliminated. Choice C correctly describes the equation $M_1V_1 = M_2V_2$, so it is likely the best answer. Choice D incorrectly pairs a statement about volume with one about pK_a. For a triprotic acid, the distance between equivalence points on the x-axis (volume) depends solely on the initial volume of acid. The distance between equivalence points on the y-axis (pH) depends on the pK_a of each proton, so choice D can be eliminated.

955. **D is the best answer.** A diprotic acid could be a strong acid like H_2SO_4 or a weak acid like H_2CO_3 meaning the pH at the equivalence point could be above or below 7, so choice D is the best answer.

956. **C is the best answer.** At the second equivalence point, the diprotic acid will have been converted into the entirely deprotonated form, which is almost certainly basic, so choice C is the best answer.

957. **A is the best answer.** The equivalence points depend upon concentration, so choice A is the best answer. The half equivalence points depend on pK_a, so choices B, C and D can be eliminated.

958. D is the best answer. The middle of the buffer region is called the half equivalence point. At this point, pH = pK_a. A weak acid is one with $pK_a > 3$, which could be pH < 7, pH = 7, or pH > 7, so choice D is the best answer.

959. A is the best answer. Carbon dioxide could be produced by neutralizing a carbonate salt or carbonic acid, a weak base or weak acid respectively. Choice A can only be the titration curve of a strong acid and strong base, making it the best answer.

960. D is the best answer. HCl, a strong acid, would cause a titration endpoint of very low pH. Only choice D does not end at a low pH, which makes it the correct choice.

961. C is the best answer. H_2SO_4 is a diprotic strong acid that is being titrated with a monoprotic strong base. Because H_2SO_4 is a diprotic acid, it will give away two protons to solution as more NaOH is added to the reaction. A strong acid has a first equivalence point at a $pK_{a1} < 3$, so the second equivalence point must be at a $pK_{a2} > 3$. pK_a = pH at the equivalence point, so the pH value must also be greater than 3 for the second equivalence point. Choices A and B can be eliminated. When a strong acid is titrated with a strong base, the equivalence point of the last proton it can release is around a pH of 7. The exact pH will depend on how strong the acid is and how many protons it can release, but the value will be near neutral. Choice C is a strong answer. A strong acid titrated with a strong base will have a nearly neutral pH for the last proton it can release, not a basic pH. Choice D can be eliminated.

962. D is the best answer. The equivalence point of a weak-acid strong base titration would normally be around a pH of 9. Because the pK_a of the indicator should be as close as possible to the equivalence point, choice D is the best answer.

963. C is the best answer. The equivalence point of a strong acid strong base titration would normally be at a pH of 7. Because the pK_a of the indicator should be as close as possible to the equivalence point, choice C is the best answer.

964. B is the best answer. The equivalence point of a strong acid-weak base titration would normally be around a pH of 5. Because the pK_a of the indicator should be as close as possible to the equivalence point, choice B is the best answer.

965. B is the best answer. In a standard titration, a few drops of indicator are added to the analyte, or the solution with unknown concentration of acid or base. However, the titrant, which is the acid or base solution that is added to the analyte, does not contain indicator. Option III, the reference solution, is not always a component of titration. This is only an optional step. Since the question says always, option III should not be included. Option II only, or choice B, is the best answer.

966. A is the best answer. The endpoint is defined as the point in titration at which the indicator changes color. This corresponds to choice A. Choice B is not the best answer because the half-equivalence point is the point at which half of the analyte has been neutralized. Choice C is not the best answer because although the equivalence point normally approximates the endpoint, they are not exactly the same. The equivalence point is the point at which the analyte is completely neutralized. Choice D is not the best answer because the buffer point is the point at which concentrations of an acid and its conjugate base are equal. Choice A is the best answer.

967. B is the best answer. The indicator should change color near the equivalence point, so choice B is the best answer. Choice A can be eliminated because the pH at the pK_a of the acid being titrated is the half equivalence point. If the indicator is active at this pH, it will change prior to the equivalence point, so choice A can be eliminated. Using an indicator that changes color at pH 7 will only work for certain acids, so choice C can be eliminated. Choice D is a common answer type on the MCAT® where the question stem is claimed to be irrelevant. Picking these types of answers should be avoided because they are usually incorrect, and choice D can be eliminated.

968. D is the best answer. Choices A and B are saying the same thing and they cannot both be true, so on those grounds those answers should be eliminated. The reason this is not measured directly in a titration is that the more base that is added, the more the acid dissociates. It is impossible to measure the dissociation, although it can be extrapolated from the curve of the entire titration. The titration is considered complete when the indicator changes color. This is called the endpoint. The equivalence point is defined as the point when the amounts of reactants are equal. When a titration is performed, the experimenter generally assumes that the equivalence point is near the endpoint, but it is not guaranteed. So, although choice C is a reasonable answer, choice D is the best answer.

969. C is the best answer. The endpoint range should cover the equivalence point, which occurs at pH 7. Use the exponents of the pK_a to estimate the best indicator. This eliminates choices A and D, which will change too late and too early respectively. Between choices B and C, choice C has a pK_a closer to 7, so choice C is the best answer.

Salts and Buffers

970. C is the best answer. This question requires an understanding of the common names of strong acids. Note that strong acids dissociate completely in water, while weak acids do not. The only weak acid in the answer choices is choice C, acetic acid.

971. C is the best answer. The results display the K_a values for four acids. Note that smaller K_a values correspond to weaker acids. The strengths of acid/conjugate base pairs are inversely related. The strongest base will be the conjugate base of the weakest acid, or the acid with the smallest K_a. Of the acids analyzed, NH_4^+ has the smallest K_a, indicating that the strongest conjugate base would be NH_3. Note that NH_4^+ is listed and not NH_3. Choice A can be eliminated. The next smallest K_a is H_2CO_3. The conjugate base, HCO_3^-, would thus be the next strongest base. Choice C is the best answer.

972. C is the best answer. NH_4Cl salt will dissociate into NH_4^+ and Cl^-. KF salt will dissociate into K^+ and F^-. Note that, following dissociation, H_2CO_3 and CH_3COOH do not share any ions with these salts, and as such, the concentrations of H_2CO_3 and CH_3COOH will not be affected. Choice A can be eliminated. NH_4Cl salt will dissociate into NH_4^+ and Cl^-. According to Le Châtelier's Principle, the addition of NH_4^+ will further promote the dissociation of NH_4^+ into NH_3 and H^+. Although more NH_4^+ will be dissociated, it is unlikely that the total NH_4^+ concentration will decrease, as the addition of the salt increased its concentration prior to dissociation. Choice B can be eliminated. KF salt will dissociate into K^+ and F^-. According to Le Châtelier's Principle, the addition of F^- will lead to the reformation of HF, increasing the concentration of HF. Choice C is the best answer. K_a determines the equilibrium ratio of acid/conjugate base at any given moment in a reaction. Note that equilibrium concentrations can change while the ratio remains the same. Although it is true that K_a is a constant that only changes with temperature, the addition of salts will in fact change equilibrium concentrations. Choice D can be eliminated. Choice C is the best answer.

973. D is the best answer. The researchers determined the K_a of 4 acids. The question is essentially asking: can the K_a values still be used after the salt is added? The K_a is the equilibrium constant of the dissociation of the acid. $K_a = [A^-][H^+]/[HA]$, where HA is the acid, and A^- is the conjugate base formed from the dissociation of the acid's hydrogen. K_a functions as a constant to determine the ratio of acid/conjugate base at any given moment in a reaction. Although the quantity of acid/conjugate base may change, K_a values will not change as more reactant/product is added, as the ratio of acid/conjugate base will remain the same. Choice A can be eliminated. CH_3COOH will dissociate to CH_3COO^- and H^+. Once dissolved, CH_3COONa will form CH_3COO^- and Na^+. According to Le Châtelier's Principle, the CH_3COO^- from the salt will force the dissociation of CH_3COOH towards the reformation of more CH_3COOH. However, the ratio of $[H^+][CH_3COO^-]/[CH_3COOH]$ will not change, so the K_a will not change. Choice B can be eliminated. The addition of salt will affect equilibrium concentrations, but it will not affect the K_a. Choice C can be eliminated. K_a is not dependent on any given concentrations; it is only dependent on temperature. The researchers' determination of K_a values can still be used. Choice D is the best answer.

974. C is the best answer. Hydrophobic residues cannot activate an acid so choice A can be eliminated. Choice B can be eliminated because the body has a relatively neutral pH. Choice C is a reasonable explanation and may be the best answer—nearby basic residues may promote deprotonation of the weak acid. If choice D where true, which it is not, the dissociation would actually decrease because increased concentration is associated with decreased dissociation, so choice D can be eliminated.

975. D is the best answer. All cations except those of alkali metals and the heavy alkaline earth metals (Ca^{2+} and heavier) form weakly acidic solutions in water. So, only Mg^{2+} is a weak acid, and choice D is the best answer.

976. B is the best answer. All cations except those of alkali metals and the heavy alkaline earth metals (Ca^{2+} and heavier) form weakly acidic solutions in water. So, only Al^{3+} is a weak acid, and choice B is the best answer.

977. C is the best answer. Nitrate is conjugate to nitric acid, a strong acid, and is thus neutral, so option I cannot be a component of the best answer, and choices A and D can be eliminated. Cyanide is conjugate to hydrocyanic acid, a weak acid, and is thus a weak base, so option II is part of the best answer. Carbonate is conjugate to the hydrogen carbonate ion, which in itself is conjugate to carbonic acid. Carbonic acid is a weak acid; therefore, its conjugates are bases, so option III is true, and choice C is the best answer.

978. D is the best answer. If the salt is more soluble in basic solutions, it must be acidic. Bases react with acids, so an acidic salt would constantly have its ions in solution disappearing. Le Châtelier's principle would then drive the solubility reaction forward. NaOH is a base and would not dissolve well in a basic solution because Le Châtelier's principle would push the reaction to the left. So, choice A is not the best answer. NaCl and KCl are salts and would not have differential solubility in acids and bases, so choices B and C can be eliminated. NH_4^+ is acidic, since it is conjugate to the weak base ammonia. So, as it dissolves and releases H^+, the OH^- will be neutralized and more NH_4Cl will dissolve. So choice D is the best answer.

979. B is the best answer. Since hydrochloric acid is a strong acid, it dissociates completely, and the resulting chloride ion must have no tendency to pick up a proton in aqueous solution. Thus, sodium chloride should be neutral, and choice B is the best answer.

980. B is the best answer. As with most organic acids, benzoic acid is a weak acid. This means it will give up its proton to solution, but not all of the benzoic acid will be deprotonated. In order to find the pH of the solution, the first step is to solve for the concentration of protons.

$$K_a = \frac{[C_6H_5CO_2^-][H^+]}{[C_6H_5CO_2H]} = 6 \times 10^{-5}$$

$$\frac{[x][x]}{[0.02\ M - x]} = 6 \times 10^{-5}$$

For the MCAT®, the value of x in the denominator is assumed to be negligible, so the equation can be reduced to:

$$\frac{[x][x]}{[0.02\ M]} = 6 \times 10^{-5}$$

$$x^2 = 1.2 \times 10^{-6}$$

$$x = 1.3 \times 10^{-3}$$

To calculate the pH, find the $-\log(1.3 \times 10^{-3}) = 2.9$.

Choice B is the best answer because it matches the calculated answer.

981. B is the best answer. This question is tricky because it involves the calculation of the pH of a weak acid, which is more complicated than a strong acid. The calculation is as follows, making reasonable estimations:

$$K_a = \frac{[H_3O^+][NH_3]}{[NH_4^+]} = 5.8 \times 10^{-10}$$

$$\frac{x^2}{0.5 - x} = \frac{x^2}{0.5} = 6.0 \times 10^{-10}$$

$$x^2 = 3.0 \times 10^{-10}$$

Since the square root of 4 is 2, it is possible to estimate that the square root of 3 is slightly less than 2.

$$x = 1.7 \times 10^{-5}$$

Now, calculate $-\log(1.7 \times 10^{-5})$. To make it simpler, estimate that it is between 4 and 5 but closer to 5. This corresponds best with choice B. Choices A and D can be eliminated automatically because they are basic pHs, and the question relates to an acid.

982. A is the best answer. The conjugate of a weak base will be more acidic than the conjugate of a strong acid is basic. So, the solution will have a pH below 7, and choice A is the best answer. Imagine the conjugate of HCl and the conjugate of NH_3. The salt formed is NH_4Cl.

983. C is the best answer. HCO_3^- is amphoteric, so it can act as both acid and base. As an acid, the pK_a is 10.25, since that would be the second dissociation of carbonic acid. As a base, it is conjugate to carbonic acid, and would thus have a pK_b of $14 - 6.37$, or about 8. Thus it is a "better" base than acid, and the pH would be greater than 7, and choice C is the best answer.

984. C is the best answer. Salts are ionic compounds that dissociate in water. The pH of a salt solution can be predicted by comparing the conjugates of the respective ions. The pH requirements of the digestive tract are pH < 7. The correct answer involves a salt that generates an acidic environment following dissociation. The conjugate of NH_4^+ is NH_3, a weak base. The conjugate of Cl^- is HCl, a strong acid. The combination of a weak base and strong acid will generate an acidic environment. Option I is correct. Choice B can be eliminated, The conjugate of Na^+ is NaOH, a strong base. The conjugate of CH_3COO^- is CH_3COOH (acetic acid), a weak acid. The combination of a strong base and weak acid will generate a basic environment. Option II is incorrect. Choice D can be eliminated. The conjugate of K^+ is KOH, a strong base. The conjugate of HSO_4 is H_2SO_4 (sulfuric acid), a strong acid. The combination of a weak base and strong acid will generate an acidic environment. Option III is correct. Choice A can be eliminated. Choice C is the best answer.

985. C is the best answer. This salt is made from the conjugates of a weak acid and a weak base. Whether the pH is acidic or basic depends upon the strengths of the conjugates. The K_a is an indicator of the acid strength, and the K_b is an indicator of the base strength. The K_b is larger, so the pH will be over 7, so choices A and B can be eliminated. Choice D incorrectly states that CN^- is an acid, so it can be eliminated, and choice C is the best answer.

986. A is the best answer. This question requires an understanding of dissociations of salts of weak acids. The question stem provides the K_a, but when the sodium bicarbonate dissociates in solution, it dissociates into Na^+, which is neutral, and HCO_3^-, which is the conjugate base of carbonic acid. The solution will therefore be basic, so choices B and C can be eliminated. Now, calculate the K_b from the K_a as follows:

$$K_aK_b = K_w$$

$$K_b = \frac{1.0 \times 10^{-14}}{4.4 \times 10^{-7}} \approx 2.5 \times 10^{-8}$$

Now, use the K_b as the dissociation constant for the equation

$$HCO_3^- + H_2O \leftrightarrow H2CO3 + OH^-:$$

$$K_b = 2.5 \times 10^{-8} = \frac{[H_2CO_3][OH^-]}{[HCO_3^-]}$$

$$2.5 \times 10^{-8} = \frac{[x][x]}{[1]} = x^2$$

Estimate the square root of K_b to be less than 2 but greater than 1:

$$1.5 \times 10^{-4} = x$$

Note that x is also about equal to the concentration of OH^- per the equation for K_b using the equation for the dissociation of $NaHCO_3$ in water. Based on this, estimate that $pOH = -\log(1.5 \times 10^{-4})$. Estimate that this value is between 3 and 4. To find the pH, subtract approximately 3.5 from 14 (because $pH = 14 - pOH$). This yields approximately 10.5, making choice A the best answer.

987. C is the best answer. NaClO dissolves into $Na^+(aq)$ and $ClO^-(aq)$. $Na^+(aq)$ is neutral because it is the conjugate of a strong base (NaOH). $ClO^-(aq)$ is the conjugate base of the weak acid HClO. To determine the pH, the aqueous interactions of $ClO^-(aq)$ must first be considered:

$$ClO^-(aq) + H_2O(l) \rightleftharpoons HClO(aq) + OH^-(aq)$$

The K_b of $ClO^-(aq)$ is as follows:

$$K_b = [HClO][OH^-]/[ClO^-].$$

Note that the K_a of HClO is 3.0×10^{-8}. The K_a and K_b of a conjugate acid/base pair are related by K_w via:

$$K_w = K_a K_b. \text{ At } 25°C, K_w = 1 \times 10^{-14}.$$

$$K_b = 1 \times 10^{-14}/3.0 \times 10^{-8} = 0.33 \times 10^{-6} = 3.3 \times 10^{-7}.$$

Because one mole of both $HClO(aq)$ and $OH^-(aq)$ will be formed, designate the quantity of both species formed as x. The quantity of $ClO^-(aq)$ remaining is thus 0.20 $M - x$. Because K_b is so small, assume that $x = 0$. The following equation can be formed:

$$3.3 \times 10^{-7} = x^2/2 \times 10^{-1}.$$

$$x^2 = 6.6 \times 10^{-8}.$$

At this point, note that $\sqrt{4} = 2$, and $\sqrt{9} = 3$. $\sqrt{6.6}$ must be between 2 and 3. Assume:

$$\sqrt{6.6 \times 10^{-8}} = 2.5 \times 10^{-4} = x = [OH^-](aq).$$

$$pOH = -\log(2.5 \times 10^{-4}).$$

This answer must be between 3 and 4, but a bit closer to 4. Assume $pOH = 3.6$. $pH = 14 - pOH = 14 - 3.6 = 10.4$. Choice C is the best answer.

988. B is the best answer. Good buffer solutions contain acids whose pK_a closely matches the pH of the solution to be buffered. Carbonic acid is the buffer found in blood, and its pK_a is 6.37. Choice B most closely matches the blood pH of 7.4 and correctly defines the pK_a of carbonic acid.

989. B is the best answer. A buffer solution's capacity can be checked by adding a known number of moles of an acid until the pH increases (or decreases) by 1. Thus, choice A, C, and D are all required. The concentration of the buffer is irrelevant to its capacity because capacity is measure in moles of acid tolerated per liter of buffer, so choice B is the best answer.

990. C is the best answer. The main regulator of blood pH is bicarbonate, which is able to donate protons when the blood pH becomes too high and is able to accept protons when the blood pH becomes too low. Thus, bicarbonate likely acts as both an acid and a base. Choices A and B are less likely to be the best answer, because bicarbonate could act as both, depending on the pH of the blood. A buffer is defined by the ability to accept and donate protons depending on the pH of the solution, which closely matches the function of bicarbonate. Choice C is most likely to be the best answer. A catalyst lowers the activation energy of a reaction. The main function of bicarbonate is to buffer the pH of the blood and carry dissolved carbon dioxide to the lungs for elimination, not to serve to decrease the activation energy of a reaction. Choice D can be eliminated, and choice C is the best answer.

991. A is the best answer. The closer pH is to pK_a, the better the buffer. This problem requires the estimation of pK_a, as well as some knowledge of biological molecules. Histidine is an amino acid for which the MCAT® requires knowledge of side chain pK_a, which is 6, making this a poor buffer. Hydrofluoric acid is a strong acid, which means it must have a pK_a below 3, making it a poor buffer at pH 8. Hydrochloric acid is also a strong acid of low pK_a. This leaves choice A, oxalic acid at pH 4, as the best answer.

992. A is the best answer. A buffer serves to minimize changes in pH by donating or accepting protons at a pH around its pK_a. At the half equivalence point, the buffer is best able to donate or accept a proton with minimal changes in pH, making choice A likely to be the best answer. At the equivalence point, minimal changes in the addition of an acid or base drastically change the reaction. Choice A is a better answer than choice B. A buffer serves to mitigate changes in pH, not indicate when a reaction is complete, eliminating choices C and D.

993. D is the best answer. An ideal buffer contains an acid whose pK_a is very close to the pH of the solution being buffered. Since the solution being buffered has a pH of 6.3, the ideal buffer acid will have a pK_a close to this value. The table provides K_a values. Remember that $pK_a = -\log(K_a)$. Acid 1 has a K_a value of 1.3×10^6. The pK_a is approximately $-6(pK_a = -\log(1 \times 10^6))$. Note the negative number. Acid 2 will also have a negative pK_a, so these two can be eliminated. Estimating from the exponent of -11 of the K_a of acid 3, it will have a pK_a of about 10, which is too high to be an ideal buffer for this solution. This leaves acid 4, which has a pK_a of about 5. This is close enough to 5.1 to be an ideal buffer.

994. B is the best answer. The definition of pH is the negative log of the H^+ ion concentration for any solution. Do not be tricked by the question referring to a buffered solution. Choice B is the best answer.

995. A is the best answer. An aqueous buffer is composed of a weak acid and its conjugate base or a weak base and its conjugate acid. HCl is a *strong* acid and therefore cannot be used in a buffer in aqueous solution, so choice A is the best answer. The other answer choices are all weak acids and their conjugate base.

996. B is the best answer. Recall from the Henderson-Hasselbalch equation that the pH of a buffer depends on the ratio of base to acid. For a buffer, diluting the solution does not change the pH, so choice B is the best answer.

997. A is the best answer. HCl is a strong acid, so this is not a buffer; however, the sodium chloride solution does dilute the HCl by a factor of 2. The HCl completely dissociates, giving $[H_3O^+] = 1$ M. Diluted by the sodium chloride solution makes it a 0.5 molar solution. Then, $pH = -\log[H_3O^+] = -\log(5 \times 10^{-1}) = 0.3$. So, choice A is the best answer.

998. C is the best answer. Ammonium is the conjugate acid of ammonia, which is a weak base. Therefore, this is a buffer. For buffers only, calculate the pH by using the following equation: $pH = pK_a + \log([\text{base}]/[\text{acid}])$. In this case, since [base] = [acid] and $\log 1 = 0$, $pH = pK_a$, so choice C is the best answer.

999. D is the best answer. This is a weak base and its conjugate acid, and is therefore a buffer. For buffers only, calculate the pH by using the following equation: $pH = pK_a + \log([\text{base}]/[\text{acid}]) = 9.26 + \log(2/0.2) = 9.26 + \log(10) = 9.26 + 1 = 10.26$, so choice D is the best answer.

1000. D is the best answer. The usual form of the Henderson-Hasselbalch equation involves pK_a, but the pK_b of the conjugate base must be used. Since $pK_a + pK_b = 14$ for conjugates, then $pK_a = 14 - pK_b$. Substitute this form into Henderson-Hasselbalch to get choice D. Choice A incorrectly swaps pK_a for pK_b. Choices B and C are algebraically identical; therefore, neither can be correct.

1001. C is the best answer. The pH of a buffer depends only on the pK_a of the acid and the ratio of base to acid. Since the ratio is the same in both cases, the pH is the same, so choices B and D can be eliminated. Solution A has greater buffer capacity because it is more concentrated, so choice A can be eliminated, and choice C is the best answer.

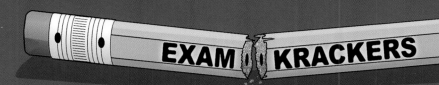
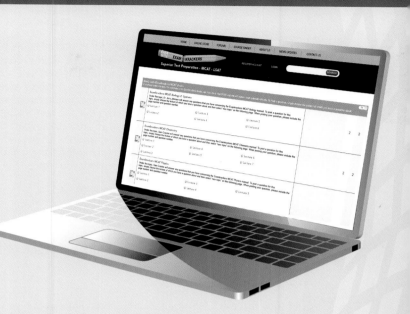
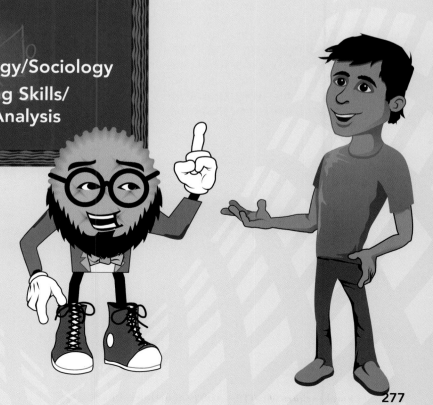

PHYSICAL SCIENCES

DIRECTIONS. Most questions in the Physical Sciences test are organized into groups, each preceded by a descriptive passage. After studying the passage, select the one best answer to each question in the group. Some questions are not based on a descriptive passage and are also independent of each other. You must also select the one best answer to these questions. If you are not certain of an answer, eliminate the alternatives that you know to be incorrect and then select an answer from the remaining alternatives. A periodic table is provided for your use. You may consult it whenever you wish.

PERIODIC TABLE OF THE ELEMENTS

1 **H** 1.0																	2 **He** 4.0
3 **Li** 6.9	4 **Be** 9.0											5 **B** 10.8	6 **C** 12.0	7 **N** 14.0	8 **O** 16.0	9 **F** 19.0	10 **Ne** 20.2
11 **Na** 23.0	12 **Mg** 24.3											13 **Al** 27.0	14 **Si** 28.1	15 **P** 31.0	16 **S** 32.1	17 **Cl** 35.5	18 **Ar** 39.9
19 **K** 39.1	20 **Ca** 40.1	21 **Sc** 45.0	22 **Ti** 47.9	23 **V** 50.9	24 **Cr** 52.0	25 **Mn** 54.9	26 **Fe** 55.8	27 **Co** 58.9	28 **Ni** 58.7	29 **Cu** 63.5	30 **Zn** 65.4	31 **Ga** 69.7	32 **Ge** 72.6	33 **As** 74.9	34 **Se** 79.0	35 **Br** 79.9	36 **Kr** 83.8
37 **Rb** 85.5	38 **Sr** 87.6	39 **Y** 88.9	40 **Zr** 91.2	41 **Nb** 92.9	42 **Mo** 95.9	43 **Tc** (98)	44 **Ru** 101.1	45 **Rh** 102.9	46 **Pd** 106.4	47 **Ag** 107.9	48 **Cd** 112.4	49 **In** 114.8	50 **Sn** 118.7	51 **Sb** 121.8	52 **Te** 127.6	53 **I** 126.9	54 **Xe** 131.3
55 **Cs** 132.9	56 **Ba** 137.3	57 **La*** 138.9	72 **Hf** 178.5	73 **Ta** 180.9	74 **W** 183.9	75 **Re** 186.2	76 **Os** 190.2	77 **Ir** 192.2	78 **Pt** 195.1	79 **Au** 197.0	80 **Hg** 200.6	81 **Tl** 204.4	82 **Pb** 207.2	83 **Bi** 209.0	84 **Po** (209)	85 **At** (210)	86 **Rn** (222)
87 **Fr** (223)	88 **Ra** 226.0	89 **Ac**⁼ 227.0	104 **Unq** (261)	105 **Unp** (262)	106 **Unh** (263)	107 **Uns** (262)	108 **Uno** (265)	109 **Une** (267)									

	58 **Ce** 140.1	59 **Pr** 140.9	60 **Nd** 144.2	61 **Pm** (145)	62 **Sm** 150.4	63 **Eu** 152.0	64 **Gd** 157.3	65 **Tb** 158.9	66 **Dy** 162.5	67 **Ho** 164.9	68 **Er** 167.3	69 **Tm** 168.9	70 **Yb** 173.0	71 **Lu** 175.0
*														
⁼	90 **Th** 232.0	91 **Pa** (231)	92 **U** 238.0	93 **Np** (237)	94 **Pu** (244)	95 **Am** (243)	96 **Cm** (247)	97 **Bk** (247)	98 **Cf** (251)	99 **Es** (252)	100 **Fm** (257)	101 **Md** (258)	102 **No** (259)	103 **Lr** (260)